Mycobacterium tuberculosis Protocols

METHODS IN MOLECULAR MEDICINE™

John M. Walker, SERIES EDITOR

METHODS IN MOLECULAR MEDICINE™

Mycobacterium tuberculosis Protocols

Edited by

Tanya Parish

St. Bartholomew's and Royal London School of Medicine and Dentistry, London, UK

and

Neil G. Stoker

London School of Hygiene and Tropical Medicine, London, UK

Humana Press **Totowa, New Jersey**

999 Riverview Drive, Suite 208
Totowa, New Jersey 07512

This publication is printed on acid-free paper. ∞
ANSI Z39.48-1984 (American Standards Institute) Permanence of Paper for Printed Library Materials.

Cover illustration: Fig. 1A from Chapter 21, *Proteomics*, by J. C. Betts and M. A. Smith.
Cover design: Patricia F. Cleary

For additional copies, pricing for bulk purchases, and/or information about other Humana titles, contact Humana at the above address or at any of the following numbers: Tel: 973-256-1699; Fax: 973-256-8341; E-mail: humana@humanapr.com, or visit our Website at www.humanapress.com

Printed in the United States of America. 10 9 8 7 6 5 4 3 2 1

Library of Congress Cataloging in Publication Data

Main entry under title:

Methods in molecular medicine™.

Mycobacterium tuberculosis protocols / edited by Tanya Parish and Neil G. Stoker.
p. cm. —(Methods in molecular Medicine; 54)
Includes bibliographical references and index.
ISBN 0-89603-776-2 (alk. paper)
1. Tuberculosis–Moleculoar aspects–Laboratory manuals. 2. Bacterial genetics–Laboratory manuals. 3. Mycobacterium tuberculosis–Laboratory manuals. I. Parish, Tanya. II. Stoker, N. G. (Neil G.) III. Series.

QR201.T6 M93 2000
579.3'74–dc21 00-040977

Preface

The aim of this book is to provide detailed protocols for studying the molecular biology of the pathogen *Mycobacterium tuberculosis*, and its interactions with host cells. As established mycobacterial laboratories move towards exploiting the genome, and laboratories with expertise in other fields apply them to mycobacteria, both traditional and novel methodologies need to be reviewed. Thus the chapters in *Mycobacterium tuberculosis Protocols* range from perspectives on storage of strains and safety issues to the application of the latest functional genomics technologies.

The last few years have been remarkable ones for research into *M. tuberculosis*. The most important landmark by far has been the completion of the genome sequence of the widely studied H37Rv strain (1). We can now predict every protein and RNA molecule made by the pathogen. This information is or will soon be enriched by the addition of genome sequences of other strains from the *M. tuberculosis* complex: a second strain of *M. tuberculosis*, *Mycobacterium bovis*, and the vaccine strain, *M. bovis* BCG. Valuable comparative data will also be provided by the genome sequences of *Mycobacterium leprae*, *Mycobacterium avium*, and *Streptomyces coelicolor*. Another recent milestone for *M. tuberculosis* has been the development of efficient mutagenesis methodologies, the lack of which has been a major handicap in functional studies. The new challenges to researchers are first to use this information and these techniques in combination with the battery of methodologies being developed around the world to exploit all genome data, so-called functional genomics research, which includes transcriptomics and proteomics. The second challenge is to integrate them with other disciplines of active research such as immunology, cell biology, and biochemistry. *Mycobacterium tuberculosis Protocols* incorporates both of these aspects in the methods described.

This book is aimed at people who are actively working on *M. tuberculosis.* However, there is much that will be relevant to work on other mycobacteria and on such phylogenetically related organisms as corynebacteria and streptomycetes. It is intended both for people with experience in handling *M. tuberculosis* and those who are new to the field.

The topics covered by the 24 chapters included are quite diverse. A major focus is the production of mutants, which plays a central role in functional studies. The recent successes in mutagenesis are reflected in the inclusion of four chapters (4–7) describing different strategies for both transposon mutagenesis and targeted allelic replacement.

Two of the most exciting recent technological developments make use of the genome sequence to allow us to look at the RNA and protein complements of the cell at a global level. Proteome analysis is described in Chapter 21, and the production and analysis of whole genome microarrays is described in Chapter 22. RNA is discussed in more detail elsewhere, with chapters on purification (Chap. 3), transcriptional start site analysis (Chap. 8), and quantitation using real-time PCR (Chap. 19).

Fractionation of the bacteria to look at protein carbohydrate and lipid components is described. The contributions focus on analysis of culture filtrates (Chap. 13), the capsule (Chap. 14), and lipids (Chap. 15). Cytological analysis of the bacteria allows the analysis of cellular properties in individual bacteria, and many of the major technological advances that have helped eukaryotic cell biology are beginning to be applied to bacteria (Chap. 9).

There is understandably enormous interest in how *M. tuberculosis* interacts with the host, and chapters discuss infection of macrophages both as a virulence assay (Chap. 17), and in order to understand the cell biology (Chap. 18). In addition, perhaps the most difficult topic to study, the persistence of bacteria, is addressed in Chap. 16.

The excitement of the post-genome era must not distract us from the fact that tuberculosis is a dreadful disease of which millions die each year, and control still suffers from difficulties in diagnosis. A relatively new method for detecting bacteria and identifying drug resistance using a cheap and sensitive phage-based method is described (Chap. 10). This method is phenotypic, in that the basis of the drug resistance need not be known. Genotypic methods are described that identify specific mutations by dot-blotting (Chap. 11) or real-time PCR (Chap. 19). Our understanding of the spread of bacteria has been revolutionized by DNA typing techniques, and the most up-to-date methodology for carrying out RFLP typing is in Chap. 12. DNA preparation from bacteria cultures and clinical isolates is discussed in Chap. 2.

Though most of *Mycobacterium tuberculosis Protocols* concentrates on laboratory methods, the genome sequence is a central resource for laboratory and bioinformatics research. A description of the main *M. tuberculosis* genome resources on the internet is therefore provided in Chap. 20.

Finally there are chapters providing basic but essential methods for work with *M. tuberculosis.* These are an up-to-date account of available cloning vectors (Chap. 1), how to store strains (Chap. 23). and last but by no means least, a discussion of some of the safety issues (Chap. 24).

This book aims to complement and update the earlier volume in this series, *Mycobacteria Protocols* (2). Some methods are deliberately complementary—for example, the computer analysis of IS*6110* fingerprints was described in the earlier book, whereas the production of the fingerprints is described here. Several diagnostic methods included in the earlier volume complement those presented here. Other topics in the earlier book that are relevant to tuberculosis research are those on pulsed field gel electrophoresis, preparation of cell-free extracts and cell wal! fractions, the use of mycobacteriophages, and the analysis of gene expression using reporter genes and RT- and RAP-PCR.

Tanya Parish
Neil G. Stoker

REFERENCES

1. Cole, S.T., R. Brosch, J. Parkhill, T. Garnier, C. Churcher, D. Harris, S.V. Gordon, K. Eiglmeier, S. Gas, C.E. Barry *et al.* (1998) Deciphering the biology of *Mycobacterium tuberculosis* from the complete genome sequence. *Nature* **393**: 537–544.
2. Parish, T. and N.G. Stoker (Eds) (1998) *Mycobacteria Protocols*. Humana Press: Totowa, NJ.

Contents

Contributors

HEIDI ALDERTON • *Department of Infectious and Tropical Diseases, London School of Hygiene & Tropical Medicine, London, UK*

PETER ANDERSEN • *Department of TB Immunology, Statens Serum Institut, Copenhagen, Denmark*

STOYAN S. BARDAROV • *Howard Hughes Medical Institute, Department of Microbiology and Immunology, Albert Einstein College of Medicine, Bronx, NY*

SVETOSLAV S. BARDAROV, JR. • *Department of Microbiology and Immunology, Albert Einstein College of Medicine, Bronx, NY*

MICHAEL R. BARER • *Department of Microbiology and Immunology, The Medical School, Newcastle upon Tyne, UK*

CLIFTON E. BARRY, 3RD • *Laboratory of Host Defenses, National Institute of Health, Rockville, MD*

WANDY BEATTY • *Molecular Microbiology, Washington University School of Medicine, St. Louis, MO*

JOANNA C. BETTS • *Respiratory Systems, Glaxo Wellcome Research and Development, Hertfordshire, UK*

ERIK C. BÖTTGER • *Institut für Medizinische Mikrobiologie, Medizinische Hochschule Hannover, Hannover, Germany*

PHILIP D. BUTCHER • *Department of Molecular Microbiology, St. George's Hospital Medical School, London, UK*

LUIS REINALDO CAMACHO • *Unité de Génétique Mycobactérienne, Institut Pasteur, Paris, France*

NICOLA CASALI • *School of Public Health, University of California at Berkeley, Berkeley, CA*

RORY P. COONEY • *Department of Marine Sciences and Coastal Management, University of Newcastle, UK*

ROBERT A. COX • *National Institute for Medical Research, The Ridgeway, London, UK*

MAMADOU DAFFÉ • *Institut de Pharmacologie et Biologie Structurale, Centre National de la Recherche Scientifique, France*

PETRA E. W. DE HAAS • *Diagnostic Laboratory for Infectious Diseases and Perinatal Screening (LIS), National Institute of Public Health and the Environment, Bilthoven, The Netherlands*

SABINE EHRT • *Department of Microbiology and Immunology, Weill Medical College of Cornell University, New York, NY*

NATALIE J. GARTON • *School of Sciences, University of Sunderland, Sunderland, UK*
BRIGITTE GICQUEL • *Unité de Génétique Mycobactérienne, Institut Pasteur, France*
JORGE A. GONZALEZ-Y-MERCHAND • *Departamento de Microbiologia, Escuela Nacional de Ciencias Biologicas, Instituto Politecnico Nacional Mexico, Mexico*
BHAVNA GORDHAN • *Molecular Biology Unit, South African Institute for Medical Research, Johannesburg, South Africa*
CHRISTOPHE GUILHOT • *Unité de Génétique Mycobactérienne, Institut Pasteur, Paris, France*
ELIZABETH U. HOOKER • *Respiratory Systems, Medicine Research Centre, Glaxo Wellcome Research and Development, Hertfordshire, UK*
KRISTIN KREMER • *Diagnostic Laboratory for Infectious Diseases and Perinatal Screening (LIS), National Institute of Public Health and the Environment, Bilthoven, The Netherlands*
TRIDIA VAN DER LAAN • *Diagnostic Laboratory for Infectious Diseases and Perinatal Screening (LIS), National Institute of Public Health and the Environment, Bilthoven, The Netherlands*
MARIE-ANTOINETTE LANÉELLE • *Institut de Pharmacologie et de Biologie Structurale, Centre National de la Recherche Scientifique, France*
MARY JACKSON • *Unité de Génétique Mycobactérienne, Institut Pasteur, Paris, France*
WILLIAM R. JACOBS, JR. • *Howard Hughes Medical Institute, Albert Einstein College of Medicine, Bronx, NY*
PAULINE T. LUKEY • *Respiratory Systems, Medical Research Centre, Glaxo Wellcome Research and Development, Hertfordshire, UK*
JOSEPH A. MANGAN • *Department of Molecular Microbiology, St. George's Hospital Medical School, London, UK*
RICCARDO MANGANELLI • *TB Center, The Public Health Research Institute, New York, NY*
RUTH MCNERNEY • *Department of Infectious and Tropical Diseases, London School of Hygiene & Tropical Medicine, London, UK*
IRENE M. MONAHAN • *Department of Molecular Microbiology, St. George's Hospital Medical School, London, UK*
FARAHNAZ MOVAHEDZADEH • *Department of Infectious and Tropical Diseases, London School of Hygiene & Tropical Medicine, London, UK*
TANYA PARISH • *Department of Infectious and Tropical Diseases, London School of Hygiene & Tropical Medicine, London, UK*

JULIAN PARKHILL • *The Sanger Centre, Wellcome Trust Genome Campus, Cambridge, UK*

IDA ROSENKRANDS • *Department of TB Immunology, Statens Serum Institut, Copenhagen, Denmark*

DAVID G. RUSSELL • *Molecular Microbiology, Washington University School of Medicine, St. Louis, MO*

PETER SANDER • *Institut für Medizinische Mikrobiologie, Medizinische Hochschule Hannover, Hannover, Germany*

DIRK SCHNAPPINGER • *Division of Infectious Diseases and Geographic Medicine, Stanford University Medical Center, Stanford, CA*

GARY K. SCHOOLNIK • *Division of Infectious Diseases and Geographic Medicine, Stanford University Medical Center, Stanford, CA*

RICHARD A. SLAYDEN • *Tuberculosis Research Section, National Institute of Health, Rockville, MD*

DEBBIE SMITH • *Department of Infectious and Tropical Diseases, London School of Hygiene & Tropical Medicine, London, UK*

ISSAR SMITH • *TB Center, The Public Health Research Institute, New York, NY*

MARJORIE A. SMITH • *Molecular Recognition, Glaxo Wellcome Medicine Research Centre, Hertfordshire, UK*

BURKHARD SPRINGER • *Institut für Medizinische Mikrobiologie, Medizinische Hochschule Hannover, Hannover, Germany*

SANJAY TYAGI • *Department of Molecular Genetics, The Public Health Research Institute, New York, NY*

TRIDIA VAN DER LAAN • *Diagnostic Laboratory for Infectious Diseases and Perinatal Screening (Lis), National Institute of Public Health and the Environment (RIVM), Bilthoven, The Netherlands*

EILEEN VAN HELDEN • *MRC Centre for Molecular and Cellular Biology, Department of Medical Biochemistry, University of Stellenbosch Medical School, Tygerberg, South Africa*

PAUL D. VAN HELDEN • *MRC Centre for Molecular and Cellular Biology, Department of Medical Biochemistry, University of Stellenbosch Medical School, Tygerberg, South Africa*

DICK VAN SOOLINGEN • *Diagnostic Laboratory for Infectious Diseases and Perinatal Screening (Lis), National Institute of Public Health and the Environment (RIVM), Bilthoven, The Netherlands*

THOMAS C. VICTOR • *MRC Centre for Molecular and Cellular Biology, Department of Medical Biochemistry, University of Stellenbosch Medical School, Tygerberg, South Africa*

MARTIN VOSKUIL • *Division of Infectious Diseases and Geographic Medicine, Stanford University Medical Center, Stanford, CA*
ROBIN M. WARREN • *MRC Centre for Molecular and Cellular Biology, Department of Medical Biochemistry, University of Stellenbosch Medical School, Tygerberg, South Africa*
LAWRENCE G. WAYNE • *Tuberculosis Research Laboratory, Department of Veterans Affairs Medical Center, Long Beach, CA*
MICHAEL WILSON • *Affymax Research Institute, Santa Clara, CA*

1

Plasmid Vectors

Nicola Casali and Sabine Ehrt

1. Introduction

Genetic manipulation of mycobacteria has historically been difficult. This is in large part due to the impenetrable nature of the cell wall, resulting in difficulty both in introducing DNA into the bacterium and subsequent isolation of intact plasmid DNA. In addition, the mycobacterial cell wall contains complex lipids and polysaccharides that can contaminate DNA preparations. The hydrophobic nature of the cell wall results in cells clumping in culture, hampering the isolation of clonal populations important for many molecular biological purposes. In spite of these obstacles, the advent of efficient mycobacterial transformation systems *(1)* resulted in an explosion of research into plasmid vectors and numerous genetic systems for *Mycobacterium tuberculosis* have now been described.

This chapter will give an overview of plasmid vectors that have been utilized in mycobacteria, focusing on those whose use has been demonstrated in *M. tuberculosis* or *M. tuberculosis* complex organisms. The first two sections will describe extrachromosomal and integrative plasmid vectors. The third section reviews selectable markers, and expression systems are discussed in the fourth section. Finally, the last section briefly describes the advantages and limitations of reporter genes for studying mycobacterial gene expression. The number of genetic tools now available prohibits a comprehensive listing; however, examples of each type of vector will be given (*see* **Table 1**).

2. Extrachromosomal Plasmid Vectors

The most commonly used extrachromosomal vectors are based on the replicon of pAL5000, a 4.8 kb cryptic plasmid from *Mycobacterium fortuitum*, originally described by Labidi et al. *(2)*. In general, these vectors also contain

From: *Methods in Molecular Medicine*, vol. 54: *Mycobacterium Tuberculosis Protocols*
Edited by: T. Parish and N. G. Stoker © Humana Press Inc., Totowa, NJ

Table 1
Mycobacterial Vectors

Vector	Replicon	Selection[a]	Description	Ref.
pYUB12	pAL5000	kan	Plasmid shuttle vector with *M. fortuitum* plasmid replicon	*(3)*
pMV261	pAL5000	kan	Plasmid shuttle vector with *hsp60* expression cassette	*(5)*
pYUB18	pAL5000	kan	Cosmid shuttle vector	*(6)*
pCG59	pAL5000	kan	Plasmid shuttle vector with temperature-sensitive replicon	*(7)*
pMB351	pLR7	kan	Plasmid shuttle vector with *M. intracellulare* plasmid replicon	*(8)*
pYT937	pMSC262	kan	Plasmid shuttle vector with *M. scrofulaceum* plasmid replicon	*(9)*
pJAZ40	pJAZ38	kan	Plasmid shuttle vector with *M. fortuitum* plasmid replicon	*(10)*
pJAZ42	pJAZ38	str	Plasmid shuttle vector	*(10)*
pBP10	pMF1	kan	Plasmid shuttle vector with *M. fortuitum* plasmid replicon	*(11)*
pCL4D	pCLP	kan	Plasmid shuttle vector with *M. celatum* plasmid replicon	*(12)*
pBL415	ϕD29	kan	Plasmid shuttle vector	*(13)*
phAE77	ϕD29	kan	Plasmid shuttle vector with temperature-sensitive replicon	*(14)*
phAE94	ϕTM4	kan	Plasmid shuttle vector with temperature-sensitive replicon	*(14)*
pEP2	pNG2	kan	Plasmid shuttle vector with *Corynebacterium* plasmid replicon	*(15)*
pEP3	pNG2	hyg	Plasmid shuttle vector	*(15)*
pJRD215	RSF1010	kan, str	Cosmid shuttle vector with IncQ plasmid replicon	*(18)*
phAE19	ϕL1	kan	Integrative shuttle vector	*(1)*

pMH94	ϕL5	kan	Integrative shuttle vector	*(20)*
pEA4	ϕMs6	kan	Integrative shuttle vector	*(21)*
pTSN39	pSAM2	kan	Integrative shuttle vector derived from *S. ambofaciens* plasmid	*(22)*
pUS702	IS900	kan	Plasmid vector with artificial transposon	*(23)*
pPE207	pAL5000	apr, hyg	Plasmid shuttle vector	*(25)*
pMH947	ϕL5	gen	Integrative shuttle vector	*(26)*
pCG76	pAL5000	str	Temperature-sensitive replicon	*(29)*
p16R1	pAL5000	hyg	Plasmid shuttle vector	*(30)*
pMD132	pAL5000	ϕL5 gene 71, kan	Plasmid shuttle vector	*(31)*
pMR001	pAL5000	mer	Plasmid shuttle vector	*(32)*
pMJ10	pAL5000	*sacB*, gen, kan	Plasmid shuttle vector with temperature-sensitive replicon for gene replacement	*(28)*
pMV361	ϕL5	kan	Integrative shuttle vector with *hsp60* expression cassette	*(5)*
pIJK-1	pAL5000	cam, kan	Plasmid shuttle vector with α-antigen leader sequence expression cassette	*(36)*
p19PS	pAL5000	kan	Plasmid shuttle vector with 19 kDa antigen leader sequence expression cassette	*(37)*
pJAM2	pAL5000	kan	Plasmid shuttle vector with inducible expression system	*(39)*

[a] cam, chloramphenicol; gen, gentamicin; hyg, hygromycin; kan, kanamycin; mer, mercury; str, streptomycin.

an origin of replication for *Escherichia coli*, facilitating manipulation of DNA in this organism before transfer into mycobacteria. Early vectors, such as pYUB12 ***(3)***, were simply chimeras of pAL5000 and *E. coli* plasmids with the addition of a gene conferring kanamycin resistance. Subsequently, regions dispensable for replication were delimited by disruption and deletion analysis ***(4)***. Finally, Stover et al. ***(5)*** defined a 1.8 kb minimal origin and engineered this region to remove restriction enzyme sites thus creating useful cloning sites. The resulting construct, pMV261, was found to transform *Mycobacterium bovis* BCG with high efficiency and had an estimated copy number of five. There are now numerous available vectors based on the pAL5000 replication origin, including shuttle cosmid vectors, such as pYUB18, which contain the lambda *cos* packaging site and can be used to clone large segments of DNA ***(6)***. Guilhot et al. ***(7)*** have isolated temperature-sensitive mutants of the plasmid pAL5000 that replicate at 30°C, but are lost from mycobacterial cells at 39°C, and can thus be used as transposon delivery systems. Vectors based on the pAL5000 replicon are able to transform a variety of mycobacterial species including *Mycobacterium smegmatis* and *M. tuberculosis*, although not members of the *Mycobacterium avium* complex.

Several replicons derived from other endogenous mycobacterial plasmids have also been used in vector construction. Beggs et al. ***(8)*** located the origin of replication of the *Mycobacterium intracellulare* plasmid, pLR7, on a 1.8 kb fragment and constructed shuttle vectors incorporating this region and a kanamycin resistance cassette. This construct was capable of transforming *M. avium* strains as well as *M. tuberculosis* and *M. bovis*. Goto et al. ***(9)*** identified a 2.3 kb fragment, from the 15 kb *Mycobacterium scrofulaceum* plasmid, pMSC262, capable of supporting autonomous replication in *M. bovis* BCG. Two further cryptic plasmids isolated from *M. fortuitum* have been described: pJAZ38 ***(10)*** and pMF1 ***(11)***. Vectors containing a 1.1 kb segment of the 16.1 kb plasmid pJAZ38 were maintained as a single-copy in *M. smegmatis*. The minimal replication region of the 9.2 kb plasmid pMF1 was delimited to a 2.1 kb fragment, and pMF1-derivatives were found to be efficiently transformed into *M. tuberculosis* and *M. smegmatis* and stably maintained as a single copy. The regions responsible for replication of pJAZ38 and pMF1 showed homology to the replication regions of pLR7 and pMSC262, although the latter two plasmids are unable to replicate in *M. smegmatis*. Like pMSC262-derived vectors, both pJAZ38 and pMF1 derivatives are compatible with pAL5000 derivatives, but pJAZ38 derivatives are not compatible with pMF1 derivatives. These results imply that pJAZ38, pMF1, pMSC262, and pLR7 are members of a single incompatibility group and that it is distinct from that of pAL5000.

Characterization of a 25 kb linear plasmid pCLP from *Mycobacterium celatum* revealed that a 2.1 kb region was able to support autonomous replication of single-copy circular plasmid forms in *M. smegmatis* ***(12)***. Vectors containing a 4 kb fragment of pCLP also replicated as circular plasmids in *M. bovis* BCG; however, these plasmids were structurally unstable and suffered rearrangements and deletions. The replication origin of pCLP shows some homology to pMF1 and related circular plasmids. However, pCLP-derived vectors were found to be compatible in *M. smegmatis* with both pJAZ38 and pAL5000 derivatives, indicating that this plasmid is a member of a third incompatibility group.

David et al. ***(13)*** established that a 2.6 kb fragment of mycobacteriophage D29 was capable of supporting autonomous plasmid replication in *M. smegmatis*. Later, Bardarov et al. ***(14)*** isolated thermosensitive mutants of similar vectors, based on the mycobacteriophages D29 and TM4. These shuttle vectors have been used as efficient transposon delivery systems to create mutant libraries of *M. bovis* BCG and *M. tuberculosis*.

Plasmids with origins from heterologous species have also been demonstrated to function in mycobacteria. Radford and Hodgson ***(15)*** established that the 1.8 kb replicon of pNG2 is able to promote plasmid replication in mycobacteria. This plasmid, which is also capable of replication in *E. coli*, was isolated from *Corynebacterium*, a genus related to *Mycobacterium*. Derivatives of pNG2, containing either kanamycin or hygromycin resistance genes, were able to transform *M. bovis* BCG with comparable efficiency to pAL5000 derivatives, and it was reported that this plasmid replicates to a high copy number in *M. bovis* BCG. Suprisingly, a number of broad host-range plasmids from Gram-negative bacteria have also been successfully transformed into fast-growing mycobacterial species. However, few of these have been tested in *M. tuberculosis*. Zainuddin et al. ***(16)*** demonstrated that the *E. coli* plasmids, pIJ666 and pSGMU37, were able to transform *M. smegmatis* to chloramphenicol resistance. Gormley and Davies ***(17)*** ascertained that RSF1010, a wide host-range IncQ plasmid expressing streptomycin resistance, which replicates in most Gram-negative bacteria, could be transferred by conjugation from *E. coli* to *M. smegmatis*. The RSF1010-derived cosmid vector pJRD215 was also successfully transformed into *M. smegmatis* and *Mycobacterium aurum*; however unlike the parental plasmid this vector was structurally unstable ***(18)***.

3. Integration Proficient Vectors

Inspired by the early observation that temperate mycobacteriophages are stably maintained in the mycobacterial genome, a number of integration proficient vectors have been constructed based on phage integration and delivery systems. In addition to stability, these vectors offer the advantage that packaged phages are able to infect mycobacteria with high efficiency. In fact, the first vectors successfully introduced into mycobacteria, were phasmids constructed by randomly inserting an *E. coli* cosmid vector into the 50 kb genome of mycobacteriophage TM4 ***(19)***. Snapper et al. ***(1)*** followed a similar approach to derive a phasmid from mycobacteriophage L1, which was shown to stably lysogenize *M. smegmatis* by integration in a site-specific fashion. Incorporation of a kanamycin resistance marker enabled the convenient selection of lysogens. Subsequently, Lee et al. ***(20)*** characterized the site-specific integration system of mycobacteriophage L5 and were able to produce refined vectors that contained the phage attachment site (*attP*) and the integrase gene (*int*) on a 2 kb fragment in an *E. coli* plasmid. In addition, they identified the mycobacterial attachment site (*attB*) in a well-conserved region of the mycobacterial genome, indicating that this plasmid might transform diverse mycobacterial species, and demonstrated its use in *M. smegmatis*, *M. bovis* BCG, and *M. tuberculosis*. Phage excision requires the phage-encoded excisionase gene, *xis*, hence vectors that do not contain this gene are stably maintained in the absence of selection.

Other integrating vectors that have been utilized in *M. smegmatis* and integrate into a conserved region of the genome may also be useful in *M. tuberculosis*. Anes et al. ***(21)*** demonstrated that a 2.7 kb fragment from mycobacteriophage Ms6 was able to support stable lysogeny in *M. smegmatis*. Martin et al. ***(22)*** designed an integration proficient vector based on a plasmid, pSAM2, originally isolated from *Streptomyces ambofaciens*, containing the *attP* region and the genes, *int* and *xis*. This plasmid integrated site-specifically into the genome of *M. smegmatis* and was reportedly stable in the absence of selection.

England et al. ***(23)*** designed an artificial transposon containing two copies of the insertion sequence IS*900*, isolated from *Mycobacterium paratuberculosis*, flanking a kanamycin resistance gene. This 1.5 kb element was inserted into an *E. coli* vector and shown to integrate into the genome of *M. smegmatis* and *M. bovis* BCG ***(24)***. While it showed some target sequence specificity, the copy number in *M. smegmatis* ranged from one to five per cell.

4. Selectable Markers

Appropriate markers are required for the selection of mycobacteria that have taken up DNA. The inherent resistance of mycobacteria to many drugs limits the choice of selectable antibiotic-resistance genes. In addition, antibiotics must be stable over the long incubation periods required for cultivation of the slow-growing mycobacteria. The first selectable genetic markers to be expressed in mycobacteria were the aminoglycoside phosphotransferase genes: *aph* from Tn*903* and *neo* from Tn*5*, conferring kanamycin resistance ***(1)***. Radford and Hodgson ***(15)*** subsequently demonstrated that a hygromycin resistance gene (*hyg*) from *Streptomyces hygroscopicus*, could be utilized in both fast- and slow-growing mycobacteria. These resistance genes still represent the most widely used selectable markers for *M. tuberculosis.*

Selection of recombinant *M. tuberculosis* with the apramycin resistance gene from *Salmonella typhimurium* has also been demonstrated; however, observed transformation frequencies were low ***(25)***. The gentamicin resistance gene *aacC1*, from transposon Tn*1696*, has been utilized in *M. intracellulare* ***(26)*** and Ho et al. ***(27)*** have demonstrated that gentamicin is bacteriostatic for *M. tuberculosis*. However, Pelicic et al. ***(28)*** report that it is not a reliable marker for *M. tuberculosis* complex organisms. Although a gene conferring both streptomycin and spectinomycin resistance has been used in *M. smegmatis* ***(29)***, the therapeutic value of these antibiotics renders their use in *M. tuberculosis* undesirable.

A number of studies suggest that transformation frequencies are highly dependent on the antibiotic resistance marker used, perhaps resulting from variable expression of heterologous genes in the mycobacterial host. For example, Garbe et al. ***(30)*** proposed that the increased frequency of transformation observed when recombinant mycobacteria were selected on hygromycin compared to kanamycin was due to more efficient expression of the *S. hygroscopicus* hygromycin resistance gene than the *E. coli*-derived kanamycin resistance gene.

Aminoglycosides act by inhibiting protein synthesis via interaction with ribosomal components and resistance is generally mediated by modification of the antibiotic. However, spontaneous resistance, arising through modification of the target, can be a significant problem for the slow-growing mycobacteria that contain a single *rrn* operon encoding ribosomal RNAs. Limiting the serial passaging of mycobacterial cultures can reduce the emergence of spontaneous resistance.

In order to circumvent the problem of dissemination of antibiotic resistance genes to the environment, the use of alternative selectable markers is highly desirable. Donnelly-Wu et al. ***(31)*** have described a selection system based on mycobacteriophage L5 gene 71 and report that selection is effective in *M. bovis* BCG. The product of gene 71 is required for maintenance of lysogeny and prevents superinfection by lytic homo-immune phage enabling the selection of phage-resistant transformants. Baulard et al. ***(32)*** demonstrated that expression of mercury resistance, from the *mer* genes of *Pseudomonas aeruginosa* Tn*501* and *Serratia marcescens* pDU1358, could be used for the selection of recombinant mycobacteria. However, the release of toxic mercury vapours may also be hazardous.

A number of counter-selectable markers, that are useful for the generation of allelic exchange mutants using a double-selection strategy, have been described. This approach employs a vector containing the target gene disrupted with a positive marker, to select for integration events, and a secondary marker with a conditionally lethal dominant effect, to select for loss of the vector sequence. For example, the *Bacillus subtilis sacB* gene has been widely used in gene replacement strategies for *M. tuberculosis* ***(33)***. This gene encodes levansucrase which catalyzes the synthesis of high-molecular weight fructose polymers and confers sucrose-sensitivity on mycobacteria.

Other counter-selectable markers that have been used in mycobacteria are *rpsL* and *katG* ***(34,35)***. However, utilization of these genes requires antibiotic-resistant strains, excluding their use for construction of attenuated *M. tuberculosis* strains as live vaccine candidates. The *rpsL* gene encodes the S12 ribosomal protein, which is the target of streptomycin, and mutation in this gene can lead to resistance. Similarly, *katG* confers isoniazid sensitivity and a mutant allele results in resistance. In a merodiploid strain, sensitivity is dominant; thus, transformation of a resistant strain with a replicating vector containing the wild-type allele renders transformants sensitive to the antibiotic. This allows subsequent selection for loss of the vector DNA, signifying a double-crossover event, by reversion to the resistant phenotype.

5. Expression Vectors

Early reports indicated that mycobacterial transcription initiation signals often functioned poorly in *E. coli*. In addition, the comparatively high G+C content of mycobacteria, reflected in the codon bias, limits translational efficiency in this organism and correct posttranslational modification may not occur. Thus, there was a need to develop expression cassettes that could be used to drive and ideally regulate the expression of cloned genes in the mycobacterial host.

The first promoters used to drive protein expression in mycobacteria were derived from genes encoding the mycobacterial heat shock proteins *hsp60* and *hsp70*. These promoters were used since heat shock genes are expressed at a high level and can be further induced under stress conditions. Stover et al. ***(5)*** found that these promoters were able to drive the expression of foreign genes to produce 10% or more of total mycobacterial protein when used on an extrachromosomal plasmid, although expression levels were highly variable between antigens. It was also noted that deregulation of promoter activity occurred when it was present on an extrachromosomal vector. Thus, although a significant increase in expression of endogenous Hsp60 was detected in response to heat shock, constitutive high-level expression was observed from the extrachromosomal *hsp60* promoter.

Other expression cassettes directing the surface expression or secretion of proteins have been designed. Matsuo et al. ***(36)*** established a mycobacterial expression system, directing secretion of the recombinant protein, based on the leader sequence of the α-antigen of *Mycobacterium kansasii*. Stover et al. ***(37)*** demonstrated the use of lipoprotein signal peptides to express membrane-associated antigens in *M. bovis* BCG, utilizing the *M. tuberculosis* 19 kDa antigen leader sequence to direct the export and surface expression of a heterologous antigen. It was noted that expression of a protein with a secretion signal often resulted in lower levels of expression than if it was expressed as a cytoplasmic protein.

Haeseleer ***(38)*** showed that expression vectors, containing the *hsp60* promoter fused to a heterologous antigen, were unstable in *M. bovis* BCG, but that equivalent plasmids without either the *hsp60* promoter or the antigen coding sequence were stable. Thus, it appeared that this instability depended on the process of antigen expression and observation of the phenomenon was increased by the growth advantage conferred on cells containing nonexpressing plasmids. Not all expression plasmids appear to be equally stable in mycobacteria; Stover et al. ***(5)*** report that pMV261 is remarkably stable and they were able to recover recombinant *M. bovis* BCG, expressing foreign antigen, from infected mice several months after immunization. In general, integrative vectors offer the advantage of relative stability ***(38)***. Lower amounts of protein are generally produced from single-copy integrative vectors than from multicopy plasmids; this may be advantageous when overexpression is lethal ***(5)***.

The development of an inducible expression system could circumvent both the problems of plasmid instability and protein toxicity. Triccas et al. ***(39)*** have constructed an expression vector based on the inducible acetamidase enzyme of *M. smegmatis* and demonstrated its use in this organism. *M. smegmatis* was grown in minimal media and the subsequent addition of acetamide resulted in the high-level induction of the recombinant protein. The authors also demonstrated the subsequent purification of His-tagged protein from *M. smegmatis* using Ni^{2+} affinity chromatography, indicating that this proven purification technique can be adapted for use in mycobacteria.

Much of the work on protein expression in mycobacteria has been directed toward the development of recombinant *M. bovis* BCG strains that express antigens from a variety of different pathogens to act as multivalent vaccines ***(5,37)***. *M. bovis* BCG represents one of the most widely administered live attenuated vaccine strains and is an excellent adjuvant, making it a suitable delivery vehicle for foreign antigen expression. In addition, recombinant *M. bovis* BCG secreting mammalian cytokines, expressed as fusions to the α-antigen leader sequence, provide a novel means to manipulate the host immune response ***(40)***.

6. Reporter Genes

Reporter genes are powerful tools for studying gene expression; they are useful for understanding transcriptional regulation including the response to environmental changes. In addition, the use of techniques developed for other pathogenic bacteria, such as in vivo expression technology (IVET) or differential fluorescence induction (DFI) may enable the identification of mycobacterial virulence factors *(41)*. In general, reporter genes encode an enzyme whose activity is easily detectable by a colorimetric or fluorimetric assay. Two types of fusions are possible: transcriptional fusions, in which the reporter gene is fused to the promoter of the gene of interest, but contains its own translational initiation signals, and translational fusions, which contain the reporter gene under both the transcriptional and translational control signals of the gene of interest.

A number of promoter probe vectors are available that can be used for the study of mycobacterial gene expression in vitro (*see* **Table 2**). Reporter vectors based on the *lacZ* gene, encoding β-galactosidase, have been widely used in mycobacteria *(42)*. Colonies can be screened on plates containing 5-bromo-4-chloro-3-indolyl β-D-galactopyranoside (X-gal), which is converted by β-galactosidase to a blue-colored product; alternatively spectrophotometric analysis can be carried out using the substrate *o*-nitrophenyl β-D-galactopyranoside (ONPG), which is cleaved to the yellow-colored *o*-nitrophenol (ONP). Although β-galactosidase activity can be measured in cells that have been permeabilized with sodium dodecyl sulfate (SDS) and chloroform *(43)*, more reproducible results may be obtained using cell-free extracts. Fluorescent substrates such as fluorescein di-(β-D-galactopyranoside) (FDG) or 4-methylumbelliferyl β-D-galactopyranoside (MUG) are especially useful when enzyme levels or bacterial numbers are low. FDG is able to cross the cell envelopes of mycobacteria as well as mammalian cells and has been used to study promoter activity of internalized *M. bovis* BCG without macrophage lysis *(43)*.

Expression of the reporter gene, *cat*, encoding chloramphenicol acetyltransferase (CAT) has been demonstrated in mycobacteria *(44,45)*. CAT activity can be estimated by growth of transformants on media containing increasing concentrations of chloramphenicol. Alternatively, CAT activity can be quantified in cell-free extracts by incubation with the radiolabeled substrate ^{14}C-chloramphenicol and detected in a scintillation counter as a function of protein concentration.

Curcic et al. *(46)* developed a promoter fusion vector, based on the *xylE* gene product, catechol 2,3-dioxygenase (CDO), which converts catechol into a product with a bright yellow color. Catechol is able to penetrate the mycobacterial wall sufficiently to screen colonies for CDO activity by spraying plates with the substrate. This does not adversely affect cell viability and subsequent spectrophotometric quantification can be carried out in cell-free extracts.

The *E. coli* periplasmic alkaline phosphatase, encoded by *phoA*, must be transported across the cytoplasmic membrane in order to be active. Thus, this reporter gene must be fused to the promoter and signal sequence of an exported

Table 2
Reporter Gene Vectors

Vector	Reporter gene and fusion	Selection[a]	Description	Ref.
pJEM12, 13, 14	*lacZ*, translational	kan	Plasmid shuttle vector	*(42)*
pJEM15	*lacZ*, transcriptional	kan	Plasmid shuttle vector	*(42)*
pUS933	*lacZ*, translational	kan	Plasmid shuttle vector	*(43)*
pSD7	*cat*, transcriptional	kan	Plasmid shuttle vector	*(44)*
pEJ108	*cat*, transcriptional	kan	Plasmid shuttle vector	*(45)*
pRCX3	*xylE*, transcriptional	kan	Plasmid shuttle vector	*(46)*
pJEM11	*phoA*, translational	kan	Plasmid shuttle vector	*(47)*
pBPnuc1	*nuc*, translational	hyg	Plasmid shuttle vector	*(48)*
pSG10	*luxA*, *luxB*, transcriptional	kan	Plasmid shuttle vector	*(50)*
pMH30	*FFlux*, transcriptional	kan	Plasmid shuttle vector	*(52)*
pMV361-lux	*FFlux*, transcriptional	kan	Integrative shuttle vector	*(52)*
pWES4	*gfp*, transcriptional	kan	Plasmid shuttle vector	*(55)*
pMV306(*hsp60/gfp*)	*gfp*, transcriptional	kan	Integrative shuttle vector	*(55)*
pFP27	*gfp*, transcriptional	kan	Plasmid shuttle vector	*(56)*

[a]kan, kanamycin; hyg, hygromycin

protein for activity. It is utilized for the identification of secreted or surface-expressed mycobacterial proteins, many of which are purported to be important for virulence ***(47)***. Activity can be determined spectrophotometrically in sonicated extracts using the substrate *p*-nitrophenyl phosphate. Alternatively, secreted proteins can be detected on plates containing 5-bromo-4-chloro-3-indolyl phosphate (X-phosphate), which is cleaved by alkaline phosphatase to a blue-colored product; however, this substrate is ineffectual in 7H10 medium precluding its use for screening slow-growing mycobacteria. A second secretion reporter system based on the *Staphylococcus aureus* nuclease has been developed for use in mycobacteria ***(48)***. Secreted mycobacterial proteins are identified by halo formation around colonies when grown on DNase agar plates containing an indicator dye. Using this system secreted proteins can be identified both in fast- and slow-growing mycobacteria without the need for surrogate hosts.

Bioluminescent reporters such as the green fluorescent protein (GFP) and luciferase are also useful for studying *M. tuberculosis* virulence since they can be assayed without cell disruption, providing the means to follow gene expression intracellularly. Thus, they can be used as reporters of changes in gene expression induced within the macrophage or even in vivo.

Both firefly luciferase, encoded by *FFlux*, and the *Vibrio harveyi* luciferase, encoded by the *luxAB* genes, have been expressed and function in mycobacteria ***(49,50)***. Luciferase emits photons during the oxidation of fatty aldehydes, which can be detected using a luminometer in whole cells, providing a highly sensitive system for the study of gene expression ***(51)***. Using the firefly luciferase, direct detection of recombinant *M. bovis* BCG in infected mouse organ homogenates was demonstrated ***(52)***. Luminescence was readily detected without lysing the mycobacteria. Bioluminescence can be used as a measure of cell viability based on the requirement of firefly luciferase for endogenous ATP production. This technology has been used to develop a sensitive technique for rapid monitoring of in vitro drug susceptibilities in *M. tuberculosis* isolates ***(50)***.

The use of GFP from the jellyfish *Aequorea victoria* offers some advantage over the systems reported above in that it is noninvasive, requiring only appropriate wavelength light for excitation fluorescence. Fluorescence emission of GFP in recombinant mycobacteria can be quantified by spectrofluorimetry and flow cytometry. GFP activity can be detected in recombinant mycobacteria inside macrophages through epifluorescence or laser scanning confocal microscopy. In addition, mycobacteria expressing GFP can be detected in infected mouse tissue and in macrophage vesicles using a fluorescence-activated cell sorter ***(53–55)***. Mutants of GFP, optimized for bacterial fluorescence, have also been utilized in mycobacteria ***(56)***. Disadvantages of GFP are its lower sensitivity compared to luciferase and its extreme stability that make it unsuitable for monitoring rapid changes of gene expression.

7. Conclusions

In recent years a large amount of work has been accomplished in the field of mycobacterial genetics, which has been greatly facilitated by the availability of a large number of plasmid vectors with different features as described in this chapter. New tools for studying mycobacterial gene expression have been developed and existing ones improved. A major advance has been the construction of vectors that enable gene replacement and efficient transposon mutagenesis in *M. tuberculosis* (*see* Chapters 4–7). However, although a variety of expression systems exist there is still a considerable need for a well-regulated system that functions in *M. tuberculosis*. The recent completion of the *M. tuberculosis* genome sequence means that future research is likely to be shaped by newly developed methods of functional genomic analysis that will allow the expression of all *M. tuberculosis* genes to be measured under a variety of environmental conditions as well as during infection of animal models (*see* Chapter 22). These data will need to be verified by the inactivation of genes or by the selective expression of genes of interest under specific conditions taking full advantage of the novel plasmid vectors now available for the genetic manipulation of *M. tuberculosis*.

References

1. Snapper, S. B., Lugosi, L., Jekkel, A., Melton, R. E., Kieser, T., Bloom, B. R., and Jacobs, W. R., Jr. (1988) Lysogeny and transformation in mycobacteria: stable expression of foreign genes. *Proc. Natl. Acad. Sci. USA* **85,** 6987–6991.
2. Labidi, A., Dauguet, C., Goh, K. S., and David, H. L. (1984) Plasmid profiles of *Mycobacterium fortuitum* complex isolates. *Curr. Microbiol.* **11,** 235–240.
3. Snapper, S. B., Melton, R. E., Mustafa, S., Kieser, T., and Jacobs, W. R., Jr. (1990) Isolation and characterization of efficient plasmid transformation mutants of *Mycobacterium smegmatis*. *Mol. Microbiol.* **4,** 1911–1919.
4. Ranes, M. G., Rauzier, J., Lagranderie, M., Gheorghiu, M., and Gicquel, B. (1990) Functional analysis of pAL5000, a plasmid from *Mycobacterium fortuitum*: construction of a "mini" mycobacterium-*Escherichia coli* shuttle vector. *J. Bacteriol.* **172,** 2793–2797.
5. Stover, C. K., de la Cruz, V. F., Fuerst, T. R., Burlein, J. E., Benson, L. A., Bennett, L. T., Bansal, G. P., Young, J. F., Lee, M. H., Hatfull, G. F., Snapper, S. B., Barletta, R. G., Jacobs, W. R., Jr., and Bloom, B. R. (1991) New use of BCG for recombinant vaccines. *Nature* **351,** 456–460.
6. Jacobs, W. R., Jr., Kalpana, G. V., Cirillo, J. D., Pascopella, L., Snapper, S. B., Udani, R. A., Jones, W., Barletta, R. G., and Bloom, B. R. (1991) Genetic systems for mycobacteria. *Methods Enzymol.* **204,** 537–555.

7. Guilhot, C., Gicquel, B., and Martin, C. (1992) Temperature-sensitive mutants of the *Mycobacterium* plasmid pAL5000. *FEMS Microbiol. Lett.* **77,** 181–186.
8. Beggs, M. L., Crawford, J. T., and Eisenach, K. D. (1995) Isolation and sequencing of the replication region of *Mycobacterium avium* plasmid pLR7. *J. Bacteriol.* **177,** 4836–4840.
9. Goto, Y., Taniguchi, H., Udou, T., Mizuguchi, Y., and Tokunaga, T. (1991) Development of a new host vector system in mycobacteria. *FEMS Microbiol. Lett.* **67,** 277–282.
10. Gavigan, J. A., Ainsa, J. A., Perez, E., Otal, I., and Martin, C. (1997) Isolation by genetic labeling of a new mycobacterial plasmid, pJAZ38, from *Mycobacterium fortuitum. J. Bacteriol.* **179,** 4115–4122.
11. Bachrach, G., Colston, M. J., Bercovier, H., Dror, B., Anderson, C., and Papavinasasundaram, K. G. (2000) A new single-copy plasmid, pMF1, from *Mycobacterium fortuitum* which is compatible with the pAL5000 replicon. *Microbiology* **146,** 297–303.
12. Picardeau, M., Le Dantec, C., and Vincent, V. (2000) Analysis of the internal replication region of a mycobacterial linear plasmid. *Microbiology* **146,** 305–313.
13. David, M., Lubinsky-Mink, S., Ben-Zvi, A., Ulitzur, S., Kuhn, J., and Suissa, M. (1992) A stable *Escherichia coli-Mycobacterium smegmatis* plasmid shuttle vector containing the mycobacteriophage D29 origin. *Plasmid* **28,** 267–271.
14. Bardarov, S., Kriakov, J., Carriere, C., Yu, S., Vaamonde, C., McAdam, R. A., Bloom, B. R., Hatfull, G. F., and Jacobs, W. R., Jr. (1997) Conditionally replicating mycobacteriophages: A system for transposon delivery to *Mycobacterium tuberculosis. Proc. Natl. Acad. Sci. USA* **94,** 10,961–10,966.
15. Radford, A. J. and Hodgson, A. L. (1991) Construction and characterization of a *Mycobacterium-Escherichia coli* shuttle vector. *Plasmid* **25,** 149–153.
16. Zainuddin, Z. F., Kunze, Z. M., and Dale, J. W. (1989) Transformation of *Mycobacterium smegmatis* with *Escherichia coli* plasmids carrying a selectable resistance marker. *Mol. Microbiol.* **3,** 29–34.
17. Gormley, E. P. and Davies, J. (1991) Transfer of plasmid RSF1010 by conjugation from *Escherichia coli* to *Streptomyces lividans* and *Mycobacterium smegmatis. J. Bacteriol.* **173,** 6705–6708.
18. Hermans, J., Martin, C., Huijberts, G. N., Goosen, T., and de Bont, J. A. (1991) Transformation of *Mycobacterium aurum* and *Mycobacterium smegmatis* with the broad host-range gram-negative cosmid vector pJRD215. *Mol. Microbiol.* **5,** 1561–1566.
19. Jacobs, W. R., Jr., Tuckman, M., and Bloom, B. R. (1987) Introduction of foreign DNA into mycobacteria using a shuttle phasmid. *Nature* **327,** 532–535.
20. Lee, M. H., Pascopella, L., Jacobs, W. R., Jr., and Hatfull, G. F. (1991) Site-specific integration of mycobacteriophage L5, Integration-proficient vectors for *Mycobacterium smegmatis, Mycobacterium tuberculosis* and bacille Calmette-Guerin. *Proc. Natl. Acad. Sci. USA* **88,** 3111–3115.
21. Anes, E., Portugal, I., and Moniz-Pereira, J. (1992) Insertion into the *Mycobacterium smegmatis* genome of the *aph* gene through lysogenization with the temperate mycobacteriophage Ms6. *FEMS Microbiol. Lett.* **74,** 21–25.

22. Martin, C., Mazodier, P., Mediola, M. V., Gicquel, B., Smokvina, T., Thompson, C. J., and Davies, J. (1991) Site-specific integration of the *Streptomyces* plasmid pSAM2 in *Mycobacterium smegmatis*. *Mol. Microbiol.* **5,** 2499–2502.
23. England, P. M., Wall, S., and McFadden, J. (1991) IS900-promoted stable integration of a foreign gene into mycobacteria. *Mol. Microbiol.* **5,** 2047–2052.
24. Dellagostin, O. A., Wall, S., Norman, E., O'Shaughnessy, T., Dale, J. W., and McFadden, J. (1993) Construction and use of integrative vectors to express foreign genes in mycobacteria. *Mol. Microbiol.* **10,** 983–993.
25. Paget, E. and Davies, J. (1996) Apramycin resistance as a selective marker for gene transfer in mycobacteria. *J. Bacteriol.* **178,** 6357–6360.
26. Marklund, B. I., Speert, D. P., and Stokes, R. W. (1995) Gene replacement through homologous recombination in *Mycobacterium intracellulare*. *J. Bacteriol.* **177,** 6100–6105.
27. Ho, Y. I., Chan, C. Y., and Cheng, A. F. (1997) In vitro activities of aminoglycoside-aminocyclitols against mycobacteria. *J. Antimicrob. Chemother.* **40,** 27–32.
28. Pelicic, V., Jackson, M., Reyrat, J. M., Jacobs, W. R., Jr., Gicquel, B., and Guilhot, C. (1997) Efficient allelic exchange and transposon mutagenesis in *Mycobacterium tuberculosis*. *Proc. Natl. Acad. Sci. USA* **94,** 10,955–10,960.
29. Guilhot, C., Otal, I., Van Rompaey, I., Martin, C., and Gicquel, B. (1994) Efficient transposition in mycobacteria: construction of *Mycobacterium smegmatis* insertional mutant libraries. *J. Bacteriol.* **176,** 535–539.
30. Garbe, T. R., Barathi, J., Barnini, S., Zhang, Y., Abou Zeid, C., Tang, D., Mukherjee, R., and Young, D. B. (1994) Transformation of mycobacterial species using hygromycin resistance as selectable marker. *Microbiology* **140,** 133–138.
31. Donnelly-Wu, M. K., Jacobs, W. R., Jr., and Hatfull, G. F. (1993) Superinfection immunity of mycobacteriophage L5, applications for genetic transformation of mycobacteria. *Mol. Microbiol.* **7,** 407–417.
32. Baulard, A., Escuyer, V., Haddad, N., Kremer, L., Locht, C., and Berche, P. (1995) Mercury resistance as a selective marker for recombinant mycobacteria. *Microbiology* **141,** 1045–1050.
33. Pelicic, V., Reyrat, J. M., and Gicquel, B. (1996) Expression of the *Bacillus subtilis sacB* gene confers sucrose sensitivity on mycobacteria. *J. Bacteriol.* **178,** 1197–1199.
34. Sander, P., Meier, A., and Beottger, E. C. (1995) *rpsL*$^+$: a dominant selectable marker for gene replacement in mycobacteria. *Mol. Microbiol.* **16,** 991–1000.
35. Norman, E., Dellagostin, O. A., McFadden, J., and Dale, J. W. (1995) Gene replacement by homologous recombination in *Mycobacterium bovis* BCG. *Mol. Microbiol.* **16,** 755–760.
36. Matsuo, K., Yamaguchi, R., Yamazaki, A., Tasaka, H., Terasaka, K., Totsuka, M., Kobayashi, K., Yukitake, H., and Yamada, T. (1990) Establishment of a foreign antigen secretion system in mycobacteria. *Infect. Immun.* **58,** 4049–4054.
37. Stover, C. K., Bansal, G. P., Hanson, M. S., Burlein, J. E., Palaszynski, S. R., Young, J. F., Koenig, S., Young, D. B., Sadziene, A., and Barbour, A. G. (1993) Protective immunity elicited by recombinant bacille Calmette-Guerin (BCG) expressing outer

surface protein A (OspA) lipoprotein: a candidate Lyme disease vaccine. *J. Exp. Med.* **178,** 197–209.

38. Haeseleer, F. (1994) Structural instability of recombinant plasmids in mycobacteria. *Res. Microbiol.* **145,** 683–687.
39. Triccas, J. A., Parish, T., Britton, W. J., and Gicquel, B. (1998) An inducible expression system permitting the efficient purification of a recombinant antigen from *Mycobacterium smegmatis. FEMS Microbiol. Lett.* **167,** 151–156.
40. Murray, P. J., Aldovini, A., and Young, R. A. (1996) Manipulation and potentiation of antimycobacterial immunity using recombinant bacille Calmette-Guerin strains that secrete cytokines. *Proc. Natl. Acad. Sci. USA* **93,** 934–939.
41. Heithoff, D. M., Conner, C. P., and Mahan, M. J. (1997) Dissecting the biology of a pathogen during infection. *Trends Microbiol.* **5,** 509–513.
42. Timm, J., Lim, E. M., and Gicquel, B. (1994) *Escherichia coli*-mycobacteria shuttle vectors for operon and gene fusions to *lacZ*: The pJEM series. *J. Bacteriol.* **176,** 6749–6753.
43. Dellagostin, O. A., Esposito, G., Eales, L. J., Dale, J. W., and McFadden, J. (1995) Activity of mycobacterial promoters during intracellular and extracellular growth. *Microbiology* **141,** 1785–1792.
44. Das Gupta, S. K., Bashyam, M. D., and Tyagi, A. K. (1993) Cloning and assessment of mycobacterial promoters by using a plasmid shuttle vector. *J. Bacteriol.* **175,** 5186–5192.
45. Parish, T., Mahenthiralingam, E., Draper, P., Davis, E. O., and Colston, M. J. (1997) Regulation of the inducible acetamidase gene of *Mycobacterium smegmatis. Microbiology* **143,** 2267–2276.
46. Curcic, R., Dhandayuthapani, S., and Deretic, V. (1994) Gene expression in mycobacteria: Transcriptional fusions based on *xylE* and analysis of the promoter region of the response regulator *mtrA* from *Mycobacterium tuberculosis. Mol. Microbiol.* **13,** 1057–1064.
47. Lim, E. M., Rauzier, J., Timm, J., Torrea, G., Murray, A., Gicquel, B., and Portnoi, D. (1995) Identification of *Mycobacterium tuberculosis* DNA sequences encoding exported proteins by using *phoA* gene fusions. *J. Bacteriol.* **177,** 59–65.
48. Downing, K. J., McAdam R. A., and Mizrahi, V. (1999) *Staphylococcus aureus* nuclease is a useful secretion reporter for mycobacteria. *Gene* **239,** 293–299.
49. Andrew, P. W. and Roberts, I. S. (1993) Construction of a bioluminescent mycobacterium and its use for assay of antimycobacterial agents. *J. Clin. Microbiol.* **31,** 2251–2254.
50. Jacobs, W. R., Jr., Barletta, R. G., Udani, R., Chan, J., Kalkut, G., Sosne, G., Kieser, T., Sarkis, G. J., Hatfull, G. F., and Bloom, B. R. (1993) Rapid assessment of drug susceptibilities of *Mycobacterium tuberculosis* by means of luciferase reporter phages. *Science* **260,** 819–822.
51. Gordon, S., Parish, T., Roberts, I. S., and Andrew, P. W. (1994) The application of luciferase as a reporter of environmental regulation of gene expression in mycobacteria. *Lett. Appl. Microbiol.* **19,** 336–340.
52. Hickey, M. J., Arain, T. M., Shawar, R. M., Humble, D. J., Langhorne, M. H., Morgenroth, J. N., and Stover, C. K. (1996) Luciferase *in vivo* expression technol-

ogy: use of recombinant mycobacterial reporter strains to evaluate antimycobacterial activity in mice. *Antimicrob. Agents Chemother.* **40,** 400–407.

53. Kremer, L., Baulard, A., Estaquier, J., Poulain-Godefroy, O., and Locht, C. (1995) Green fluorescent protein as a new expression marker in mycobacteria. *Mol. Microbiol.* **17,** 913–922.
54. Dhandayuthapani, S., Via, L. E., Thomas, C. A., Horowitz, P. M., Deretic, D., and Deretic, V. (1995) Green fluorescent protein as a marker for gene expression and cell biology of mycobacterial interactions with macrophages. *Mol. Microbiol.* **17,** 901–912.
55. Parker, A. E., and Bermudez, L. E. (1997) Expression of the green fluorescent protein (GFP) in *Mycobacterium avium* as a tool to study the interaction between mycobacteria and host cells. *Microb. Path.* **22,** 193–198.
56. Barker, L. P., Porcella, S. F., Wyatt, R. G., and Small, P. L. (1999) The *Mycobacterium marinum* G13 promoter is a strong sigma 70-like promoter that is expressed in *Escherichia coli* and mycobacteria species. *FEMS Microbiol. Lett.* **175,** 79–85.

2

Isolation of DNA from *Mycobacterium tuberculosis*

Paul D. van Helden, Thomas C. Victor, Robin M. Warren, and Eileen G. van Helden

1. Introduction

Research into and identification of *Mycobacterium tuberculosis* can take on a number of facets, many of which involve the use of DNA at one stage or another. The quality and quantity of DNA required will depend on the end-use requirement. For example, good yields of pure, high-molecular-weight DNA uncontaminated by DNA from other sources (i.e., homogeneous) are optimal for the generation of cosmid libraries and sequencing ***(1)***, Southern hybridization ***(2–6)***, or microarray analysis ***(7)*** for genome studies, whereas relatively crude DNA (fragmented DNA or DNA from multiple sources [i.e., heterogeneous]) may be adequate for PCR-based diagnosis ***(8–12)*** or amplification of regions of the genome for other purposes, e.g., identification of mutations conferring drug resistance ***(13,14)***.

The source of material and the method selected for DNA preparation will define the purity and yield. It is important to bear in mind the aim of the project when deciding on the process to be followed. For example, strain genotyping using Southern hybridization ***(2–6)*** would generally require highly purified high-molecular-weight DNA from live cultures, whereas PCR-based examination of small areas of the genome can be done from archival material, such as formalin-fixed granulomas or Ziehl-Neelsen (ZN) slides ***(8–12)***. If fresh or frozen material is available, it may be preferable to establish a culture of *Mycobacterium tuberculosis* in liquid or on solid medium prior to attempting DNA recovery. This will facilitate recovery of high yields of clean, homogeneous high-molecular-weight DNA.

The tough cell wall of *Mycobacterium tuberculosis* can be both an advantage and a hindrance. The tough and complex cell wall ***(15)*** complicates purification

From: *Methods in Molecular Medicine*, vol. 54: *Mycobacterium Tuberculosis Protocols*
Edited by: T. Parish and N. G. Stoker © Humana Press Inc., Totowa, NJ

in comparison to that of bacteria with relatively fragile walls. The mycobacteria have cell walls with copious amounts of polysaccharides, which can adversely influence subsequent manipulation of DNA. This cell wall can, however, allow the recovery of intact bacteria from a variety of sources and therefore help to remove much contaminating material, but the subsequent lysis of the bacterium and removal of the wall components to recover purified DNA is not trivial.

The extent to which purification needs to be done will also be a function of the starting material, since many biological samples contain unknown but potent inhibitors of enzymes ***(16)***, which may hamper further manipulation of the DNA.

Here we describe protocols for the preparation of DNA from *M. tuberculosis*. We have focused on the recovery of DNA from clinically derived samples, which can be used for diverse purposes, such as DNA fingerprinting, cloning, or PCR diagnostic work. Note that many of the appropriate methods for DNA purification from clinical material may result in a heterogeneous DNA preparation, which contains both mycobacterial and human genomic DNA ***(8–12,17)***. The sample preparation method always represents a trade-off between the requirements for the optimal methods, the source material and the aim of the procedure. In this regard, the number of organisms per volume of sample is critical. Factors to consider during sample preparation include the efficiency of target recovery, maintenance of intact DNA, the removal of known and unknown inhibitors, and safety factors for the worker. If DNA purification for diagnostic purposes is envisaged, care must be taken to avoid cross-contamination during all preparative stages ***(19)***. These are not the only methods that can be used or have been described; however, in our laboratory these methods are used on a regular basis and yield good quality material for further manipulation. For example, methods involving mechanical lysis ***(20)*** or use of guanidinium salts ***(21)*** have been described, but these harsher methods can yield sheared DNA, which may not be useful for purposes such as Southern blotting or cloning of larger fragments ***(22)***. The recovery of sheared or heterogeneous DNA does not necessarily exclude obtaining typing data, however, since PCR-based methods may still be useful in these cases ***(23)***.

Good quality and high yields of DNA can be obtained when *M. tuberculosis* is cultured in BACTEC vials, on Lowenstein-Jensen (LJ) slants, on 7H11 agar, or in 7H9 broth. The description of the culturing of the organism is not the objective of this chapter and the reader should refer to the relevant literature for further information ***(20)***. Clinical isolates of *M. tuberculosis* for DNA purification will frequently be established as cultures on LJ slants or in BACTEC vials. If the latter, a small aliquot can be streaked and grown on LJ or in liquid medium for further DNA isolation. DNA may also be recovered from other clinical sources, such as microscopy slides (ZN-stained), biopsy material, biological fluids (e.g., sputum, blood, urine, cerebrospinal fluid [CSF], or in vitro cultures [e.g., macrophages]). The preparation and recovery of these is described, since the diagnosis and rapid characterization of clinical strains may play an important role in future strategies to curb the spread of the disease.

2. Materials

2.1. Recovery of Bacteria from Various Sources

Many sources of mycobacteria can be used for DNA preparation including: ZN- or auramine-stained microscopy slides, cultures on solid or in liquid medium, and biological specimens, e.g., sputum, biopsies, urine, CSF, in vitro cultures (*see* **Note 1**).

2.1.1. From Liquid Medium

1. Phosphate buffered saline (PBS): 8 m*M* NaCl, 2.6 m*M* KCl, 1.4 m*M* K_2HPO_4, 8 m*M* Na_2HPO_4, pH 7.4.
2. Oven or water bath set at 80°C.
3. Extraction buffer: 50 m*M* Tris-HCl, 25 m*M* EDTA, 5% mono-sodium glutamate, pH 7.4.
4. 50 mL Polypropylene tubes containing ±30 glass balls (5 mm).

2.1.2. From Solid Medium

1. Oven or water bath set at 80°C.
2. Extraction buffer: (*see* **Subheading 2.1.1., item 3**).
3. Disposable inoculation loops.
4. 50 mL polypropylene tubes containing ±30 glass balls (5 mm).

2.1.3. Formalin-Fixed Tissue

1. Xylene.
2. Absolute ethanol.
3. Speedy-vac (Savant, New York).
4. Sterile distilled water.

2.1.4. Frozen or Fresh Tissue Sample

1. Mortar and pestle.
2. Dounce glass homogenizer with loose pestle.
3. Cell lysis buffer: 32 m*M* sucrose, 1% Triton X-100, 5 m*M* $MgCl_2$, 10 m*M* Tris-HCl, pH 7.6.

2.1.5. Microscopy Slides

1. PBS (*see* **Subheading 2.1.1., item 1**).
2. Scalpel and blades.
3. 10% Saponin.
4. Sterile distilled water.
5. 20% Chelex 100 (Sigma, Poole, Dorset, UK).

2.1.6. Sputum

1. Decontamination solution: 4% (w/v) NaOH, 1% (w/v) *N*-acetyl-L-cysteine.
2. Extraction buffer (*see* **Subheading 2.1.1., item 3**).
3. Lysozyme stock: 50 mg/mL, make immediately prior to use.
4. 10X proteinase K buffer: 100 m*M* Tris-HCl, 50 m*M* EDTA, 5% SDS, pH 7.8.
5. Proteinase K stock solution: 10 mg/mL. Store in aliquots at –20°C.
6. Buffer-saturated phenol *(22)*: gently warm phenol to 68°C (place the bottle in extra container to contain spillages). Add hydroxyquinoline to 0.1%. Add an equal volume of 0.5 *M* Tris-HCl, pH 8.0. Stir for at least 10 min, then allow phase separation. Aspirate upper aqueous phase. Add an equal volume of 0.1 *M* Tris-HCl (pH 8.0). Repeat mixing and aspiration until pH of aqueous phase is >7.8. Add 0.1 vol of 0.1 *M* Tris-HCl, pH 8.0, containing 0.2% mercaptoethanol. Keep the solution in the dark at 4°C for up to 4–5 wk (*see* **Note 2**).
7. Phenol/chloroform/isoamylalcohol (25:24:1). Prepare with the buffer-saturated phenol (*see* **Note 2**).

2.1.7. Bone Marrow or Whole Blood

1. Histopaque 1077 (Sigma).
2. PBS (*see* **Subheading 2.1.1., item 1**).
3. Lysis buffer: 10 m*M* Tris-HCl, pH 8.2, 400 m*M* NaCl, 2 m*M* EDTA. Add 50 µL of 10% SDS and 50 µL of 10 mg/mL proteinase K per mL of buffer before use.
4. 6 *M* NaCl.
5. Sterile distilled water.

2.1.8. Infected Macrophages

1. 10 m*M* EDTA, pH 7.5.
2. PBS (*see* **Subheading 2.1.1., item 1**).
3. 10% SDS.

2.2. Enzymatic Lysis of Cells and Isolation of Genomic DNA

1. DNAse free RNAse: 10 mg/mL stock (*see* **Note 3**).
2. 50 mg/mL lysozyme stock: make immediately prior to use.

2.3. Removal of Protein and Cellular Contaminants

1. 10X proteinase K buffer.
2. Proteinase K stock solution: 10 mg/mL. Store in aliquots at –20°C.
3. Phenol/chloroform/isoamylalcohol (25:24:1) (*see* **Subheading 2.1.6., item 7**).
4. Chloroform/isoamylalcohol (24:1)

2.4. DNA Precipitation and Recovery

1. 3 *M* sodium acetate, adjust to pH 5.5 with acetic acid.
2. Ice-cold isopropanol.
3. 70% ethanol.
4. 1X TE-buffer: 10 m*M* Tris-HCl, 1 m*M* EDTA, pH 8.0.

2.5. Quantitation and Purity of Genomic DNA

1. TE (*see* **Subheading 2.4., item 4**).
2. Restriction enzyme and buffer.
3. Agarose gel electrophoresis equipment.
4. 3 *M* Na acetate, pH 5.5.
5. Absolute ethanol (at –20°C).

3. Methods

3.1. Recovery of Bacteria from Various Sources

Note that DNA recovered from pure cultures will be homogeneous, whereas clinical samples may yield heterogeneous DNA (*see* **Note 1**).

3.1.1. From Liquid Medium

1. Cells from liquid samples, including cultures ***(24)***, urine, and CSF (*see* **Note 4**) may be recovered by centrifugation in a category 3 biosafety laboratory. Centrifuge samples in sealed tubes (*see* **Note 5**) for 5 min in a microfuge or at 3000*g* in a bench centrifuge for 15 min.
2. Wash cells once with 1 mL of PBS without resuspending cells.
3. Heat-kill cells by placing in oven or water-bath at 80°C for 1 h (*see* **Note 6**).
4. Resuspend cells in extraction buffer and proceed with DNA extraction as described below (**Subheading 3.1.2., step 3**). Use approx 6 mL of buffer for every 100 µL of cell pellet.

3.1.2. From Solid Medium

The example given is for isolation of DNA from *M. tuberculosis* grown on solid medium ***(20)***, for example, use an LJ slant culture of *M. tuberculosis* which has clearly visible colonies. Pure cultures will yield high molecular weight homogeneous DNA.

1. Heat sealed tube at 80°C for 1 h to kill bacteria (*see* **Note 6**). Subsequent steps can be carried out in a class 2 or 3 laminar flow cabinet.
2. Add 3 mL of extraction buffer and carefully scrape the colonies off the slant, using a disposable loop (estimated colony volume up to 100 µL).
3. Pour the buffer and bacteria into a 50 mL polypropylene tube containing approx 30 glass balls (5 mm diameter).
4. Add 3 mL of extraction buffer to the slant and remove remaining colonies — pool both extracts into polypropylene tube.
5. Vortex the suspension in a tightly sealed polypropylene tube at full speed for 2–3 min to disrupt the bacterial colonies. All clumps should be broken up. Proceed with DNA extraction by lysis of cells (*see* **Subheading 3.2.**).

3.1.3. Tissue (Formalin Fixed)

Heterogeneous DNA will be obtained from this source.

1. Collect one 10 μm tissue section from each paraffin block in a sterile 1.5 mL tube and deparaffinize as follows *(25)* (*see* **Note 7**).
2. Add 0.5 mL of xylene to the tube and vortex.
3. Incubate at room temperature for 5 min.
4. Centrifuge at 11,000*g* for 5 min.
5. Remove the supernatant and wash the pellet twice with ethanol.
6. Dry on a Speedy-vac sample concentrator.
7. Resuspend the pellet in 20 μL of sterile distilled water and boil for 10 min.
8. Proceed as in **Subheading 3.2.** (*see* **Note 8**).

3.1.4. Frozen or Fresh Tissue Samples

If it is not necessary to establish a culture prior to DNA extraction, the following procedure may be followed. The following steps should be done in a laminar flow cabinet in a class 3 biosafety facility.

1. Homogenize (grind) sample under liquid nitrogen in a mortar and pestle.
2. Add 6 vol of lysis buffer and homogenize with three strokes of a loose pestle in a Dounce glass homogenizer.
3. Treat as for sputum (*see* **Subheading 3.1.6.**).

3.1.5. Microscopy Stained Slide

1. Pipet 100 μL of PBS onto stained area of slide (*see* **Note 9**).
2. Scrape the material off with a scalpel and transfer to a 1.5 mL tube containing 900 μL of PBS and 50 μL of 10% Saponin.
3. Invert several times and incubate overnight at 4°C.
4. Centrifuge at 11,000*g* for 5 min, remove the supernatant and resuspend the pellet in 1 mL of PBS.
5. Incubate at 4°C for 2 h.
6. Centrifuge at 11,000*g* and discard the supernatant.
7. Add 50 μL of distilled water and 50 μL of 20% Chelex.
8. Incubate for 10 min at 95°C. Vortex every 2 min.
9. Spin for 5 min at 11,000*g* and recover the supernatant. Proceed as in **Subheading 3.2.** (*see* **Note 8**).

*3.1.6. Sputum (see **Note 8**)*

1. Liquefy sputum by adding an equal volume of decontamination solution to a sputum sample in a sealable centrifuge tube (*see* **Note 10**).
2. Centrifuge at 11,000*g* for 10 min.
3. Aspirate supernatant (at this stage the pellet may be stored at –20°C for future use).
4. Heat for 10 min at 95°C (or 80°C for 1 h).
5. Resuspend the pellet in 100 μL of extraction buffer (*see* **Subheading 2.2.7.**).
6. Add 10 μL of 10 mg/mL lysozyme (*see* **Note 11**).
7. Incubate at 37°C for 2 h, with occasional mixing.

8. Add 10 µL of proteinase K buffer and 10 µL of proteinase K stock solution.
9. Incubate overnight (16 h) at 45°C.
10. Add an equal volume (150 µL) of phenol/chloroform/isoamylalcohol (25:24:1) and mix gently by inverting tube 6 times, ensuring that liquid remaining in the bottom of the tube is also mixed ("flick" with finger).
11. Centrifuge in a microfuge at 10,000*g* for 5 min.
12. Remove upper aqueous phase (approx 100 µL). Proceed to **Subheading 3.4.**

3.1.7. Bone Marrow or Whole Blood

1. Layer 1 mL of bone marrow aspirate or blood onto 3 mL of Histopaque 1077 in a conical tube and centrifuge at 400*g* for 30 min at room temperature.
2. Aspirate the upper layer to within 0.5 cm of the opaque interface containing mononuclear cells, and discard.
3. Pipet off the opaque interface into a conical centrifuge tube containing 5 mL PBS, taking care not to transfer any Histopaque. Centrifuge at 250*g* for 10 min.
4. Discard the supernatant and wash the pellet again with PBS.
5. Resuspend the pellet in 1 mL of lysis buffer.
6. Incubate at 65°C for 1 h.
7. Add 0.2 mL of 6 *M* NaC1 and mix.
8. Centrifuge at 2000*g* for 15 min.
9. Recover the supernatant and add 2 vol of cold ethanol. Incubate at –70°C for 30 min. Recover the DNA by "fishing out" or by centrifugation at 12,000*g* for 10 min.
10. Dry the DNA pellet on a Speedy-vac sample concentrator.
11. Redissolve the DNA in 30 µL of water or TE (*see* **Note 12**).

3.1.8. Infected Macrophages (in vitro)

1. Aspirate the culture medium from adherent cells in dish.
2. Add sufficient cold 10 m*M* EDTA pH 7.5 per well (for a 1 cm diameter well, use 110 µL) to just cover cells and incubate for 10 min.
3. Add 2 vol of PBS and 0.2 vol of 10% SDS and incubate at 4°C for 10 min.
4. Remove the suspension and proceed as in **Subheading 3.1.6., step 4**, or **Subheading 3.1.1.**

3.2. Lysis of Bacterial Cells

This step is used primarily for cultures of *M. tuberculosis* (*see* **Subheading 3.1.2.**) and in this case yields high-quality homogeneous DNA. DNA from other starting material is also obtainable using this method, but may be contaminated with other DNA (e.g., from the host source) (*see* **Note 13**).

1. Add 400 µL of 50 mg/mL lysozyme stock and 10 µL of 10 mg/mL RNAase (*see* **Note 11**).
2. Incubate at 37°C for 2 h. Mix occasionally by gentle agitation.
3. Proceed to **Subheading 3.3.**

3.3. Removal of Protein and Cellular Contaminants

Cell lysates obtained by enzymatic, mechanical or other means of lysis or a crude preparation can be processed using this method. The volumes given are for 6 mL of cell suspension (*see* **Note 14**).

1. Add 0.1 vol (600 µL) of 10X proteinase K Buffer.
2. Add 150 µL of 10 mg/mL proteinase K.
3. Mix gently and incubate at 45°C for 16 h.
4. Add 5 mL of phenol/chloroform/isoamylalcohol and mix gently by inverting tube five times. Repeat the inversion steps four times over 30 min (*see* **Note 15**).
5. Centrifuge at 3000*g* at room temperature for 20 min.
6. Remove upper aqueous phase. If viscous, use a plastic pipet tip with narrow end cut off to enlarge aperture.
7. Add 5 mL of chloroform/isoamylalcohol, mix gently and centrifuge at 3000*g* at room temperature for 20 min.
8. Recover the upper aqueous phase and proceed to **Subheading 3.4.**

3.4. DNA Precipitation and Recovery

1. Add 0.1 vol (700 µL) of 3 *M* Na acetate, pH 5.5, to the supernatant (from **Subheading 3.3.**).
2. Add an equal volume of isopropanol.
3. Gently mix by inverting tube 2–4 times.
4. "Fish" the DNA out with a sealed tip Pasteur pipet (*see* **Note 16**).
5. Alternatively, incubate at –20°C for 30 min and centrifuge at 3000*g* for 30 min (*see* **Notes 17** and **18**).
6. Wash the pellet in 5 mL of 70% ethanol.
7. Air dry at 55°C until dry.
8. Dissolve the DNA pellet in 500 µL of TE. Incubate at 65°C until dissolved and store at –20°C (*see* **Note 12**).

3.5. Quantitation and Purity of Genomic DNA

3.5.1. Spectrophotometric Quantitation of DNA

1. Make a 1/50 dilution of an aliquot of the DNA stock in TE.
2. Read the absorbance at A_{260} and A_{280}.
3. Calculate the concentration of DNA using the formula (A_{260}) × (50 µg/mL) × (dilution fold) = concentration (µg/µL) of undiluted genomic DNA (*see* **Note 19**).
4. The A_{260}/A_{280} ratio should be 1.8 (*see* **Note 20**).

3.5.2. Electrophoretic Estimation of Quantity and Purity

1. Pipet approx 6 µg (estimated by spectrophotometry or other means) of DNA into a small tube.
2. Add 10 µL of 10X concentrate buffer appropriate for the restriction enzyme to be used, 3 µL of a 10 U/µL restriction enzyme stock and water to a final volume of 100 µL.

3. Incubate the mixture at the appropriate temperature (usually 37°C) for 3–16 h.
4. Electrophorese 1/10 of the sample (10 µL), as well as 100 ng of uncut DNA on a 1% agarose gel, using high molecular weight standards.
5. Stain the gel with ethidium bromide and visualize by UV transillumination (*see* **Note 21**).
6. Precipitate the cut DNA solution by adding 0.1 vol of 3 *M* sodium acetate, pH 5.5, and 3 vol of 100% ethanol at –20°C. Keep at –20°C overnight.
7. Spin at 10,000*g* and aspirate. Wash DNA with 70% ethanol. Dry and redissolve the DNA such that the final concentrations of cut DNA are all equal (*see* **Note 21**).

4. Notes

1. *M. tuberculosis* is a human pathogen, which requires extensive therapy to cure. Drug-resistant strains may be common and may be difficult, if not impossible to deal with once disease has progressed in an individual. Therefore all samples should be regarded as potentially hazardous and not be removed from a category 3 biosafety facility until inactivated. Work with live (or potentially live) organisms should be done only by properly trained persons, following appropriate safety guidelines.
2. Phenol and chloroform are corrosive, toxic and phenol may cause burns. Work should be done in an adequately ventilated environment (preferably fume hood) and appropriate safety measures taken (goggles, gloves, laboratory coat). The best quality phenol should always be used.
3. DNAse-free RNAse is best purchased commercially. Alternatively, it may be prepared by heating the enzyme to 100°C for 15 min ***(22)***.
4. Centrifugation of biological samples (e.g., CSF) will also pellet eukaryotic cells and result in a DNA preparation of mixed sources. This can be avoided by centrifugation over sucrose ***(26)***.
5. Centrifugation of samples containing live *M. tuberculosis* should be carried out in holders which seal with O-rings to minimize danger of creating aerosol suspensions.
6. Heat treatment at 80°C for 1 h will effectively kill the pathogen ***(18)***. Nevertheless, for added safety, subsequent steps (up to the phenol extraction step) should be carried out in a laminar flow cabinet. Extending the period of heating may lead to DNA degradation.
7. Decontamination of the microtome knife can be done with 70% ethanol after sectioning each block.
8. This preparation is not necessarily pure or homogeneous DNA, but is useful for direct PCR-based amplification.
9. The stained material (in the case of a ZN-slide) or microtome section cannot be scraped off while dry, as the material crumbles and shatters and is easily lost. The addition of PBS allows the scraped material to be easily recovered from the liquid.
10. A 10 µL aliquot of the liquefied sputum sample can be used directly for PCR analysis. The following method provides good reproducibility: overlay 0.5 mL of

the liquefied sputum sample onto 1 mL of sterile 50% (w/v) sucrose. Centrifuge at 12,000*g* for 5 min and wash the pellet in 100 µL of sterile saline, finally resuspend in 50 µL of saline. Use 10 µL of this suspension (with or without lysis of cells) directly for PCR amplification. This method may also be used for other samples, e.g., CSF, urine. The partial purification of the bacteria often improves results, as inhibitors of PCR are present in many fluids, whether of plant or animal origin. Prior to PCR-based analysis, lyse the bacteria by boiling and use the solution directly as the PCR substrate.

11. Lysozyme and RNAse A digestions must be done prior to addition of SDS and proteinase K.
12. If the DNA pellet fails to dissolve easily in TE or water, add a further volume and repeat 65°C heating step until dissolved.
13. Mechanical lysis results in sheared DNA which is not as useful as DNA prepared in this way.
14. Use tubes which seal to avoid spillage or generation of aerosols. Tubes should be polypropylene, which is resistant to the organic solvents used.
15. Hexadecyltrimethylammonium bromide (CTAB) treatment prior to the first phenol/chloroform extraction step can be carried out. This helps to remove polysaccharides which can copurify with DNA. Add 5 *M* NaCl or 3 *M* Na acetate, followed by addition of CTAB ***(20)*** to a final concentration of 10–12%. Mix and incubate for 10 min at 65°C. Proceed with extraction.
16. It is desirable to be able to recover a stringy precipitate with a rod or pipet tip, since this represents high molecular weight, good-quality DNA.
17. Isopropanol precipitation of DNA usually yields a large fluffy DNA conglomerate. If the cell number is low or for other reasons no conglomerate is seen, DNA may still be recovered by centrifugation and washing in 70% ethanol. If an oily residue is seen at these stages, discard prep and begin again. Usually, if the fluffy precipitate is not seen it is indicative of smaller fragments of DNA, which will give background problems if restriction fragment length polymorphism (RFLP) analysis or cloning of large fragments is planned.
18. DNA quantity is also dependent on the confluency of culture. Inadequate starting material will not yield sufficient DNA for "spooling" from alcohol precipitation.
19. This calculation is based on the approximation that 20 A_{260} U of DNA represents a concentration of 1 mg/mL. The dilution factor is 50, if 20 µL is pipeted into 1000 mL.
20. Pure double-stranded DNA has an A_{260}/A_{280} ratio of 1.8 ***(20,22)***. Ratios of 1.7 to 2.0 are acceptable, but indicate some degree of contamination, which may lead to inhibition of subsequent procedures. Further purification can be done by reextracting with phenol/chloroform/isoamylalcohol as described in **Subheading 3.3**.
21. Uncut DNA should show a band larger than 50kb. Diffuse material below this indicates sheared DNA. The digested DNA should be seen as a series of fragments over a broad size-range. There should be no DNA remaining in the intact genomic DNA zone. Quanititation is estimated on the basis of comparable fluo-

rescence intensity, between samples or with an accurately measured standard. For RFLP or dot-blot analysis, the concentration of DNA is important and should be determined as described.

References

1. Cole, S. T., Brosch, R., Parkhill, J., Garnier, T., Churcher, C., Harris, D., Gordon, S. V., Eiglmeier, K., Gas, S., Barry, C. E., 3rd, Tekaia, F., Badcock, K., Basham, D., Brown, D., Chillingworth, T., Connor, R., Davies, R., Devlin, K., Feltwell, T., Gentles, S., Hamlin, N., Holroyd, S., Hornsby, T., Jagels, K., and Barrell, B. G. (1998) Deciphering the biology of *Mycobacterium tuberculosis* from the complete genome sequence. *Nature* **393,** 537–544.
2. Van Embden, J. D., Cave, M. D., Crawford, J. T., Dale, J. W., Eisenach, K. D., Gicquel, B., Hermans, P., Martin, C., McAdam, R., and Shinnick, T. M. (1993) Strain identification of *Mycobacterium tuberculosis* by DNA fingerprinting: recommendations for a standardized methodology. *J. Clin. Microbiol.* **31,** 406–409.
3. Van Soolingen, D., de Haas, P. E., Hermans, P. W., and van Embden, J. D. (1994) DNA fingerprinting of *Mycobacterium tuberculosis. Methods Enzymol.* **235,** 195–205.
4. Wiid, I. J. F., Werely, C., Beyers, N., Donald, P., and van Helden, P. D. (1994) Oligonucleotide $(GTG)_5$ as a marker for *Mycobacterium tuberculosis* strain identification. *J. Clin. Microbiol.* **32,** 1318–1321.
5. Warren, R., Hauman, J., Beyers, N., Richardson, M., Schaaf, H. S., Donald, P., and van Helden, P. (1996) Unexpectedly high strain diversity of *Mycobacterium tuberculosis* in a high-incidence community. *S. Afr. Med. J.* **86,** 45–49.
6. Warren, R., Richardson, M., van der Spuy, G., Victor, T., Sampson, S., Beyers, N., and an Helden, P. (1999) DNA fingerprinting and molecular epidemiology of tuberculosis: use and interpretation in an epidemic setting. *Electrophoresis* **20,** 1807–1812.
7. Behr, M. A., Wilson, M. A., Gill, W. P., Salamon, H., Schoolnik, G. K., Rane, S., and Small, P. M. (1999) Comparative genomics of BCG vaccines by whole-genome DNA microarray. *Science* **284,** 1520–1523.
8. Shankar, P., Manjunath, N., Mohan, K. K., Prasas, K., Behari, M., Shriniwas, and Ahuji, G. K. (1991) Rapid diagnosis of tuberculosis meningitis by PCR. *Lancet* **337,** 5–7.
9. Lombard, E. H., Victor, T., Jordaan, A., and van Helden, P. D. (1994) The detection of *Mycobacterium tuberculosis* in bone marrow aspirates using the polymerase chain reaction. *Tuberc. Lung Dis.* **75,** 65–69.
10. Donald, P. R., Victor, T. C., Jordaan, A. M., Schoeman, J. F., and van Helden, P. D. (1993) Polymerase chain reaction in the diagnosis of tuberculous meningitis. *Scand. J. Infect. Dis.* **25,** 613–617.
11. Victor, T., Jordaan, H. F., van Niekerk, D. J. T., Louw, M., Jordaan, A., and van Helden, P. D. (1992) Papulonecrotic tuberculid identification of *Mycobacterium tuberculosis* DNA by polymerase chain reaction. *Am. J. Dermatopathol.* **14,** 491–495.

12. Van Vollenhoven, P., Heyns, C. F., de Beer, P. M., Whitaker, P., van Helden, P. D., and Victor, T. (1996) Polymerase chain reaction in the diagnosis of urinary tract tuberculosis. *Urol. Res.* **24,** 107–111.
13. Victor, T. C., Pretorius, G. S, Telix, J. V., Jordaan, A. M., and van Helden, P. D. (1996) KatG mutations in isoniazid-resistant strains of *Mycobacterium tuberculosis* are not infrequent. *Antimicrob. Agents Chemother.* **40,** 1572.
14. Victor, T. C., Warren, R., Butt, J. L., Jordaan, A. M, Felix, J. V., Venter, A, Sirgel, F. A., Schaaf, H. S., Donald, P. R., Richardson, M., Cynamon, M. H., and van Helden, P. D. (1997) Genome and MIC stability in *Mycobacterium tuberculosis*: indications for continuation of usage of INH in MDR-TB. *J. Med. Microbiol.* **46,** 847–857.
15. Brennan, P. J. and Nikaido, H. (1995) The envelope of mycobacteria. *Ann. Rev. Biochem.* **64,** 29–63.
16. Victor, T., du Toit, R., and van Helden, P. D. (1992) Purification of sputum samples through sucrose improves the detection of *Mycobacterium tuberculosis* by PCR. *J. Clin. Microbiol.* **30,** 1514–1517.
17. Wright, D. K. and Manos, M. M. (1990) Sample preparation from paraffin-embedded tissues, in PCR Protocols: A guide to methods and applications. Academic Press, New York. Chapter **19,** 153–158.
18. Bemer-Melchor, P., and Drugeon, H. B. (1999) Inactivation of *Mycobacterium tuberculosis* for DNA typing analysis. *J. Clin. Microbiol.* **37,** 2350–2361.
19. Victor T., Jordaan, A., du Toit, R., and van Helden, P. (1993) Laboratory experience and guidelines to avoid false PCR results. *Eur. J. Clin. Chem. Clin. Biochem.* **31,** 531–533.
20. Belisle, J. T. and Sonnenberg, M. G. (1998) Isolation of genomic DNA from mycobacteria, in *Methods in Molecular Biology*, vol. 101, *Mycobacteria Protocols* (Parish, T. and Stoker, N. G., eds.), Humana, Totowa, NJ, pp. 31–44.
21. Boom, R., Sol, C. J., Solimons, M. M., Jansen, C. L., Wetheim-van-Dillen, P. M., and van der Noordaa, J. (1990) Rapid and simple method for purification of nucleic acids. *J. Clin. Microbiol.* **28,** 495–503.
22. Sambrook, J., Fritsch, E. F., and Maniatis, T. (1989) *Molecular Cloning: A Laboratory Manual*, 2nd ed. Cold Spring Harbor Laboratory, Cold Spring Harbor, NY.
23. Richner, S., Meiring, J., and Kirby, R. (1999) DNA profiling of *Mycobacterium tuberculosis* from the Eastern Province of South Africa and the detection of a high level of genetic diversity. *Electrophoresis* **20,** 1800–1806.
24. Meyer, P. R., Bourn, W. R., Steyn, L. M., van Helden, P. D., Beyers, A. D., and Brown, G. D. (1998) Novel method for rapid measurement of growth of mycobacteria in detergent-free media. *J. Clin. Microbiol.* **36,** 2752–2754.
25. Claas, E. C., Melchers, W. J., van der Linden, H. C., Lindeman, J., and Quint, W. G. (1989) Human papillomavirus detection in paraffin-embedded cervical carcinomas and metastases of the carcinomas by the polymerase chain reaction. *Am. J. Pathol.* **135,** 703–709.

3

Extraction of RNA from Intracellular *Mycobacterium tuberculosis*

Methods, Considerations, and Applications

Irene M. Monahan, Joseph A. Mangan, and Philip D. Butcher

1. Introduction

Pathogenicity in *Mycobacterium tuberculosis* may be thought of as a multifactorial process with both pathogen and host-response effector molecules contributing to the process of infection, leading either to immunopathology and disease or control of infection and long-term persistence. Little is known about this at a genetic level, but it is becoming recognized that bacterial virulence constitutes the correct temporal and spatial regulation of many genes that may be necessary for a particular phase in infection in response to specific environmental cues.

The complete genome sequence of *M. tuberculosis* is now available ***(1)*** and will facilitate the understanding of the complex biology of host-pathogen interactions that lead to tuberculosis. We can now move toward a functional understanding of the genome sequence, where the patterns of gene expression in different environments are defined and linked with the structure and function of the protein products, and other molecules in the cell. Thus, monitoring the expression of mRNA for specific genes or on a whole genome scale using microarrays is fast becoming a major and tractable component of functional genomics of *M. tuberculosis* (*see* Chapter 22). In this respect, analysis of gene expression after exposure to antibiotics for all 3924 predicted open reading frames (ORFs) of the *M. tuberculosis* genome using microarrays has recently been described ***(2)***, and several reports have used subtraction hybridization analysis to define a more limited set of differentially regulated mRNA transcripts after exposure to isoniazid ***(3)*** or after phagocytosis by macrophages ***(4)***.

From: *Methods in Molecular Medicine*, vol. 54: *Mycobacterium Tuberculosis Protocols*
Edited by: T. Parish and N. G. Stoker © Humana Press Inc., Totowa, NJ

There is a growing interest in the study of gene expression at the mRNA level in mycobacterial research. One imperative, therefore, is the availability of efficient, reliable, and simple technologies for the extraction of mRNA for subsequent analysis by methods such as Northern blotting, primer extension, RNAse protection, reverse transcription (RT)-polymerase chain reaction (PCR), random arbitrarily primed (RAP)-PCR, RNA fingerprinting, subtractive cDNA hybridization, and microarray hybridization. Any RNA extraction method must be rapid enough to prevent degradation of short half-life mRNA (approx 2 min), and must prevent artifactual changes in transcription during the bacterial recovery and extraction processes. Such effects may not be apparent when studying a single gene, which fortuitously may not be differentially regulated by that condition. However, for whole genome transcript analysis by microarrays, the issue is clearly critical. In the case of infection models or natural disease (e.g., murine models of infection; in vitro macrophage infection; human tuberculosis), it would be advantageous to be able to remove excess host RNA effectively so as not to swamp the bacterial mRNA. These criteria are difficult to meet with organisms such as *M. tuberculosis*, which have complex cell walls that cannot easily be disrupted by standard detergent or chaotropic solutions used for the rapid lysis of other bacteria. Removal of host cell RNA is especially important for gene expression studies utilizing randomly primed approaches to generating cDNA where the preponderance of host RNA would effectively compete for the available primers, thus reducing the specific activity of the bacterial component. Although beneficial, removal of host cell RNA is less of an issue where gene specific priming is used, such as RT-PCR, which is less affected by nontarget sequences.

We have developed simple, quick, and reproducible methods over the past few years to extract intact RNA from pure mycobacterial cultures ***(5–7)***. We have extended these methods to rapidly isolate mycobacterial total RNA from macrophage infection models free from host RNA through differential lysis with simultaneous protection from degradation of the bacterial mRNA ***(8)***. We have also shown that these preparation methods prevent transcriptional changes during extraction ***(9)***. As most bacterial mRNA is not polyadenylated, it is difficult to purify it away from the much more abundant ribosomal RNA. However, it has been shown that total bacterial RNA can be used for cDNA synthesis for microarray analysis due to the low hybridization volume and the relatively low complexity of the bacterial mRNA ***(2,10)***.

The protocol described in this chapter uses a guanidinium thiocyanate (GTC)-based lysis solution to extract total RNA from bacteria either grown in broth or recovered from inside adherent macrophage cell lines. The GTC solution penetrates the mycobacteria without causing bacterial lysis, immediately protects the labile mRNA from degradation and at the same time blocking any further transcriptional changes during the process of bacterial harvesting. Furthermore, this method allows the recovery of mycobacteria from within macrophages, because of a differential lysis effect. Since it completely lyses the macrophage but not the mycobacteria, this allows the now chemically stabilized bacteria to be recovered from the lysate by centrifugation, without changes in mRNA representation due to altered environmental conditions. Thus, this method ensures that the bacterial mRNA transcript profile associated with the condition under study remains unchanged during the subsequent manipulations and is essentially free of host RNA, thus facilitating approaches to monitoring mRNA transcription during infection.

2. Materials

2.1. Culture of Mycobacteria

1. Dubos broth: dissolve 1.3 g Dubos broth base (Difco, West Molesy, Surrey, UK) in 180 mL of water, autoclave and cool below 50°C.
2. Albumin-dextrose complex supplement (ADC): 10 g bovine serum albumin, fraction V (BSA), 15 g D-glucose, 1.6 g NaCl in 200 mL water. Filter sterilize with 0.45 micron filter.
3. Dubos/ADC: aseptically add 20 mL of ADC to 180 mL of Dubos broth. Leave at 37°C for 24 h to test for sterility (*see* **Note 1**).
4. Thoma chamber (Hawksley, London, UK).
5. 30 mL plastic V-bottom universals (Bibby Sterilin LTD, Stone, Staffordshire, UK).

2.2. Macrophage Cell-Line Culture and Infection

1. THP-1 cells: a human acute monocytic leukemic cell line of macrophage lineage ($CD14^+$, $CD15^+$). Source: Dr. G. Farrar and MRC AIDS Directed Program Reagent Project *(11)*.
2. Fetal calf serum (FCS) (Life Technologies, Paisley, UK): heat inactivate at 56°C for 30 min. Store at –20°C in 50 mL aliquots.
3. 200 m*M* glutamine stock solution (Life Technologies). Note that glutamine is unstable and will only last 5 d once reconstituted.
4. RPMI 1640 medium (without glutamine) containing 2 g/L bicarbonate (Life Technologies).
5. Complete RPMI medium without antibiotics: add 50 mL of FCS and 5 mL of glutamine stock solution to one 500 mL bottle of RPMI.
6. Antibiotic stock solution: penicillin 5000 U/mL and 5 mg/mL Streptomycin (ICN, Basingstoke, UK). Final concentration of 100 U/mL and 100 µg/mL respectively.
7. Complete RPMI medium plus antibiotics: add 50 mL of FCS, 5 mL of glutamine stock and 10 mL of antibiotic stock solution to one 500 mL bottle of RPMI.
8. Phorbol 12-myristate-13-acetate (PMA) stock solution: 2 µ*M* (24 µg/mL); dissolve 1 mg of PMA in 1 mL of dimethyl sulphoxide (DMSO) and add 40.67 mL of RPMI medium. Store at –20°C in 1 mL aliquots. Do not repeatedly thaw and refreeze.

9. Neubauer hemocytometer counting chamber (Weber Scientific, Teddington, Middlesex, UK).
10. 25 cm^2 tissue culture flasks.
11. 175 cm^2 tissue culture flasks.
12. Sonicator with 2 mm probe (Ultrasonics Engineering, London, UK).

2.3. RNA Extraction

1. GTC solution 1 (for RNA extraction from *M. tuberculosis* infected macrophage monolayers): 4 *M* guanidine thiocyanate (Fluka Company, Gillingham, Dorset, UK), 0.5% sodium N-lauryl sarcosine, 25 m*M* tri-sodium citrate, 0.1 *M* 2-mercaptoethanol, 0.5% Tween-80, pH to 7.0 with 1 *M* HCl (*see* **Note 6**).
2. GTC solution 2 (for RNA extraction from *M. tuberculosis* broth cultures): 5 *M* guanidine thiocyanate, 0.5% sodium N-lauryl sarcosine, 25 m*M* tri-sodium citrate, 0.1 *M* 2-mercaptoethanol, 0.5% Tween-80, pH to 7.0 with 1 *M* HCl.
3. 0.5% w/v Tween-80.
4. RNAse-free distilled water.
5. 2 mL skirted, screw-capped, microcentrifuge tubes with O-ring seal containing 0.5 mL of 0.1 mm silica/ceramic beads (Ribolyser blue tubes from Hybaid Ltd, Ashford, Middlesex, UK or Fast RNA blue matrix tubes from Bio101, Vista, CA).
6. Ribolyser reciprocal shaker (Ribolyser from Hybaid or Fastprep FP120 cell disruptor from Bio101).
7. 500 m*M* sodium acetate pH 4: add 4.1 g of sodium acetate (anhydrous) to 80 mL of water, titrate to pH 4.0 using glacial acetic acid and adjust the final volume to 100 mL. Recheck the pH periodically as it can drift.
8. Acid phenol: water saturated phenol (Biophenol; Camlab, Cambridge, UK). Equilibrate by shaking with 2 vol of 50 m*M* sodium acetate, pH 4.0, after first removing the water phase (*see* **Note 4**).
9. Detergent solution: 9.6 mL of neat DivoLab No. 1 detergent solution (Weston Favell Centre, Northampton, UK or Lever Institutional and Laundry Products, Southfield, MI), 24 mL of 500 m*M* sodium acetate pH 4.0, and 66.4 mL RNAse-free distilled water.
10. Chloroform/isoamyl alcohol 24:1.
11. Isopropanol solution: add 49.7 mL isopropanol to 0.3 mL 3 *M* sodium acetate, pH 5.2.

3. Methods

3.1. Growth of Mycobacteria

When working with hazard group 3 microorganisms like *M. tuberculosis*, it is essential to perform all the work in a Class I biological safety cabinet in a Category III laboratory according to local Health and Safety Regulations.

1. Take a colony from an agar plate or slope and inoculate 10 mL of Dubos/ADC. Culture for 7–10 d at 37°C with gentle shaking (*see* **Note 1**).

2. Inoculate 200 mL of Dubos/ADC with the 10 mL culture and incubate with gentle shaking for 7–10 d until the bacterial count reaches no more than 10^8/mL. For an estimate of growth, count in a Thoma chamber after treating an aliquot with 10% formalin for 1 h.
3. Take 20 mL of this culture and inoculate 200 mL of Dubos/ADC. Incubate for 5–7 d at 37°C; this should provide a mid-log phase culture (*see* **Note 3**). Aliquots (2 mL) of this culture can be frozen at –70°C for future stocks.
4. Every 7 d, subculture 20 mL into 200 mL Dubos/ADC. This can be repeated for six passages, after which time it should be discarded and a fresh culture started from frozen culture (1 mL aliquots at –70°C) (*see* **Note 2**).
5. Thaw 1 mL of frozen bacteria and add to 9 mL Dubos/ADC and incubate for 10 d. Add this to fresh 200 mL Dubos/ADC and culture as above.

3.2. RNA Extraction from In Vitro Grown Broth Cultures of M. tuberculosis

1. Prepare in advance a 2 mL skirted, screw-capped, microcentrifuge tube with an "O" ring seal containing 0.5 mL of 0.1 mm silica/ceramic beads. Add 500 μL of detergent solution (*see* **Note 7**), 500 μL acid-phenol and 100 μL of chloroform/isoamyl alcohol (24:1) for later use.
2. Add 4 vol of 5 *M* GTC lysis solution 2 to the mycobacteria in liquid culture, i.e., 400 mL of 5 *M* GTC to 100 mL of bacteria in broth culture, and mix rapidly by swirling. This produces a final concentration of 4 *M* GTC.
3. Transfer to 30 mL plastic V-bottom universals and centrifuge at 5000*g* for 30 min to pellet the mycobacteria (*see* **Note 5**). Decant the supernatant carefully without disturbing the pellet which is often very small and sometimes difficult to see. Resuspend the mycobacterial pellet from one universal in 1 mL of 4 *M* GTC solution 1. Use this 1 mL GTC to resuspend the pellets from other universals.
4. Pellet bacteria in a microcentrifuge at 15,000*g* for 20 s.
5. Rapidly resuspend pellet in 1 mL of 0.5% Tween-80. This is essential for certain types of culture media which for unknown reasons cause low yields without this wash step. Spin again. The whole procedure should take less than 2 min.
6. Resuspend the washed bacterial pellet in 200 μL of RNAse-free distilled water and immediately add to the RNA extraction solution in the ribolyser tube from **step 1** and immediately process in the ribolyser reciprocal shaker at 6.5 power setting for 45 s (*see* **Note 8**).
7. The bacteria will be completely disintegrated and solubilized in the detergent/solvent solution. Remove tube from the reciprocal shaker and spin in a microcentrifuge at 15,000*g* for 10 min to pellet the bacterial debris, and separate the phases.
8. Carefully remove the upper aqueous layer (about 500 μL) containing the RNA, without contamination with the phenol phase or interphase, and put in a fresh microfuge tube and reextract with 500 μL of chloroform/isoamyl alcohol (24:1), again removing the aqueous phase to a fresh microfuge tube.

9. Precipitate the RNA by the addition of an equal volume (approx 500 µL) of isopropanol solution. Leave at –70°C for at least 30 min or may be kept for long-term storage; spin in microcentrifuge for 15 min to pellet the precipitated RNA and carefully remove the isopropanol supernatant.
10. Briefly dry the pellet in a vacuum drier for a few minutes and redissolve the RNA in RNAse-free water (*see* **Note 9**).
11. Store at –70°C (*see* **Note 7**).

3.3. Macrophage Cell Line Culture

All tissue culture work should be carried out under suitable conditions in a Class II biological safety cabinet. When infecting cells with hazard group 3 microorganisms like *M. tuberculosis*, the tissue culture is performed in a Class I safety cabinet in a Category III laboratory according to local Health and Safety Regulations.

3.3.1. Recovery of Frozen Cell Stocks

Cells can be stored in liquid nitrogen in 1 mL aliquots in 90% FCS, 10% DMSO at a cell density of 10^7/mL. To reconstitute cells from frozen stocks:

1. Rapidly thaw 1 mL aliquots in a 37°C water bath.
2. Add to 25 mL of prewarmed complete RPMI medium containing antibiotics.
3. Spin at 75*g* for 10 min to collect cells. Remove supernatant and resuspend cell pellet in 20 mL of complete RPMI + antibiotics and place in a 25 cm^2 tissue culture flask in a humidified 37°C incubator containing 5% CO_2 in air.
4. After 24 h, remove the medium and replace with fresh complete RPMI medium containing antibiotics (*see* **Note 10**).
5. Count the cells to estimate cell density and grow until 1×10^6 cells/mL is reached (approx 3 d) at which stage cells are ready to be passaged.

3.3.2. Enumeration of Macrophages

1. Resuspend cells in medium and place in a Neubauer hemocytometer counting chamber.
2. The average number of cells in four big squares (each containing 16 small squares) $\times 10^4$ = total cells/mL.

3.3.3. Maintenance, Passage and Expansion of THP–1 Cell Line

1. Grow THP-1 cells in suspension and passage every 5 d as follows:
2. Grow THP-1 cells to 1×10^6/mL in 20 mL of complete RPMI with antibiotics at 37°C in a humidified 5% CO_2/air incubator.
3. Add 1 mL of cell suspension to 10 mL of complete RPMI with antibiotics in a new 25 cm^2 tissue culture flask and repeat passage every 5 d.
4. To expand the cells into 175 cm^2 tissue culture flasks that hold 30 mL culture medium, add 3 mL of grown cells per flask and 27 mL of complete RPMI medium.

5. Culture for 5 d and then split again to expand the number of flasks required (*see* **Note 12**).

3.3.4. Preparation of Cells for Infection

1. Passage cells at least three times in medium without antibiotics (*see* **Note 10**).
2. Dilute the PMA stock 1/100 in complete RPMI medium and add 0.5 mL to each 175 cm^2 flask containing cells at 1×10^6/mL in 30 mL of culture medium. The final PMA concentration is 20 n*M* or 12 ng/mL) (*see* **Note 16**).
3. Leave for 24 h.
4. Remove nonadherent cells by washing twice with warmed complete RPMI (by tipping off supernatant medium and replace with 30 mL fresh medium). Be gentle so as not to disturb the monolayer.

3.4. Infection of Macrophage Monolayers

1. For each 175 cm^2 flask required spin 10 mL (approx 5×10^8 bacteria) of mid log phase mycobacteria in Dubos/ADC at 5000*g* for 10 min (*see* **Note 12**).
2. Resuspend in 1 mL of RPMI complete medium without antibiotics and sonicate at 70% amplitude with the 2-mm probe for 5×3 s bursts to disperse clumps.
3. Add sonicated bacteria onto cell monolayer in 175 cm^2 flasks (contain approx $2–5 \times 10^7$ macrophages) and leave for 12 h to phagocytose in CO_2 incubator at 37°C (*see* **Note 11**).
4. Decant medium and wash away extracellular bacteria and non adhered cells by adding 20 mL of warmed complete media. Gently rock the flask, tip off medium and repeat washing twice.
5. Replace with 30 mL of fresh medium.
6. Leave for desired time intervals before RNA extraction (*see* **Note 12**).

3.5. RNA Extraction from intracellular M. tuberculosis (see Note 13)

1. Tip off medium from infected macrophage monolayer in a 175 cm^2 flask and wash twice with 20 mL of warmed complete RPMI media. Then pour on 100 mL of 4 *M* GTC lysis solution and immediately rock the flask to lyse cells (*see* **Note 14**).
2. Pipet quickly up and down without making bubbles with a long nose, plastic Pasteur pipet at least 20 times until viscosity is reduced. Alternatively, pour the cell lysate into 30 mL plastic universal containers and vortex for 2 min (*see* **Note 15**).
3. Centrifuge at 5000*g* for 20 min in 30 mL plastic universals with V-bottoms to pellet mycobacteria (which do not lyse).
4. Tip away the supernatant and resuspend the mycobacterial pellet from one universal (which is often very small and sometimes difficult to see) in 1 mL of 4 *M* GTC solution. Use this 1 mL GTC to resuspend the pellets from other universals. Thus, all the pellets from 30 flasks are now resuspended in 1 mL of GTC solution.
5. Pellet bacteria in a microcentrifuge at 15,000*g* for 20 s.

6. Rapidly resuspend pellet in 1 mL of 0.5% Tween-80. This is essential for certain types of culture media that for unknown reasons cause low yields without this wash step. Spin again. The whole procedure should take less than 2 min.
7. Resuspend the washed bacterial pellet in 200 µL of RNAse-free distilled water and immediately add to the RNA extraction solution in the ribolyser tube from **step 1** and immediately process in the Ribolyser reciprocal shaker at 6.5 power setting for 45 s (*see* **Note 8**).
8. The bacteria will be completely disintegrated and solubilized in the detergent/solvent solution. Remove tube from the reciprocal shaker and spin in a microcentrifuge at 15,000*g* for 10 min to pellet the bacterial debris, and separate the phases.
9. Carefully remove the upper aqueous layer (about 500 µL) containing the RNA, without contamination with the phenol phase or interphase, and put in a fresh microfuge tube and reextract with 500 µL of chloroform/isoamyl alcohol (24:1), again removing the aqueous phase to a fresh microfuge tube.
10. Precipitate the RNA by the addition of an equal volume (approx 500 µL) of isopropanol solution. Leave at –70°C for at least 30 min or may be kept for long-term storage; spin in microcentrifuge for 15 min to pellet the precipitated RNA and carefully remove the isopropanol supernatant.
11. Briefly dry the pellet in a vacuum drier for a few minutes and redissolve the RNA in RNAase-free water (*see* **Note 9**).
12. Store at –70°C or below (*see* **Note 7**).

4. Notes

1. Several liquid culture media are available for mycobacteria, such as Middlebrook 7H9, but we use Dubos/ADC. One major issue is to minimize clumping, thus improving quantitation of bacterial numbers and achieving more consistent phagocytosis of mycobacteria by macrophages. We see little difference between 7H9 and Dubos media, since both contain Tween-80, which minimizes clumping.
2. Continual passage of bacteria in liquid culture may result in phenotypic changes due to selection of natural subtypes/mutants. Precautions to prevent this involve minimizing the number of passages by returning to a frozen stock of bacteria. Frozen stocks can be prepared simply by freezing a mid-log phase culture in Dubos broth (containing ADC supplement) at –70°C.
3. For a more accurate determination of the growth curve of *M. tuberculosis*, colony forming units (cfu) can be estimated by plating out dilutions of broth culture onto Middlebrook 7H11 agar plates containing 10% v/v OADC supplement (Difco) and 0.5% glycerol. Cfu may be estimated after 3 wk of incubation at 37°C. In liquid culture a true mid-log phase is achieved within 2–4 d, after which the curve starts to flatten out with stationary phase after about 15 d. Small variations in culture conditions can affect the growth phase and hence may affect gene expression profiles.
4. The pH of the phenol is critical for the efficient phase partitioning of DNA into the organic phase.

5. Use only these V-bottom universals, as the angle aids the formation of a tight bacterial pellet. We have tried larger plastic screw-capped centrifuge tubes (50 mL) with conical bottoms to minimize the number of tubes to be spun, but the bacterial pellet is easily lost.
6. The inclusion of Tween-80 in the GTC solution aids the sedimentation of mycobacteria.
7. General precautions when handling RNA. RNA should not be thawed and frozen repeatedly. Store the RNA in small volumes; thaw, use once and discard any remainder. RNA is best stored at –70°C or below; –20°C is not recommended. RNA should be handled with great caution; it is highly susceptible to degradation by trace amounts of ribonucleases. All precautions to prevent ribonuclease contamination of all buffers, tubes, and tips must be taken. Wear gloves at all times to minimize the transfer of ribonucleases from skin. Observe strict hygiene with gloves and change them frequently. Do not use autoclaved tips or tubes, since this can introduce ribonucleases that renature on cooling. Use them directly from the manufacturers' packages and do not handle them except with clean gloves. All water should be deionized, glass distilled and collected directly into RNAse-free plasticware. We do **not** use diethylpyrocarbonate (DEPC) treated water as trace amounts persist even after autoclaving and can inhibit some enzyme reactions.
8. During processing, the tubes increase in temperature due to the large frictional forces being generated; if further processing is necessary, the tubes should first be cooled on ice. If the tubes become too hot, they may fracture in the machine causing sample loss. Tubes should not be over filled as the solutions expand upon processing and again cause tube failure and sample loss.
9. A cloudy precipitate is sometimes seen during resuspension of the RNA pellet. We believe this to be a component of the detergent solution which coprecipitates with the RNA. Although noninhibitory to reverse transcriptase, *Taq* polymerase or Klenow enzymes, the precipitate causes unacceptably high background fluorescence for microarray hybridizations. The precipitate may be removed by spinning the RNA, once completely dissolved, at full speed in a microcentrifuge for 2 min and carefully removing the aqueous phase which contains the RNA. For microarray hybridizations, we do not recommend the use of detergent-based lysis methods for RNA extractions. Methods based on acid-phenol *(2)* or acid phenol/GTC, and their commercial derivatives (TRIzol from Life Technologies, Paisley, Scotland; RNAzol B from Cinna/Biotecx Labs, Inc., Friendswood, TX) may prove to be suitable alternatives.
10. The use of antibiotics in tissue culture should be minimized since streptomycin builds up inside cells and may affect gene expression or even kill mycobacteria. For routine maintenance of cells we include antibiotics, but exclude them for at least three passages during expansion of cell numbers prior to infection. Good sterile technique is therefore essential.
11. An infection ratio (multiplicity of infection) of 10 mycobacteria per cell is used here. Too many bacteria can kill the cells and too few may not result in sufficient RNA for analysis. Gene expression patterns may also vary according to MOI as

the number of intracellular mycobacteria may influence the nature of host-pathogen interaction; this must be considered when interpreting or comparing results. Another factor that may influence apparent changes in mRNA is the kinetics of interaction of cohorts of phagocytosed mycobacteria. During a 12 h period of phagocytosis some mycobacteria will be phagocytosed early, whereas others may be phagocytosed later. The longer the period of phagocytosis, the less likelihood of a single cohort of bacteria with similar gene expression patterns being analyzed. This assumes that the gene expression patterns change in response to a changing environment within the cell (i.e., cell adhesion and entry, phagolysosome fusion, adaption, escape to cytoplasm, and growth, and so on). However, this has not yet been clearly demonstrated for mycobacteria, but should be considered in the design of experiments such as this. For THP-1 cells, we use a 12 h period of phagocytosis and 12, 24, 48, and 72 h time points after infection. These times may be reduced but this will result in the recovery of fewer intracellular mycobacteria and therefore the number of THP-1 cells infected (flasks) will need to be increased to obtain sufficient mycobacterial RNA for analysis.

12. The number of flasks of macrophages required is dependent on the efficiency of phagocytosis of the macrophage cell line, the multiplicity of infection (MOI), the yield of intracellular mycobacteria recovered from infected macrophages, the efficiency and yield of the RNA extraction method. In this protocol, we describe the use of THP-1 macrophage cell line which has efficiencies of phagocytosis over a 12 h period of 30% of added mycobacteria at an MOI of 10. For THP-1 cells, we see > 80% of cells containing mycobacteria with 2–3/cell at 12 h after infection. The RNA extraction method described yields about 20 μg of total RNA per 10^9 mycobacteria. Thirty tissue culture flasks (175 cm^2) each containing 2–3 × 10^7 THP-1 cells, when infected with 5 × 10^8 *Mycobacterium bovis* BCG/flask (MOI = 10) yielded approx 100 μg of total RNA with no visible macrophage RNA.
13. We have shown that penetration of mycobacteria by the GTC lysis solution used in this protocol occurs in less than 1 min but without bacterial lysis, that mRNA is stabilized intact and that no changes in mRNA transcription occur during this process ***(9)***. Thus, lysis of macrophages in GTC allows separation of bacteria from the macrophage cell lysate at leisure without compromising the mRNA. Unlysed, but mRNA-stabilized mycobacteria, are simply separated from macrophage lysate by centrifugation and washing in GTC. Intact mycobacterial RNA, free from macrophage RNA, is thus recovered. **Warning:** an RNA extraction method that does not immediately inactivate transcription and prevent degradation of mRNA will be of no value and will generate data that is not biologically relevant to the questions asked.
14. It is essential to have a sufficient volume of GTC lysis solution to quickly and efficiently lyse the macrophages. If there is insufficient lysis solution, contaminating macrophage RNA will be extracted along with the mycobacterial RNA. We use 35 mL of GTC solution per 175 cm^2 tissue culture flask containing approx 2 × 10^7 cells.

15. Reducing viscosity with Pasteur pipeting is an effective technique but may not be used safely for pathogenic mycobacteria due to the high risk of generating aerosols. For pathogenic mycobacteria, transferring the lysate to universal containers followed by vigorous vortexing is the safest effective method. Failure to reduce the viscosity sufficiently will result in inefficient sedimentation of the mycobacteria and reduced yields of RNA.
16. When THP-1 cells are grown and infected in suspension, it is difficult to separate extracellular mycobacteria from infected macrophages using centrifugation and washing methods. When monitoring intracellular gene expression, it is essential to remove extracellular bacteria so that mRNA is only extracted from intracellular mycobacteria. The addition of PMA to stimulate the differentiation of THP-1 alters their phenotype to an adhered cell type. Extracellular bacteria may simply be washed off the cell monolayer. However, THP-1 cells adhere only weakly and excessive fluid flow will wash the cells off. Some loss after infection during washing is inevitable and we lose about 20–50% of cells at 24 h and 72 h after infection, respectively.

References

1. Cole, S. T., Brosch, R., Parkhill, J., Garnier, T., Churcher, C., Harris, D. et al. (1998) Deciphering the biology of *Mycobacterium tuberculosis* from the complete genome sequence. *Nature* **393,** 537–544.
2. Wilson, M., DeRisi, J., Kristensen, H. H., Imboden, P., Rane, S., Brown, P. O., and Schoolnik, G. K. (1999) Exploring drug-induced alterations in gene expression in *Mycobacterium tuberculosis* by microarray hybridization. *Proc. Natl. Acad. Sci. USA* **96,** 12,833–12,838.
3. Alland, D., Kramnik, I., Weisbrod, T. R., Cerny, R., Miller, L. P., Jacobs, Jr., W. R., and Bloom, B. R. (1998) Identification of differentially expressed mRNA in prokaryotic organisms by customized amplification libraries (DECAL): the effect of isoniazid on gene expression in *Mycobacterium tuberculosis. Proc. Natl. Acad. Sci. USA* **95,** 13,227–13,232.
4. Graham, J. E., and Clark-Curtiss, J. E. (1999) Identification of *Mycobacterium tuberculosis* RNAs synthesized in response to phagocytosis by human macrophages by selective capture of transcribed sequences (SCOTS). *Proc. Natl. Acad. Sci. USA* **96,** 11,554–11,559.
5. Mangan, J. A., Sole, K. M., Mitchison, D. A., and Butcher, P. D. (1997) An effective method of RNA extraction from bacteria refractory to disruption, including mycobacteria. *Nucleic Acids Res.* **25,** 675–676.
6. Butcher, P. D., Sole, K. M., and Mangan, J. A. (1999) RNA extraction, in *Molecular Mycobacteriology: Techniques and Clinical Applications* (Ollar, R. A. and Connell, N. D., eds.), Marcel Dekker Inc. USA, pp. 325–350.
7. Patel, B. K. R., Banerjee, D. K., and Butcher, P. D. (1991) Extraction and characterisation of mRNA from mycobacteria: implication for virulence gene identification *J. Microbiol. Methods* **13,** 99–111.
8. Butcher, P. D., Mangan, J. A., and Monahan, I. M. (1998) Intracellular gene expression: Analysis of RNA from mycobacteria in macrophages using RT-PCR, in *Meth-*

ods in Molecular Biology, vol. 101: *Mycobacteria Protocols* (Parish, T. and Stoker, N. G., eds.), Humana, Totowa, NJ, pp. 285–306.

9. Monahan, I. M. (1997) PhD Thesis. University of London.
10. de Saizieu, A., Certa, U., Warrington, J., Gray, C., Keck, W., Mous, J. (1998) Bacterial transcript imaging by hybridization of total RNA to oligonucleotide arrays. *Nat. Biotechnol.* **16,** 45–48.
11. Tsuchiya S., Yamabi, M., Yamaguchi, Y., Kobayashi, Y., Konno, T., and Tada, K. (1980) Establishment and characterisation of a human acute monocyte cell line (THP-1). *Int. J. Cancer* **26,** 171–176.

4

Transposon Mutagenesis in Mycobacteria Using Conditionally Replicating Mycobacteriophages

Stoyan S. Bardarov, Svetoslav S. Bardarov, Jr., and William R. Jacobs, Jr.

1. Introduction

Genetic analyses of pathogenic mycobacteria such as *Mycobacterium tuberculosis* and *Mycobacterium bovis* required improvement of existing methodologies for the generation of large representative libraries of mutants. Two basic methodologies have been used to generate mutant libraries in both fast- and slow-growing mycobacteria: chemical mutagenesis and transposon mutagenesis. Chemical mutagenesis has successfully been used to produce different auxotrophic mutants in the fast growing mycobacteria *Mycobacterium phlei* ***(1,2)*** and *Mycobacterium smegmatis* ***(3,4)***. A detailed chemical mutagenesis protocol for the generation of mutant libraries in the fast-growing mycobacteria can be found in the previous volume of this manual ***(5)***. Chemical mutagenesis is not the ideal method for producing large representative mutant libraries for the slow-growing mycobacteria because: (1) the mutation frequency is relatively low, (2) multiple mutations may occur in the same cells, (3) clumping of the mycobacteria makes the identification and purification of the mutant clones very difficult, and (4) no generalized transducing phage has been described for the slow-growing mycobacteria to allow transfer of the point mutations and construction of isogenic strains.

Transposon mutagenesis has successfully been used in diverse genera of bacteria ***(6,7)*** including both fast- and slow-growing mycobacteria ***(8–12)***. Transposons are an extremely useful tool in the molecular genetics of mycobacteria, as the insertion of a transposable element into a gene most often leads to its inactivation. The reversion frequency of the resulting "null" mutations is relatively low since the frequency of the precise excision of the transposon and

From: *Methods in Molecular Medicine*, vol. 54: *Mycobacterium Tuberculosis Protocols*
Edited by: T. Parish and N. G. Stoker © Humana Press Inc., Totowa, NJ

restoration of the gene function is low. Transposon mutagenesis is useful in the analysis of operon structure because of the strong polar effects on the genes located downstream of the transposon insertion point. Upon integration, transposons introduce new genetic markers, such as antibiotic resistance genes, which makes the isolation and clonal purification of the mutants on selective media relatively very easy. Transposons also provide a starting point for DNA sequencing and rapid identification of the mutated gene.

1.1. Structure and Classification of the Mobile Genetic Elements

Transposable elements are mobile DNA fragments that move within the bacterial chromosome by a mechanism that is independent of the general homologous recombination systems of the host bacterium. Most of the transposable elements move to their new target location (chromosome, plasmids, or phages) with relatively low frequencies ranging between 10^{-7} and 10^{-4}. These elements exhibit little preference for the location of the target site, although some members of the Tn*3* family of transposons (γδ and Tn*1721*) transpose more readily into plasmids than to the host chromosome. The transposition process leading to integration of the mobile genetic elements does not require extensive DNA homology between the ends of the element and the chromosomal target site.

Transposable elements are diverse in size, structure, mechanism of transposition, specificity of the insertion site, and regulation with respect to their movement ***(13)***. Based on the structure and complexity, all mobile genetic elements can be classified into three broad classes ***(14)***. The first class is represented by the simple insertion sequence (IS) elements. Their size usually does not exceed 2 kb in length. IS-elements encode a transposase, an enzyme required for the transposition process, which is flanked by inverted repeat DNA sequences (IR). In the recombination process these sequences serve as a substrate for the transposase and certain host factors. Depending on the type of the IS element and the mechanism of its integration, a duplication of the target DNA sequence may occur, generating direct repeats of different length. More complex structures referred to as transposons (Tn) represent the second class of mobile genetic elements. In addition to the basic IS element encoding the transposase, transposons also carry genes encoding different traits such as antibiotic resistance, heavy metal resistance, or genes encoding virulence determinants. Class III mobile genetic elements are represented by the "transposable" bacteriophages such as the temperate phage λ and bacteriophage μ of *Escherichia coli*. Besides encoding genes necessary for their transposition into the host chromosome, these more complex mobile genetic elements carry genes responsible for their replication, phage development, and cell lysis.

1.2. Transposable Elements in Mycobacteria

After the discovery of the first mobile genetic elements, namely IS*900* in *Mycobacterium paratuberculosis* ***(15)*** and IS*6110* in *M. tuberculosis* ***(16–18)***, numerous IS elements have been identified and characterized in both fast- and slow-growing mycobacteria ***(19,20)***. Most of the insertion sequences have been identified in an attempt to develop molecular probes for diagnosis ***(17,21)***, by hybridization to drug resistance markers ***(22)***, or in "transposon trap" experiments using different reporter genes ***(23,24)***. It has been found that most of the mycobacterial insertion sequences exhibit species-specificity or very narrow host range distribution. The complete *M. tuberculosis* genome sequence data enable the precise determination of the number and position of the numerous copies of IS*6110* and IS*1081* in the genome of *M. tuberculosis* H37Rv ***(25–27)***. Interestingly, these insertion sequences are present in different numbers and locations in the genomes of most clinical isolates of *M. tuberculosis*, which makes them very useful probes for fingerprinting for epidemiological purposes ***(28,29)***. More information about the transposable genetic elements in mycobacteria can be found in the recently published extensive reviews on that subject ***(19,20)***.

Tn*610* was the first naturally occurring transposon identified in *Mycobacterium fortuitum* FC1. It has been isolated and characterized at the molecular level ***(22)*** using a DNA probe specific for the site-specific integrase gene of Tn*1696*, a member of Tn*21* family of integrons. Tn*610* is a class II composite insertion element composed of the gene *sul3* (encoding sulfonamide resistance) flanked by two copies of IS*6100*. An artificial transposon based on Tn*610* (named Tn*611*) was engineered in which the gene encoding sulfonamide resistance (*sul3*) was replaced by a gene encoding kanamycin resistance (*aph*). In *M. smegmatis* it has been shown that these transposons move by a replicative mechanism leading to the formation of cointegrate structures ***(22)***.

1.3. *IS*1096/*Tn*5367

IS*1096* is an insertion element isolated from *M. smegmatis* in a "transposon trap" experiment using β-galactosidase as a reporter gene ***(24)***. This insertion sequence is 2260 bp long, flanked by 26 bp imperfect inverted repeats. IS*1096* contains two open reading frames: *tnpA*, encoding a transposase, and *tnpR*, the product of which has a low homology to the resolvases of Tn*1000* and Tn*552*. However, the participation of *tnpR* in the recombination process is unclear. Tn*5367* was engineered from IS*1096* by insertion of the *aph* gene (encoding kanamycin resistance) between the two open reading frames ***(9)***. Tn*5367* transposes in a relatively random fashion in both fast- and slow-growing mycobacteria by a nonreplicative ("cut-and-paste") mechanism with a frequency of 10^{-5} ***(8,9)***.

1.4. Transposon Delivery Systems in Mycobacteria

1.4.1. Plasmids

Transposon mutant libraries of mycobacteria have been generated using two methods for plasmid-mediated transposon delivery. The first approach utilizes a "suicide" plasmid vector consisting of a composite transposon located on a plasmid that is unable to replicate in mycobacteria. Transposon mutants are isolated in two steps after transformation of cells with such a plasmid. First, transformants are selected for the phenotype encoded by the transposon (usually antibiotic resistance marker) and then in a second step they are screened for the desired mutant phenotype caused by the insertional inactivation of a particular gene(s) ***(9)***. Although this is a useful method for delivery of transposons, it is of limited value for the generation of large representative libraries of transposon mutants since the frequency of the transposition events will be directly proportional to the plasmid transformation efficiency, which in mycobacteria is relatively low. The second approach for plasmid delivery of transposons in mycobacteria utilizes a conditionally replicating plasmid vector based on a temperature-sensitive pAL5000 origin of replication (*oriM*) ***(10)***. Transformants are first selected at the permissive temperature for plasmid replication (32°C). Transposon mutants are isolated in a second step by shifting the bacterial culture to the nonpermissive temperature (39°C). A detailed protocol for the generation of representative *M. smegmatis* insertion libraries using this approach can be found in the previous volume of this manual ***(30)***. The disadvantage of the conditionally replicating plasmid system is that it is best used in the fast-growing mycobacteria able to grow at a wide growth temperature interval (32°C–42°C). Slow-growing mycobacteria such as *M. bovis* BCG and *M. tuberculosis* grow very slowly at 32°C, thus lengthening the already long procedure. Another disadvantage is that unless the transposition event is regulated, there is no means to select against the propagation of the transposon mutants during the outgrowth stage resulting in many siblings among the mutants selected.

1.4.2. Conditionally Replicating Mycobacteriophages

Conditionally replicating phage systems have proven to be very efficient systems for transposon mutagenesis in numerous bacterial species ***(7)***. One of the great advantages of a phage delivery system is that essentially every cell in the bacterial population can be infected with the transposon-carrying phage, thereby allowing the potential generation of large numbers of independent mutants. Transposon mutants are selected in one step simply by their ability to grow on selective media under conditions in which the donor phage vector cannot persist.

Recently we described the development of the conditionally replicating shuttle phasmid phAE94, a derivative of mycobacteriophage TM4, which enables the efficient delivery of Tn*5367* in both fast- and slow-growing mycobacteria ***(8)***. PhAE94 consists of a recombinant *E. coli* cosmid vector containing Tn*5367* inserted into a nonessential region of the genome of a conditionally replicating thermosensitive derivative of mycobacteriophage TM4. The resulting shuttle phasmid can replicate at 30°C but cannot replicate and lyse the host cells at 37°C. Using this system it was possible to generate, in one step, large representative transposon libraries containing more than 10^4 independent mutants of *M. bovis* BCG and *M. tuberculosis*.

Below we describe a detailed protocol for the generation of Tn*5367* transposon libraries in *M. bovis* BCG and *M. tuberculosis* using the conditionally replicating mycobacteriophage phAE94 as delivery vector. Detailed protocols for growth of mycobacteriophages and preparation of high titer lysates are described previously ***(29)***.

2. Materials

2.1. Mycobacterial Strains

1. *M. smegmatis* strain mc^{2}155: A high-frequency transformation (*ept*) derivative of *M. smegmatis* mc^{2}6 ***(31)***.
2. *M. bovis* BCG sub-strains Pasteur, Copenhagen, and Moreau: attenuated vaccine strains of *M. bovis* BCG (Statens Serum Institute, Copenhagen, Denmark).
3. *M. tuberculosis* strain Erdman: virulent isolate of *M. tuberculosis*.

These strains are available from Stoyan Bardarov, Department of Microbiology and Immunology, Albert Einstein College of Medicine, 1300 Morris Park Ave., Bronx, NY.

2.2. Growth of Mycobacteria

1. 20% w/v Tween-80: dissolve 20 g of Tween-80 in 80 mL of deionized water. Heat at 56°C and bring into solution with thorough mixing on a magnetic stirrer. Filter sterilize through 0.2 µm filter. Store at room temperature.
2. 50% v/v glycerol: mix 250 mL glycerol with 250 mL deionized water and stir thoroughly until in solution. Sterilize by autoclaving.
3. ADS enrichment (10X stock): dissolve 50 g bovine serum albumin-Fraction V, 20 g dextrose and 85 g NaCl in 800 mL deionized water. Adjust the volume to 1 L and then filter sterilize through 0.2 µm filter. Store at 4°C (*see* **Note 3**).
4. 10% w/v casein hydrolysate (Difco, Detroit, MI): dissolve 10 g of casein hydrolysate powder in 80 mL deionized water and adjust the volume to 100 mL. Filter sterilize through 0.2 µm filter. **Do not autoclave.** Store in dark at 4°C.
5. Kanamycin sulfate (Sigma, St. Louis, MO): Prepare a 50 mg/mL stock solution. Filter sterilize and store at –20°C.

6. Middlebrook 7H9 broth (10X stock): dissolve 47 g Middlebrook 7H9 powder (Difco) in 920 mL deionized water, add 40 mL of 50% Glycerol (2% v/v final concentration) and filter sterilize using 0.2 µm filter membrane. Store in dark at 4°C. To prepare 1X 7H9 broth, add 100 mL of 10X 7H9 stock, 100 mL of 10X ADS stock and 2.5 mL of 20% Tween-80 (0.05% final) to 800 mL of deionized water. Filter sterilize through 0.2 µm filter. Store in dark at 4°C (*see* **Note 1**).
7. Middlebrook 7H9 agar: add 15 g agar Noble (Difco) to 800 mL deionized water, and autoclave. Cool to 56°C and then add 100 mL of sterile preheated 10X 7H9 broth and 100 mL of 10X ADS enrichment. Add 2.5 mL 20% Tween-80 (0.05% final concentration) if desirable. When necessary (growth of transposon mutants), add the proper amounts from the stock antibiotics, L-amino acids or casein hydrolysate (Difco) enrichments (*see* **Note 2**).

2.3. Mycobacteriophage Transposon Delivery Vector

1. phAE 94: Temperature sensitive phasmid derivative of mycobacteriophage TM4 *(8,32)*. Genotype: TM4 *ts* (pYUB552::Tn*5367* (kan)). At 30°C it behaves as virulent phage but it is unable to replicate at 37°C. Reversion frequency of the *ts* mutation(s) is 10^{-9} PFU/mL.
2. This phasmid is available from Stoyan Bardarov, Department of Microbiology and Immunology, Albert Einstein College of Medicine, 1300 Morris Park Ave., Bronx, NY.

2.4. Preparation of High Titer Phage Lysates

1. Middlebrook 7H9 bottom agar: add 12 g Bacto-agar (Difco) to 900 mL of deionized water and autoclave. Cool to approx 56°C and then add 100 mL of 10X 7H9 broth preheated to 56°C with stirring. **Do not add ADS** (*see* **Note 4**).
2. Top agar: add 3 g Bacto-Agar (Difco), 1 mL of 50% glycerol and 1 mL of 1 *M* $CaCl_2$ to 500 mL of deionized water. Sterilize by autoclaving. Store batches of top agar in solidified form. Top agar can be stored in a melted form at 56°C for up to one week (*see* **Note 4**).
3. LB (Luria-Bertani) agar plates: Dissolve 25 g Luria-Bertani broth base (Difco) in 1 L of distilled water. Add agar (Difco) at 15 g/L. Sterilize by autoclaving.
4. 1 *M* Tris-HCl, pH 7.4: add 121.1 g Trizma-base to 800 mL deionized water. Adjust pH to 7.4 with hydrochloric acid. Adjust the volume to 1 L with deionized water. Dispense into convenient volumes and sterilize by autoclaving.
5. 1 *M* $MgSO_4$: Dissolve 24.6 g $MgSO_4$ in 80 mL deionized water. Adjust the volume to 100 mL with deionized water. Sterilize by autoclaving.
6. 1 *M* $CaCl_2$: Dissolve 55.5 g $CaCl_2$ in 400 mL deionized water. Adjust the volume to 500 mL with deionized water. Sterilize by autoclaving.
7. Phage buffer (MP buffer): Add 50 mL of 1 *M* Tris-HCl, pH 7.4, 10 mL of 1 *M* $MgSO_4$, 2 mL of 1 *M* $CaCl_2$ and 30 mL 5 *M* NaCl to 800 mL of deionized water. Adjust the volume to 1 L with deionized water. Dispense into convenient volumes and sterilize by autoclaving.

8. Glass test tubes: 16X 100 mm round-bottom borosilicate with autoclavable cap (Fisher Scientific, Pittsburgh, PA).
9. 0.45 µm filter units.

2.5. Transposon Mutagenesis

1. Enriched Middlebrook 7H9 broth: Middlebrook 7H9 broth (*see* **Subheading 2.2., item 6**) enriched with 0.2% casein hydrolysate or with any particular L-amino acid at the recommended concentration.
2. Wash medium: add 50 mL of 10X Middlebrook 7H9 broth stock and 50 mL of 50% glycerol (5% final concentration) to 400 mL distilled water. **Do not add Tween-80** (*see* **Note 5**). Filter sterilize through 0.2 µm filter. Store at 4°C.
3. Phage adsorption medium: add 50 mL of 10X Middlebrook 7H9 stock and 20 mL of 50% glycerol (2% final concentration) to 430 mL distilled water. Do not add Tween-80 (*see* **Note 5**). Filter sterilize through 0.2 µm filter. Store at 4°C.
4. "Inkwell" square 30 mL culture bottles (Nalgene, Rochester, NY).
5. 500 mL tissue culture roller bottles.

2.6. Growth of the Transductants and Selection for Transposition Events

1. Complete medium: enriched Middlebrook 7H9 agar plates (*see* **Subheading 2.2., item 7**) containing 25 µg/mL kanamycin.
2. Phosphate buffered saline (PBS) 10X stock: add 12.36 g Na_2HPO_4, 1.80 g $NaH_2PO_4.H_2O$ and 85 g NaCl to 800 mL of distilled water. When completely dissolved, adjust the volume to 1 L. Sterilize by autoclaving.
3. Phosphate buffered saline-Tween-80 (PBST): add 100 mL of PBS 10X stock solution and 10 mL of 20% stock solution of Tween-80 to 890 mL distilled water. Filter sterilize through 0.2 µm filter.
4. 30 mL "Inkwell" square culture bottles (Nalgene).

2.6. Analysis of the Transposon Mutants

1. Plastic loops.
2. Primers: the following primers are used to generate a 541 bp DNA fragment used for detection of the presence of the kanamycin resistance gene in the transposon mutants:

   Aph 1: 5'-AGGTAGCGTTGCCAATGATG-3'

   Aph 2: 5'-CTCACCGAGGCAGTTCCATA-3'
3. dNTP's: 25 m*M* stock solutions of dATP, dCTP, dGTP, and dTTP (Perkin-Elmer, Branchburg, NJ). Working stock of 2.5 m*M* is prepared by mixing equal volumes of each dNTP.
4. GeneAmp PCR kit containing Ampli*Taq* polymerase, 10X PCR buffer, and 25 m*M* $MgCl_2$ (Perkin Elmer).

2.7. Storage of Libraries of Transposon Mutants

1. Middlebrook 7H9 wash medium (*see* **Subheading 2.5., item 2**).

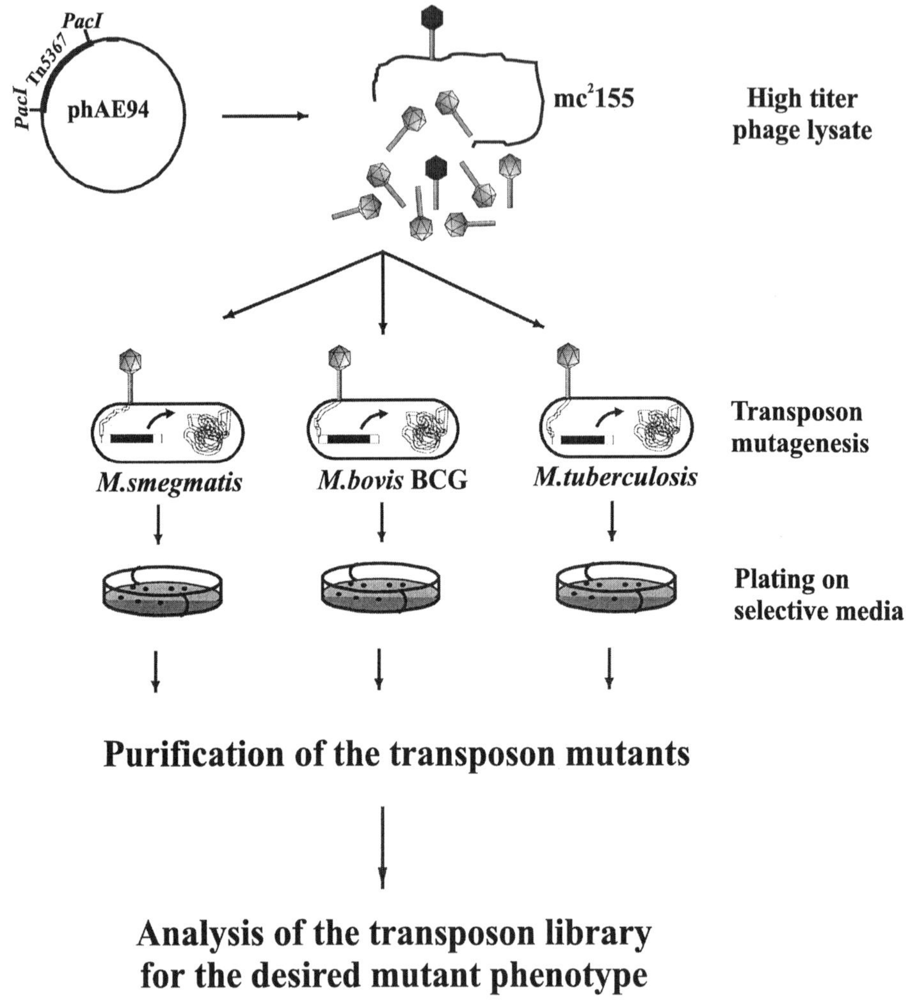

Fig. 1. An outline of the major steps for the generation of transposon libraries in mycobacteria using conditionally replicating mycobacteriophage phAE94.

2. Cryogenic vials (Nalgen).
3. Tissue culture scrapers.
4. Water bath sonicator.

3. Methods

Figure 1 presents an outline of the major steps for transposon mutagenesis in mycobacteria using conditionally replicating shuttle phasmids as a molecular vector.

3.1. Preparation of High Titer Phage Stocks from phAE94

3.1.1. Growth of M. smegmatis *mc²155 Competent for Phage Infection*

1. Starter culture: inoculate 1.5 mL of Middlebrook 7H9 broth (without ADS enrichment) with a well-isolated single colony of *M. smegmatis* mc^2155 grown on Middlebrook 7H9 agar plate. Incubate the culture at 37°C with shaking or on a roller apparatus until late-log phase is reached.
2. Inoculate 50 mL Middlebrook 7H9 broth–0.05% Tween-80 (without ADS) with 0.5 mL from the starter culture (1/100 dilution) and incubate with a slow shaking (80–100 rpm) to an OD_{600} of 0.8 to 1.0 (*see* **Note 6**).
3. Wash the cell pellet twice with wash medium (*see* **Note 5**) by centrifugation at 3000*g* at room temperature. Gently resuspend the cell pellet avoiding blowing air in the cell suspension with the pipet, which leads to generation of air bubbles (*see* **Note 7**).
4. After the final wash resuspend the cell pellet in phage adsorption medium in 0.8X of the original volume. The OD_{600} of the cell suspension should be in the range of 1.2 to 1.5.

3.1.2. Determination of the Phage Titer

1. Grow and prepare a culture of *M. smegmatis* mc^2155 competent for phage infection as described in **Subheading 3.1.1.**
2. Prepare 10-fold serial dilutions of the phage stock in 1 mL of phage buffer generating serial dilutions of 10^{-7} to 10^{-1}.
3. Carefully add 0.1 mL from each phage dilution to 0.3 mL of the cells in a sterile disposable glass test tube.
4. Incubate the phage-cells mix at 30°C for 30 min to allow for adsorption of the phage to the bacterial cells.
5. To each dilution tube add 3.5 mL molten top agar (56°C), gently mix and quickly pour onto prewarmed (30°C) bottom agar plates. Spread the top agar evenly by tilting the plate in a circular motion until the entire surface of the plate is covered.
6. Allow the top agar to solidify and incubate the plates at 30°C in an inverted position to avoid condensation on the lid of the plates.
7. Count the phage plaques on each dilution plate containing well-separated individual phage plaques.
8. The titer of the lysate is expressed as:

$$\text{PFU/mL} = 10 \times (\text{number of the plaques}) \times (\text{dilution factor})$$

3.1.3. Confirming the Phage ts Phenotype

1. Plate the phage at permissive temperature (30°C) (as described in detail in **Subheading 3.1.2.**) such that 50 to 100 well-separated plaques are obtained.
2. Aliquot 0.3 mL of the competent *M. smegmatis* mc^2155 cells (*see* **Subheading 3.1.1.**) into disposable glass tubes.

3. Add 3.5 mL of top agar (56°C) to the tubes, gently mix, and quickly pour onto prewarmed (30°C) bottom agar plates. Spread the top agar by tilting the plate in a circular motion until the whole surface of the plate is evenly covered.
4. Using sterile toothpicks transfer individual phage plaques onto two replica plates in an orderly fashion using a 50 square grid. Test 20 to 50 phage plaques.
5. Incubate one set of plates at permissive temperature (30°C) and the other at nonpermissive temperature (37°C).
6. Isolate a plaque from the plate grown at the permissive temperature that corresponds to a plaque, which fails to grow (no clearance in the cell lawn) at the nonpermissive temperature by using sterile Pasteur pipet (or a precut 1 mL plastic pipet tip). Soak the plug in 0.5 mL of phage buffer.
7. Expand the phage to a high titer as described below in **Subheading 3.1.4.** (*see* **Note 8**).

3.1.4. Preparation of High Titer Phage Stocks from Plate Lysate

1. Grow and prepare a culture of *M. smegmatis* mc^2155 competent for phage infection as described in **Subheading 3.1.1.**
2. Prepare 10-fold serial dilutions of the phage using 2 mL phage buffer and titer the phage as described in **Subheading 3.1.2.** Save the phage dilutions at 4°C for later use.
3. Incubate the plates from each phage dilution at 30°C until well-formed individual plaques appear at the high dilution plates.
4. Inspect the plates from the different phage dilutions and choose the one giving confluent lysis of the bacterial lawn.
5. Prepare 10 to 15 phage plates from that particular dilution using the saved serial dilutions from **step 2**.
6. Incubate the plates in upright position at 30°C until complete lysis of the bacterial lawn is observed.
7. Cover the surface of each plate with 4 mL phage buffer and incubate for 30 min at room temperature.
8. Scrape the top agar of each plate with glass spreader and transfer it into 50 mL high-speed centrifuge tube.
9. Remove the agar and the cell debris by centrifugation at 30,000*g* for 30 min.
10. Filter the supernatant through a 0.45 μm filter and store the lysate at 4°C.
11. Check for contamination by streaking a loop full of the lysate on LB agar plate (*see* **Subheading 2.4., step 3**).
12. Determine the titer as described in **Subheading 3.1.2.**

3.2. Transposon Mutagenesis

3.2.1. Growth of M. tuberculosis and M. bovis BCG Substrains for Transposon Mutagenesis

1. Starter culture: inoculate 10 mL of complete Middlebrook 7H9 medium with 1 mL frozen stock of the mycobacterial strain to be mutagenized in a 30 mL square media bottle. Grow the culture until the mid- to late log-phase is reached.

2. Inoculate 50 mL of complete Middlebrook 7H9 medium with 1 mL of the starter culture in a 500 mL roller bottle and grow at 37°C in a roller apparatus at 5 rpm for 3 to 7 d until the mid- to late log-phase is reached (OD_{600} 0.8 to 1.0 equivalent to 2–5 × 10^8 cfu/mL).
3. Centrifuge 10 mL sample of the culture at 3000*g* in a 15 mL centrifuge tube at room temperature.
4. Wash the cells twice with 10 mL of wash medium.
5. Carefully resuspend the cell pellet in 10 mL phage adsorption medium and transfer the cell suspension into 30 mL square media bottle.
6. Incubate the cell suspension standing at 37°C for at least 24 h.
7. Centrifuge the cell suspension at room temperature and carefully resuspend the cell pellet in 1 mL of phage adsorption medium. Heat the cell suspension at 37°C.
8. Add the proper amount from the high titer phage stock preheated at 37°C to obtain multiplicity of infection (MOI) of 10.
9. Incubate the tube containing the cell-phage mix standing at 37°C for 3 h to allow for adsorption of the phage.
10. Transfer the suspension to the prerolled culture bottle at 37°C containing 50 mL Middlebrook 7H9 complete medium. Incubate for 18–24 h.
11. Include a "no phage" control by adding 1 mL of phage buffer to the cell suspension. Process this control in parallel with the experimental.
12. Spin down the cells at 3000*g* at room temperature. Resuspend the cell pellet in 2 mL of complete Middlebrook 7H9 medium.

3.2.2. Selection for Transposon Mutants

1. Plate 0.2 mL per plate using the appropriate enriched Middlebrook 7H9 medium plus 25 μg/mL kanamycin.
2. Remove 0.1 mL from the "no phage" control and prepare serial dilutions from 10^{-7} to 10^{-4} using PBST. Plate for viable counts on complete Middlebrook 7H9 medium containing no antibiotic.
3. Plate 200 μL from the remaining 0.9 mL of the "no phage" control onto kanamycin-containing complete Middlebrook 7H9 agar plates to determine the frequency of spontaneous resistance to kanamycin.
4. Transposition frequency is determined as a ratio between the number of kanamycin resistant cells and the total number of input cells minus the number of the spontaneous kanamycin resistant cells.

3.2.3. Analysis of the Transposon Mutants

1. Using a plastic loop pick 10 well-separated, randomly chosen kanamycin-resistant colonies and resuspend each one in 50 μL of sterile water in an 1.5 mL tube.
2. Boil the cell suspensions for 15 min and then immediately chill on ice.
3. Centrifuge at 3000*g* for 10 min to pellet the cell debris.
4. Use 2–5 μL of the supernatant as a template in a 50 μL PCR reaction mix containing 5 μL of 10X PCR buffer, 8 μL of 2.5 m*M* dNTPs, 1 U of Ampli*Taq* poly-

merase, 0.5 µL of Primer 1 (20 pmol final), 0.5 µL of Primer 2 (20 pmol final) and 3 µL of 25 m*M* $MgCl_2$ stock.

5. Carry out the PCR reaction using the following cycling conditions: an initial denaturing step at 96°C for 5 min, followed by 35 cycles of 95°C for 1 min, 58°C for 10 s, 72°C for 45 s and a final extension step of 30 min at 72°C. Store at 4°C.

3.2.4. Preservation of the Transposon Libraries

1. Add 5 mL of the wash medium to each plate containing kanamycin-resistant colonies and carefully scrape the colonies using a tissue culture scraper.
2. Pellet the cells by centrifuging at 3000*g* for 10 min.
3. Carefully resuspend the cell pellet in 5 mL wash medium.
4. Sonicate the cell suspension in a water bath sonicator until smooth cell suspension is obtained.
5. Aliquot 300 µL of the cells into 2 mL cryogenic vials freeze in a dry-ice-ethanol bath and store at –70°C.
6. To expand the library of transposon mutants use the frozen stocks to start 10 mL of culture in complete 7H9 medium containing kanamycin and 0.05% Tween-80.
7. Use this culture to screen for the desired transposon mutant by plating on the selective media.

4. Notes

1. Upon autoclaving, Middlebrook 7H9 medium precipitates, primarily due to the formation of insoluble phosphate salts. We find an improvement in the growth rate of the slow-growing mycobacteria when using filter-sterilized Middlebrook 7H9 medium, in which the essential nutrients and microelements are preserved in a soluble form. Growth of *M. bovis* BCG and *M. tuberculosis* in filter-sterilized 7H9 medium also increases the efficiency of phage infection as judged by the kinetics of light accumulation when using luciferase reporter mycobacteriophages ***(33)***.
2. Unpurified regular agar brands, such as Bacto-agar (Difco) are contaminated with traces of low molecular weight fatty acids — one of the major inhibitors of the growth of slow-growing mycobacteria ***(34)***. We find that when grown on solid media prepared with Agar-Noble (Difco) slow-growing mycobacteria form colonies much faster than when plated on solid media prepared with Bacto-Agar (Difco).
3. Always add the albumin powder to the water since the reverse leads to the formation of a very sticky clump, which is difficult to dissolve. Prechilling the water to 4°C facilitates solubilization. Add the measured amount of dextrose and NaCl when albumin is completely dissolved. Centrifuge at 10,000*g* for 30 min to remove undissolved albumin aggregates and then filter sterilize the supernatant using 0.2 µm filter unit. Always use the prefilter supplied with the filter units.
4. Higher mycobacteriophage titers are obtained when *M. smegmatis* is grown on minimal ("hungry") agar media. The lower concentration of the agar in the bottom agar plates helps the phage particles to diffuse more readily thus forming

larger morphologically uniform plaques. Prolonging the doubling time of the infected cells allow the phages to replicate and reach their full burst size before the cell division occurs. Rich undefined media such as Luria-Bertani agar, Tryptic soy agar or Middlebrook 7H11 decrease the doubling time of the infected cells, thus the bacterial lawn outgrows the phage which leads to the formation of turbid, difficult to observe, morphologically uneven phage plaques.

5. The presence of Tween-80 or oleic acid in the growth media or in the phage adsorption medium inhibits the infection of mycobacterial cells by most of the presently used mycobacteriophages. A known exception is mycobacteriophage I3 that is also resistant to chloroform treatment *(35)*. Some mycobacterial species such as *M. smegmatis* are able to metabolize Tween-80. Therefore late-log or stationary phase culture of *M. smegmatis* grown in the presence of 0.05% Tween-80 is sensitive to phage infection.
6. The addition of Tween-80 (up to 0.2%) in the growth medium in combination with slow shaking of the *M. smegmatis* culture reduces the amount of clumping and helps produce more homogenous cell suspensions.
7. Care should be taken to resuspend the cell pellets very gently, avoiding the generation of air bubbles by blowing air in the cell suspension. The high surface tension and the cohesive forces at the surface of the air bubbles increase the chances for the formation of large cell aggregates.
8. phAE94 is a thermosensitive derivative of mycobacteriophage TM4 with a reversion frequency to the wild-type phage of 10^{-9}. High titer phage lysates of 10^{10} or 10^{11} PFU/mL will contain a small proportion of wild-type phages. Therefore it is important that new batches of high titer phage lysates are always started from a single plaque tested for the thermosensitive phenotype.

Acknowledgments

We thank Marty Pavelka, Miriam Braunstein, and Michelle Larsen for their critical reading of the manuscript.

References

1. Konickova-Radochova, M., et al. (1969) The use of ethyl methanesulfonate for the induction of mutants in *Mycobacterium phlei* PA. *Folia Microbiol.* (Praha). **14,** 470–474.
2. Konickova-Radochova, M., et al. (1974) Mutagenesis by N-methyl-N-nitroso-N'-nitroguanidine in synchronized cultures of *Mycobacterium phlei. Folia Microbiol.* (Praha). **19,** 16–23.
3. Hinshelwood, S. and Stoker, N. G. (1992) Cloning of mycobacterial histidine synthesis genes by complementation of a *Mycobacterium smegmatis* auxotroph. *Mol. Microbiol.* **6,** 2887–2895.
4. Holland, K. T. and Ratledge, C. (1971) A procedure for selecting and isolating specific auxotrophic mutants of *Mycobacterium smegmatis. J. Gen. Microbiol.* **66,** 115–118.

5. Brooks, L. A. (1998) Chemical mutagenesis of mycobacteria, in *Mycobacteria Protocols: Methods in Molecular Biology*, vol. 101 (Parish, T. and Stoker, N. G., eds.), Humana, Totowa, NJ, pp. 175–186.
6. Kleckner, N., Roth, J., and Botstein, D. (1977) Genetic engineering in vivo using translocatable drug-resistance elements. New methods in bacterial genetics. *J. Mol. Biol.* **116,** 125–159.
7. Kleckner, N., Bender, J., and Gottesman, S. (1991) Uses of transposons with emphasis on Tn*10*. *Methods Enzymol.* **204,** 139–180.
8. Bardarov, S., Kriakov, J., Carriere, C., Yu, S., Vaamonde, C., McAdam, R. A., Bloom, B. R., Hatfull, G. F., and Jacobs, W. R., Jr. (1997) Conditionally replicating mycobacteriophages: a system for transposon delivery to *Mycobacterium tuberculosis*. *Proc. Natl. Acad. Sci. USA* **94,** 10,961–10,966.
9. McAdam, R. A., Weisbrod, T. R., Martin, J., Scuderi, J. D., Brown, A. M., Cirillo, J. D., Bloom, B. R., and Jacobs, W. R., Jr. (1995) In vivo growth characteristics of leucine and methionine auxotrophic mutants of *Mycobacterium bovis* BCG generated by transposon mutagenesis. *Infect. Immunol.* **63,** 1004–1012.
10. Guilhot, C., Otal, I., Van Rompaey, I., Martin, C., and Gicquel, B. (1994) Efficient transposition in mycobacteria: construction of *Mycobacterium smegmatis* insertional mutant libraries. *J. Bacteriol.* **176,** 535–539.
11. Fomukong, N. G., et al. (1993) Transpositional activity of IS*986* in *Mycobacterium smegmatis*. *Gene* **130,** 99–105.
12. England, P. M., Wall, S., and McFadden, J. (1991) IS*900*-promoted stable integration of a foreign gene into mycobacteria. *Mol. Microbiol.* **5,** 2047–2052.
13. Berg, C. M. and Berg, D. E. (1996) Transposable element tools for microbial genetics, in *Escherichia coli and Salmonella: Cellular and Molecular Biology*, 2nd ed., vol. 2. (Niedhardt, F. C., et al., eds.) ASM Press, Washington, DC, pp. 2588–2612.
14. De Bruijn, F. J. and Rosenbach, S. (1994) Transposon mutagenesis, in *Methods in General and Molecular Bacteriology*, vol. 1 (Gerhardt, P., ed.), American Society of Microbiology, Washington, DC, pp. 387–405.
15. Green, E. P., Tizard, M. L., Moss, M. T., Thompson, J., Winterbourne, D. J., McFadden, J. J., and Hermon-Taylor, J. (1989) Sequence and characteristics of IS*900*, an insertion element identified in a human Crohn's disease isolate of *Mycobacterium paratuberculosis*. *Nucleic Acids Res.* **17,** 9063–9073.
16. Thierry, D., Brisson-Noel, A., Vincent-Levy-Frebault, V., Nguyen, S., Guesdon, J. L., and Gicquel, B. (1990) Characterization of a *Mycobacterium tuberculosis* insertion sequence, IS*6110*, and its application in diagnosis. *J. Clin. Microbiol.* **28,** 2668–2673.
17. Thierry, D., Cave, M. D., Eisenach, K. D., Crawford, J. T., Bates, J. H., Gicquel, B., and Guesdon, J. L. (1990) IS*6110*, an IS-like element of *Mycobacterium tuberculosis* complex. *Nucleic Acids Res.* **18,** 188.
18. McAdam, R. A., Hermans, P. W., van Soolingen, D., Zainuddin, Z. F., Catty, D., van Embden, J. D., and Dale, J. W. (1990) Characterization of a *Mycobacterium tuberculosis* insertion sequence belonging to the IS*3* family. *Mol. Microbiol.* **4,** 1607–1613.
19. McAdam, R. A., Guilhot, C., and Gicquel, B. (1994) Transposition in Mycobacteria, in *Tuberculosis: Pathogenesis, Protection and Control* (Bloom, B. R., ed.) American Society for Microbiology, Washington, DC, pp.

20. Dale, J. W. (1995) Mobile genetic elements in mycobacteria. *Eur. Respir. J. Suppl.* **20,** 633s–648s.
21. Eisenach, K. D., Crawford, J. T., and Bates, J. H. (1988) Repetitive DNA sequences as probes for *Mycobacterium tuberculosis*. *J. Clin. Microbiol.* **26,** 2240–2245.
22. Martin, C., Timm, J., Rauzier, J., Gomez-Lus, R., Davies, J., and Gicquel, B. (1990) Transposition of an antibiotic resistance element in mycobacteria. *Nature* **345,** 739–743.
23. Guilhot, C., Gicquel, B., Davies, J., and Martin, C. (1992) Isolation and analysis of IS*6120*, a new insertion sequence from *Mycobacterium smegmatis*. *Mol. Microbiol.* **6,** 107–113.
24. Cirillo, J. D., Barletta, R. G., Bloom, B. R., and Jacobs, W. R., Jr. (1991) A novel transposon trap for mycobacteria: isolation and characterization of IS*1096*. *J. Bacteriol.* **173,** 7772–7780.
25. Cole, S. T., Brosch, R., Parkhill, J., Garnier, T., Churcher, C., Harris, D., et al. (1998) Deciphering the biology of *Mycobacterium tuberculosis* from the complete genome sequence. *Nature* **393,** 537–544.
26. Gordon, S. V., Heym, B., Parkhill, J., Barrell, B., and Cole, S. T. (1999) New insertion sequences and a novel repeated sequence in the genome of *Mycobacterium tuberculosis* H37Rv. *Microbiology* **145,** 881–892.
27. Philipp, W. J., Schwartz, D. C., Telenti, A., and Cole, S. T. (1998) Mycobacterial genome structure. *Electrophoresis* **19,** 573–576.
28. van Soolingen, D., de Haas, P. E., Hermans, P. W., and van Embden, J. D. (1994) DNA fingerprinting of *Mycobacterium tuberculosis*. *Methods Enzymol.* **235,** 196–205.
29. van Soolingen, D. and Hermans, P. W. (1995) Epidemiology of tuberculosis by DNA fingerprinting. *Eur. Respir. J. Suppl.* **20,** 649s–656s.
30. Perez, E., Gavigan, J. A., Otal, I., Guilhot, C., Pelicic, V., Giquel, B., and Martin, C. (1998) Tn*611* transposon mutagenesis in *Mycobacterium smegmatis* using a temperature-sensitive delivery system. *Methods Mol. Biol.* **101,** 187–198.
31. Snapper, S. B., Melton, R. E., Mustafa, S., Kieser, T., and Jacobs, W. R., Jr. (1990) Isolation and characterization of efficient plasmid transformation mutants of *Mycobacterium smegmatis*. *Mol. Microbiol.* **4,** 1911–1919.
32. Carriere, C., Riska, P. F., Zimhony, O., Kriakov, J., Bardarov, S., Burns, J., Chan, J., and Jacobs, W. R., Jr. (1997) Conditionally replicating luciferase reporter phages: improved sensitivity for rapid detection and assessment of drug susceptibility of *Mycobacterium tuberculosis*. *J. Clin. Microbiol.* **35,** 3232–3239.
33. Bardarov, S. S., Jr, Bardarov, S., and Jacobs, W. R., Jr. (unpublished).
34. Wards, B. J. (1996) Evaluation of defined media suitable for isolation of auxotrophic mutants of mycobacteria. *J. Basic Microbiol.* **36,** 355–362.
35. Rado, T. A. and Bates, J. H. (1980) Mycobacteriophage structure and function: a review. *Adv. Tuberc. Res.* **20,** 64–91.

5

Gene Replacement and Transposon Delivery Using the Negative Selection Marker *sacB*

Mary Jackson, Luis Reinaldo Camacho, Brigitte Gicquel, and Christophe Guilhot

1. Introduction

1.1. Common Themes in Gene Replacement and Transposon Mutagenesis

Gene replacement and transposon mutagenesis are two complementary tools that have been widely used to perform genetic studies in various living organisms. In mycobacteria, and especially in the *Mycobacterium tuberculosis* complex, the lack of these tools has severely hampered the genetic studies of these organisms, especially regarding the identification and characterization of virulence genes of these important pathogens.

Site-directed mutagenesis by gene replacement is an important genetic technique which allows the production of defined mutations in a specific gene. This occurs by replacement of a wild-type allele of a gene by a mutated allele through homologous recombination. For the characterization of *M. tuberculosis* protein functions and identification of virulence factors, gene replacement represents a unique approach to: (1) check that a gene suspected to be involved in a specific biological activity indeed possesses this characteristic and (2) measure the qualitative and quantitative importance of this biological activity both in the physiology of the bacteria and in vivo during the infection of the host. Transposon mutagenesis is an equally important tool allowing the introduction of large numbers of random mutations into a chromosome. The resulting mutants may be screened for those exhibiting an interesting phenotype. It allows the identification of genes involved in a biological process of interest without previous assumptions on the gene's nature.

From: *Methods in Molecular Medicine*, vol. 54: *Mycobacterium Tuberculosis Protocols*
Edited by: T. Parish and N. G. Stoker © Humana Press Inc., Totowa, NJ

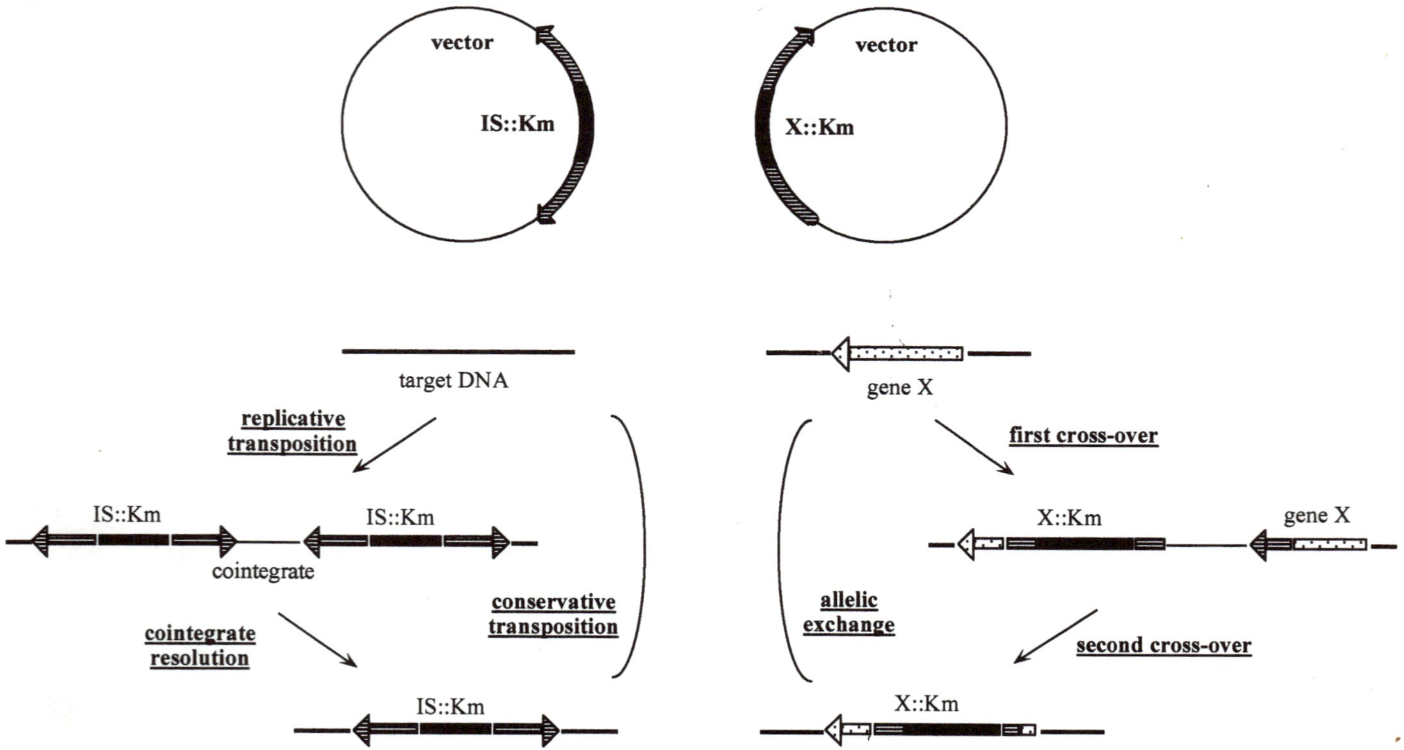

Fig. 1. Common theme in allelic exchange and transposon delivery. In both mutagenesis methods, a DNA fragment is transferred from one molecule, the vector, to a second DNA molecule, the target. In both case, this transfer may occur in two sequential steps, the entire vector being integrated into the target molecule during the first step and this cointegrate being resolved during the second step. In spite of this common theme, these two transfers rely upon different mechanisms, homologous recombination being catalyzed by the recombination function of the host whereas transposition is catalyzed by a protein, the transposase, encoded by the transposon itself.

These two mutagenesis methods rely upon two different biological processes. Gene replacement takes advantage of the host's functions allowing recombination between two stretches of homologous DNA. Transposon mutagenesis uses mobile DNA elements which encode functions catalyzing their transfer from one DNA molecule to another. In spite of these differences, both methods exhibit common themes: (1) a DNA fragment is transferred from a vector onto a target DNA, (2) this transfer is extremely inefficient, requiring very powerful vector systems to become detectable events, and (3) intermediates in the process may be produced in which the entire donor molecule is integrated into the target molecule (**Fig. 1**). These common themes explain why common strategies were developed to perform both kind of mutagenesis. These strategies are described in the following sections.

1.2. Gene Replacement in M. tuberculosis

In mycobacteria, and especially in the mycobacteria of the *M. tuberculosis* complex, homologous recombination has been shown to occur at low frequencies, below 10^{-3} events/cell (for a review, *see* **ref. *1***), often preventing the construction of defined mutants of *M. tuberculosis*. In the first attempts at allelic exchange in *M. tuberculosis* and *Mycobacterium bovis* BCG, linear DNA molecules or suicide vectors were used to deliver a copy of the target gene disrupted by an antibiotic cassette to the recipient strain. After electroporation, antibiotic-resistant transformants were selected on plates. Theoretically, these clones may result from three types of genetic events (**Fig. 2**); (1) a double cross-over between the disrupted copy of the target gene and the wild-type copy of the gene located on the bacterial chromosome (allelic replacement) (**Fig. 2C**), (2) a single cross-over between the disrupted copy of the target gene and the chromosomal wild-type allele leading to the insertion of the entire delivery vector at the target gene's locus (**Fig. 2A**), (3) an illegitimate recombination event leading to the insertion of the entire delivery vector into the chromosome of the bacteria at a nonhomologous locus (**Fig. 2B**). Although the application of this gene replacement procedure generally yields an easily detectable frequency of allelic exchange in the fast-growing *Mycobacterium smegmatis (2,3)*, only in a very limited number of cases has allelic exchange been achievable in *M. tuberculosis* and *M. bovis* BCG *(4–6)*. Even in those cases, the population of allelic exchange did not exceed 6% of the total transformants. Generally, the great majority of the selected transformants is found to have undergone illegitimate recombination events — 80 to 100% of the transformants according to the studies by Aldovini et al. *(7)* and Kalpana et al. *(3)*, thus hampering the detection of allelic exchange mutants. Although different hypotheses have been proposed to explain this high proportion of illegitimate recombination events in slow-growing mycobacteria (for a review, *see*

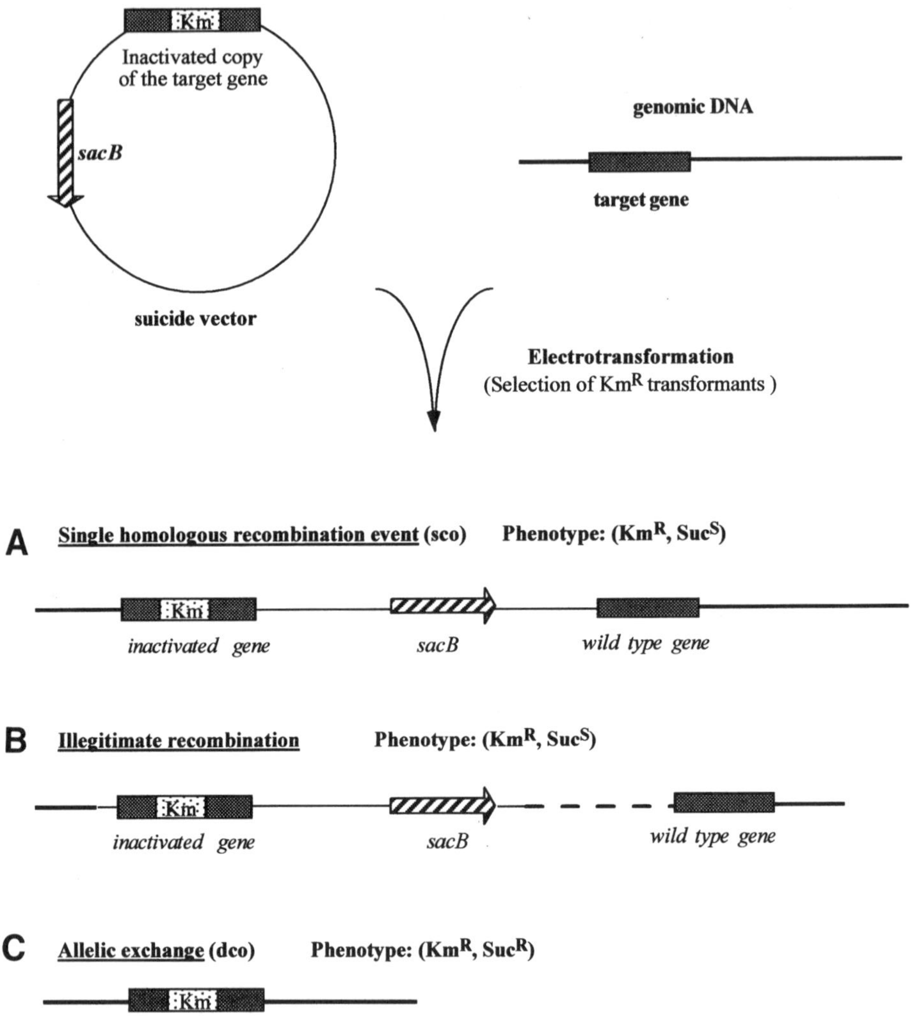

Fig. 2. Expected products following transformation of bacteria of the *M. tuberculosis* complex with a suicide vector carrying a mutated allele of a gene. Following electroporation of a mutated gene carried on a suicide vector in *M. tuberculosis* or *M. bovis* BCG, three kind of events can lead to the incorporation of the mutated allele into the chromosome: a) a single cross-over event between the wild-type gene and the mutated allele, b) illegitimate recombination between any part of the plasmid and the chromosome in a nonhomologous fashion, c) allelic exchange (double cross-over event). When a marker is present in the body of the vector, outside the mutated allele, the resulting transformants will have different phenotypes.

ref. *1*) the genetic mèchanisms underlying this phenomenom remain unknown. The relatively low electro-transformation efficiencies of *M. tuberculosis* strains (10^2 to 10^4 transformants per microgram DNA) are a further obstacle to the generation of allelic exchange mutants.

In conclusion, it appears that the successful isolation of allelic exchange mutants of *M. tuberculosis* is dependent on the ability of the genetic tools and protocols used to: (1) compensate for the low transformation efficiencies and, (2), enable the efficient detection or selection of allelic exchange mutants among the total population of transformants which have integrated the disrupted copy of the target gene. Recently, it has been shown that UV pretreatment of DNA or use of single-stranded DNA increases the frequency of homologous recombination in different mycobacterial species, including *M. tuberculosis* ***(8,9)***. This helps to overcome the problem of the low transformation efficiency. For selection of mutants, the major breakthrough has come from the use of counterselectable markers.

1.3. Transposon Mutagenesis in M. tuberculosis

A transposon mutagenesis system requires two different components: a mobile DNA element (the transposon) and a delivery vector. An ideal mobile element should (1) have a high (or at a least detectable) transposition frequency, (2) have a low specificity of insertion and (3) be absent from the target DNA molecule to avoid problems of recombination. For mycobacteria of the *M. tuberculosis* complex, three mobile elements appear to be good candidates: IS*6100*, IS*6120*, and IS*1096* ***(10)***. To date only IS*1096* derivatives have been used to produce insertional mutants libraries of *M. tuberculosis* and *M. bovis* BCG. Regarding the delivery vector, suicide plasmids were first used to demonstrate transposition ***(11)***. However, in these systems, the low transposition frequency of the elements used was not compensated for by a sufficiently high transformation efficiency to get large numbers of transposition events. In the best cases, only 100 insertional mutants per experiment were obtained with *M. bovis* BCG ***(11)***. Therefore this delivery system appears unsuitable for constructing large libraries of insertional mutants. To circumvent the problem of the low transformation efficiency, thermosensitive plasmids were used in *M. smegmatis* ***(12)***. However, these vectors appeared only partially thermosensitive in slow-growing mycobacteria hampering their use in *M. tuberculosis*. As for allelic exchange, a major breakthrough came from the use of counter-selectable markers.

1.4. Counter-Selectable Markers

Counter-selectable markers are placed on the body of the delivery vectors and allow, upon application of a counter-selective pressure, for the selection of the only transformants which have integrated the mutated allele of the gene and lost the body of the vector carrying the counter-selectable marker, i.e., allelic exchange mutants (**Fig. 2**). One such counter-selectable marker is the *rpsL*$^+$ gene which has been successfully used in *M. smegmatis* ***(13)*** (*see* Chapter 7). Another counter-selectable marker is the *katG* gene which was successfully used in *M. bovis* BCG ***(14)***. A common drawback of these two counter-selectable markers is that they rely upon the use of antibiotic-resistant strains (streptomycin- and izoniazid-resistant strains, respectively). This is not the case with the counter-selectable marker *sacB*, which allowed allelic exchange and transposon mutagenesis to be achieved in both fast and slow-growing mycobacteria ***(15–18)***. The expression of the *sacB* gene is lethal to mycobacteria in the presence of sucrose in the culture medium ***(19)***. The levan sucrase from *Bacillus subtilis* (encoded by the *sacB* gene) catalyzes the formation of polymers of fructose in the cell envelope that are then released into the culture medium. In Gram-negative bacteria such as *E. coli*, where the envelope comprises an outer membrane and a periplasmic space, the expression of the *sacB* gene in the presence of sucrose presumably leads to the accumulation of polymers of fructose in the periplasmic space finally resulting in the lysis of the bacteria ***(20)***. In corynebacteria and mycobacteria, toxicity is thought to be due to the unusual structure of the envelope of these bacteria which resembles more that of Gram-negative bacteria than that of Gram-positive bacteria ***(21)***.

1.5. Main sacB*-Based Protocols Used to Perform Insertional Mutagenesis in* M. tuberculosis

Two main protocols relying upon the use of the counter-selectable marker *sacB* have been designed to perform insertional mutagenesis in *M. tuberculosis* in a reliable way. For allelic exchange, both suicide and conditionally-replicating delivery plasmids have been used successfully. For the generation of large libraries of mutants (containing more than 10^4 mutants) by transposition, only replicating plasmids have been found to be suitable so far.

1.5.1. Protocols Based upon the Use of Suicide Vectors Carrying the Counterselectable Marker sacB *for Allelic Exchange*

1.5.1.1. The One-Step Procedure

As when using a classical allelic exchange protocol, *M. tuberculosis* is electro-transformed with a suicide vector (unable to replicate in mycobacteria) carrying an antibiotic cassette-disrupted copy of a target gene and the counter-selectable marker *sacB* on the plasmid. The transformation mix is then plated onto antibiotic plus sucrose plates at 37°C in order to directly select for allelic exchange mutants. Alternatively, antibiotic-resistant transformants can first be selected on antibiotic-containing plates and then screened for growth on sucrose plates ***(18)***. Although this approach has been successfully used in *M. bovis* BCG ***(18)***, to our knowledge, no such successful use has yet been reported in *M. tuberculosis*, presumably because of the low transformation efficiencies encountered in this species.

1.5.1.2. Two-Step Procedure

M. tuberculosis is electro-transformed with a suicide vector carrying an antibiotic cassette-disrupted copy of a target gene and the counter-selectable marker *sacB*. In the first step of the experiment, an antibiotic resistant transformant that has undergone a single homologous recombination event is selected and propagated at 37°C in liquid medium. In the second step of the experiment, this culture is plated onto antibiotic-sucrose plates to select for clones which have undergone a second intrachromosomal crossover leading to the excision of the vector and to the replacement of the wild-type copy of the gene by the disrupted one. This procedure allowed allelic exchange to be achieved in both *M. smegmatis* ***(15)*** and *M. bovis* BCG ***(16)***.

It is worth noting that the two-step procedure is the only one to allow for the generation of unmarked mutations ***(15,22)***. In this case, the antibiotic marker is included in the vector and not in the mutated allele of the target gene. During the second step, the culture is plated onto sucrose containing plates without antibiotic. This approach is also of particular interest for studying the essentiality of mycobacterial genes ***(23)***. If single cross-over events are easily achievable at a specific locus, but allelic exchange mutants cannot be isolated upon application of the second selection step of the procedure, then the gene may be essential. The putative essentiality of the target gene can then be assessed by providing a single cross-over transformant with an extra-copy of the wild-type gene to form a mero-diploid strain. If the second cross-over event then occurs, it provides evidence that the inability to isolate an allelic exchange mutant is not due to the impossibility for cross-over events to occur at this locus of the chromosome, but to the essentiality of the target gene.

1.5.2. Protocols Based upon the Use of a Thermosensitive Replicative Vector Carrying the Counterselectable Marker sacB

In order to circumvent the problem of low transformation efficiencies often encountered with *M. tuberculosis* strains, conditionally-replicating vectors can be used to deliver a disrupted copy of a target gene or a transposon. A thermosensitive (*ts*) derivative of pAL5000, able to replicate at 30°C but not at 39°C in fast-growing mycobacteria has been isolated by Guilhot and collaborators ***(24)***. This vector was used in conjunction with the *sacB* counter-selectable marker to successfully achieve allelic replacement and transposon mutagenesis in *M. tuberculosis* ***(17)***. The principle of the gene replacement procedure based on the use of such *ts-sacB* vectors is as follows: *M. tuberculosis* is transformed by electroporation with a *ts-sacB* vector carrying an antibiotic-disrupted copy of a target gene or a mobile element. A transformant is selected on antibiotic containing plates and propagated in liquid medium at permissive temperature (32°C). At this temperature, the *ts-sacB* delivery vector replicates in *M. tuberculosis*, allowing time for allelic exchange or transposition events to occur. The bacteria are then cultured on plates containing antibiotic and sucrose at the nonpermissive temperature (39°C). As the *ts-sacB* vector is unable to replicate at 39°C, the shift in temperature from 32°C to 39°C, although maintaining an antibiotic selective pressure, results in the selection of integration events. The simultaneous application of sucrose counterselective pressure results in the direct selection for the transformants which have integrated the disrupted copy of the gene or the transposon into their chromosome and lost the body of the vector, i.e., allelic exchange or transposition mutants. Since these vectors were shown to be only partially thermosensitive in *M. tuberculosis* and *M. bovis* BCG ***(17)***, the use of sucrose also allows the counterselection of *M. tuberculosis* clones still retaining copies of the *ts-sacB* delivery vector in their cytoplasm.

2. Materials

2.1. Vectors

All these plasmids are available upon request to J. Rauzier, Unité de Génétique Mycobactérienne, Institut Pasteur, 25 rue du Dr. Roux, 750 15 Paris, France.

1. Thermosensitive vectors carrying the counter-selectable marker *sacB*; e.g., pPR27 and pPR23 ***(17)*** (**Fig. 3**).
2. Transposon mutagenesis plasmids: pPR28, pPR29, pPR30 and pPR32 ***(17)*** (**Fig. 3**).
3. Suicide vector carrying the counter-selectable marker *sacB*; e.g., **ref. *25***.
4. Plasmid pCG106.

2.2. Culture Media

1. Liquid medium: Middlebrook 7H9 medium (Difco, West Mosley, Surrey, UK) supplemented with 10% v/v ADC (Difco) and 0.05% Tween-80.
2. Solid medium: Middlebrook 7H10 or 7H11 agar supplemented with 10% v/v OADC (Difco).
3. Antibiotics stock solutions: 20 mg/mL kanamycin or 200 mg/mL hygromycin, sterilize by filtering and store at –20°C. Add to the culture medium when required at the following concentrations, kanamycin 20–50 µg/mL, hygromycin 50 µg/mL.

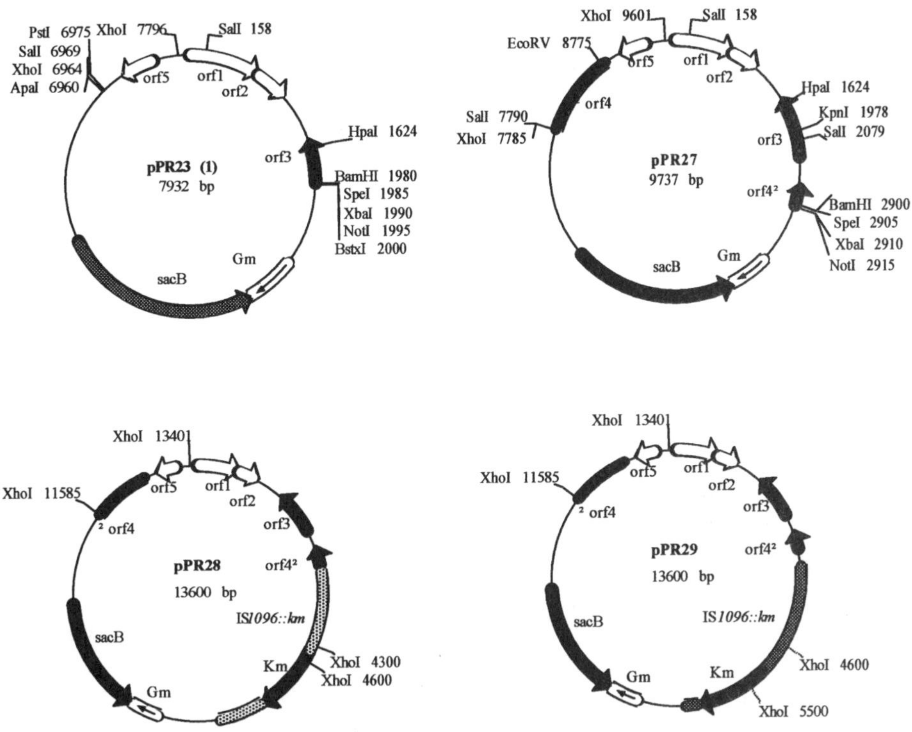

Fig. 3. Plasmids used to perform insertional mutagenesis in *M. tuberculosis*. Plasmids pPR23 and pPR27 are *ts-sacB* vectors used for allelic exchange. Plasmids pPR28 and pPR29 carry transposons Tn*5366* and Tn*5368* respectively ***(11,17)***. The *Xho*I restriction sites are shown because they are convenient to analyze the transposition products by Southern blot.

4. Sucrose: add to the culture medium to a final concentration of 2% w/v.
5. Incubators set at 32°C, 37°C, and 39°C.
6. Restriction enzyme *Xho*I.

3. Methods

*3.1. Two-Step Procedure Using a Suicide-*sacB *Vector for Allelic Exchange*

1. Clone copy of the target gene disrupted with an antibiotic resistance gene (kanamycin or hygromycin resistance) into a suicide vector carrying the counter-selectable marker *sacB*, e.g., pJQ200 (*see* **Notes 1** and **2**).
2. Electroporate *M. tuberculosis* electrocompetent cells with approx 2 μg of this construct.

3. Transfer into 5 mL 7H9 medium (without antibiotic) and incubate at 37°C for 24 h with agitation.
4. Plate serial dilutions onto solid medium containing the appropriate antibiotic (according to the antibiotic marker chosen) and incubate for 2 to 3 wk at 37°C.
5. Pick a few antibiotic resistant transformants and grow them in 5 mL liquid medium containing antibiotic for 2 wk at 37°C (*see* **Note 3**).
6. Analyze transformants by Southern blotting and select one that has undergone a homologous single cross-over event.
7. Plate serial dilutions of the liquid culture of this selected transformant onto solid medium containing antibiotic and 2% sucrose.
8. Incubate at 37°C for 2 to 3 wk to allow for the second cross over event.
9. Pick a few antibiotic and sucrose resistant clones and culture in 5 mL of liquid medium at 37°C
10. Analyze these clones by Southern blot analysis and/or PCR analysis to find the allelic exchange mutants (*see* **Notes 3** and **4**).

3.2. One Step Procedure Using a Suicide-sacB Vector (see Note 5)

1. Clone copy of the target gene disrupted with an antibiotic resistance gene (kanamycin or hygromycin resistance) into a suicide vector carrying the counter-selectable marker *sacB*, e.g., pJQ200 (*see* **Notes 1** and **2**).
2. Electroporate *M. tuberculosis* electrocompetent cells with approx 2 μg of this construct.
3. Transfer into 5 mL 7H9 medium (without antibiotic) and incubate at 37°C for 24 h with agitation.
4. Plate serial dilutions onto solid medium containing 2% sucrose and the appropriate antibiotic (according to the antibiotic marker chosen) and incubate for 2 to 3 wk at 37°C (*see* **Note 6**).
5. Pick the antibiotic and sucrose resistant clones and culture in 5 mL liquid medium at 37°C.
6. Analyze by Southern blot analysis and/or PCR analysis to isolate the clones that are allelic exchange mutants (*see* **Note 4**).

3.3. Gene Replacement Using a Thermosensitive-sacB Replicative Vector

1. Clone an antibiotic (kanamycin or hygromycin)-disrupted copy of the target gene into a *ts-sacB* vector, e.g., pPR27, pPR23 (*see* **Note 1**).
2. Electroporate *M. tuberculosis* electrocompetent cells with approx 2 μg of this construct.
3. Transfer into 5 mL liquid medium (without antibiotic) and incubate at 32°C with agitation for 48 h (*see* **Note 7**).
4. Plate serial dilutions onto solid medium containing antibiotic (according to the antibiotic marker chosen).
5. Incubate plates for 5 to 7 wk at 32°C.

6. Pick a few antibiotic resistant transformants (3 to 5 colonies) and grow them in 5 mL liquid medium containing antibiotic for about 3 wk at 32°C.
7. Plate serial dilutions of these liquid cultures onto solid media containing antibiotic and 2% sucrose. Incubate at 39°C for 2 to 3 wk.
8. Pick a few antibiotic-resistant, sucrose-resistant clones and culture in 5 mL of liquid medium at 37°C (*see* **Note 3**).
9. Analyze by Southern blot analysis and/or PCR analysis to isolate the clones that are allelic exchange mutants (*see* **Note 8**).

*3.4. Transposon Delivery Using a Thermosensitive-*sacB *Replicative Vector*

1. Electroporate *M. tuberculosis* electrocompentent cells with 1 μg of transposon mutagenesis plasmid (pPR28, pPR29, pPR30, or pPR31). Transfer into 5 mL of liquid medium (without antibiotic) and incubate at permissive-temperature (32°C) with agitation for 3 d (*see* **Note 7**).
2. Prepare serial dilutions of cells and plate 200 μL of each onto solid medium containing 50 mg/L of kanamycin in order to obtain single colonies.
3. Incubate for 5 to 7 wk at 32°C (*see* **Note 9**).
4. Pick several single kanamycin-resistant transformants and grow them in 5 mL of liquid medium containing 20 mg/L of kanamycin until saturation at 32°C.
5. Check by PCR analysis that these clones contain the plasmid (*see* **Notes 3** and **10**).
6. Prepare serial dilutions of the liquid cultures and plate 100 μL of each dilution onto solid medium containing antibiotic and 2% sucrose and 100 μL onto solid medium containing antibiotic alone.
7. Incubate the set of plates containing 2% sucrose at the nonpermissive temperature (39°C) for 2 to 3 wk to select for the insertion mutants (*see* **Note 7**).
8. Incubate the other set of plates containing antibiotic alone at 32°C for 5 wk. These serve to evaluate the frequency of transposition (*see* **Note 11**).
9. Perform Southern hybridization using the transposon as a probe ***(26)*** on the chromosomal DNA of a few insertion mutants to ensure that they result from random transposition (*see* **Subheading 3.5.**).

3.5. Southern Analysis of Transposon Mutants

1. Inoculate the parental strain and several antibiotic-resistant sucrose-resistant clones in 5 mL liquid medium and allow to grow for 3 wk at 37°C (*see* **Note 3**).
2. Isolate genomic DNA and digest approx 1 μg of it with the restriction enzyme *Xho*I, which cleaves IS*1096* at 2 sites.
3. Run the digested DNA on an agarose gel, transfer the DNA to a membrane, and hybridize with the DNA probe from plasmid pCG106 (*see* **Note 12**).
4. Label the probe and hybridize to the *Xho*I digested genomic DNAs. Visualize the hybridization pattern (**Fig. 4**) (*see* **Notes 13** and **14**).

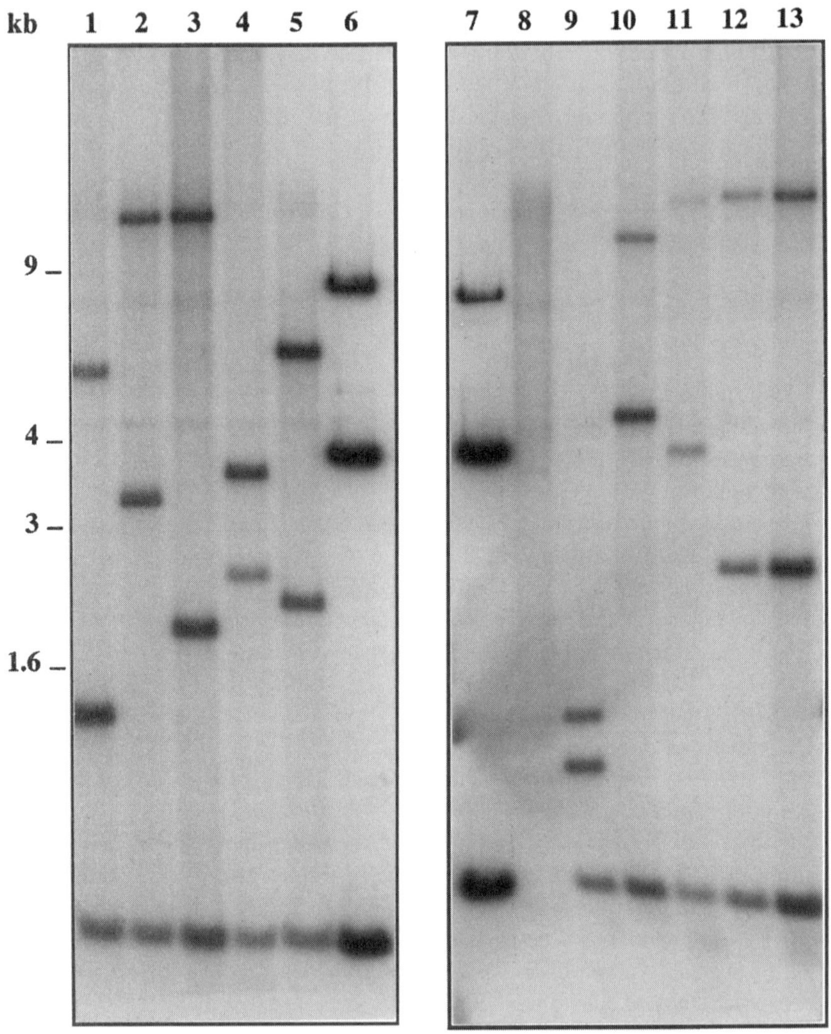

Fig. 4. Result of a Southern blot analysis of ten randomly picked transposon mutants. *Xho*I digested genomic DNAs from 10 randomly picked insertional mutants were hybrized with a radiolabeled IS*1096*::Km probe. Lane 1–6, insertional mutants obtained with plasmid pPR32; lane 6, plasmid pPR32; lane 7, plasmid pPR30; lane 8, *M. tuberculosis* MT103 (parental strain); lane 9–13, insertional mutants obtained with plasmid pPR30.

4. Notes

1. The minimal length of homologous DNA to be used in gene replacement experiments in *M. tuberculosis* is not known and is probably dependent (among other things) on the gene that is targeted. However, from the published examples of

successful gene replacement in slow-growing mycobacteria, it seems reasonable to consider using about 1 kilobase of homologous DNA on each side of the inserted antibiotic cassette (about 2 kilobases of homologous DNA in all).

2. It is also possible using this protocol to generate unmarked mutations. In this case, the antibiotic resistance cassette is placed on the body of the vector to allow for the selection of a transformant having undergone a single cross-over event at **steps 3** and **4** of the procedure. The antibiotic is then omitted from the culture medium in all the subsequent steps of the protocol. Selection on sucrose plates at **step 5** results in the selection of both revertants and allelic exchange mutants *(15)*.
3. About 10 colonies are usually picked and analyzed.
4. Due to mutations in the *sacB* gene that can arise at frequencies as high as 10^{-4}, the detection of allelic exchange mutants among the antibiotic- and sucrose-resistant colonies might be hampered. We thus recommend that another marker (for instance a colored marker such as the *xylE [27]* or the *gfp* genes *[28,29]*) is included in the delivery vector. Since this second marker should be excised at the same time as the body of the delivery vector during the second intra-chromosomal cross-over, allelic exchange mutants (phenotypically antibiotic- and sucrose-resistant, colored marker negative) can be distinguished from clones carrying mutations in *sacB* (phenotypically antibiotic and sucrose resistant, colored marker positive). In addition, the colored marker can be useful to check that the antibiotic-resistant colonies obtained from the electroporation result from the integration of the delivery vector and that they are not "spontaneous" antibiotic-resistant strains. Kanamycin resistant colonies of *M. tuberculosis* which do not result from the expression of the antibiotic resistance cassette carried by the delivery vector have sometimes been shown to represent the majority of the antibiotic resistant colonies.
5. Alternatively, plate the electroporation onto solid medium containing the appropriate antibiotic and incubate for 2 to 3 wk at 37°C. Culture the antibiotic-resistant transformants in liquid medium with antibiotic for 2 wk at 37°C. Then test transformants for sucrose resistance by plating cultures onto solid medium containing 2% sucrose and antibiotic. Incubate for 2 to 3 wk at 37°C.
6. Although this one-step procedure has been successfully used in *M. bovis* BCG *(18)*, to our knowledge no successful report of its utilization exists in *M. tuberculosis*. Gene replacement using this protocol might be difficult to achieve in *M. tuberculosis* due to the low transformation efficiencies in this species.
7. The *ts-sacB* plasmids are thermosensitive for replication in mycobacteria. The permissive temperature for isolation of these plasmids is 32°C and the restrictive temperature routinely-used is 39°C. Thus, it is very important to control the temperature of growth, which must be 32°C before transposition. When the temperature is shifted up to 39°C, the replication of the plasmid is inhibited, and only the cells in which transposition has occurred into the *M. tuberculosis* chromosome will be able to grow in the presence of kanamycin.
8. Due to the mutations in the *sacB* gene mentioned in **Note 4,** it is also of great use to add to the *ts-sacB* delivery vector a colored marker such as *xylE* or *gfp* that will

Table 1
Number of Colonies Obtained Using the Transposition Protocol with IS*1096* Derivatives

Strain	Plasmid (transposon)	cfu/mL 32°C Km	cfu/mL 39°C Km+Suc
M. tuberculosis MT103	pPR28	9×10^6	9×10^3
	(Tn*5366*)	2×10^7	8×10^3
		6×10^7	4×10^3
		4×10^7	1×10^4
M. tuberculosis MT103	pPR29	2×10^7	1×10^5
	(Tn*5368*)	5×10^7	2×10^5
		3×10^7	1×10^5
M. tuberculosis MT103	pPR30	6×10^7	9×10^3
	(Tn*5367*)	2×10^7	3×10^4
M. tuberculosis MT103	pPR32	1×10^7	3×10^4
	(Tn*5368*)	7×10^7	1×10^4
M. bovis BCG	pPR30	5×10^7	3×10^5
M. bovis BCG	pPR32	3×10^7	6×10^5

enable allelic exchange mutants to be distinguished from clones carrying mutations in the *sacB* gene at the last step of the protocol. This colored marker is also useful for checking that the antibiotic-resistant colonies picked contain the delivery vector and are not antibiotic spontaneous resistant clones.

9. Kanamycin-resistant colonies of *M. tuberculosis* that do not result from the expression of the antibiotic resistance cassette carried by the delivery vector have sometimes been shown to represent the majority of the antibiotic resistant colonies. Therefore we recommend using 50 mg/L of kanamycin as selection for mycobacteria as well as to include a plate with untransformed cells as a control for the occurrence of spontaneous mutants.
10. Colonies exhibiting resistance to kanamycin may be screened rapidly by PCR using primers pAL1 and pAL2 derived from the delivery plasmids (pAL1 5'GTCCCGGACCGCTACC3' and pAL2 5'GATAGCCGCGTCGCTTAACG3'). A single PCR product of 500 bp indicates the presence of the plasmid in the transformants. PCR reactions are usually carried out directly on crude DNA extracts from lyzed bacteria obtained after 5 cycles of rapid freezing (in a dry ice/ethanol bath) and boiling of a 1 mL of a liquid culture. About 2 to 4 µL of the crude DNA extract are enough for the PCR reaction.
11. **Table 1** shows the number of colonies obtained under optimal conditions.
12. Plasmid pCG106 is a pBluescript derivative in which a 4.0 kb *Hin*dIII fragment from pYUB285 ***(11)*** containing IS*1096*::Km has been inserted at the *Hin*dIII restriction site. This 4.0 kb *Hin*dIII restriction fragment is used as a probe to analyze by Southern hybridization the integration of the transposon in insertion mutants.

13. We use ^{32}P-α-dCTP to label our probes using the Megaprime DNA-labeling system (Amersham). Many other commercial kits can be obtained for labeling the probes.
14. It should be noted that several clones can exhibit the same hybridization patterns, which is not unexpected since there are several culture steps in the library construction protocol at which duplication events might have occurred. The Southern analysis of several transposon mutants picked randomly will give an idea of the proportion of siblings in the library.

References

1. McFadden, J. (1996) Recombination in mycobacteria. *Mol. Microbiol.* **21,** 205–211.
2. Husson, R. N., James, B. E., and Young, R. A. (1990) Gene replacement and expression of foreign DNA in mycobacteria. *J. Bacteriol.* **172(2),** 519–524.
3. Kalpana, G. V., Bloom, B. R., and Jacobs, Jr., W. R. (1991) Insertional mutagenesis and illegitimate recombination in mycobacteria. *Proc. Natl. Acad. Sci. USA* **88,** 5433–5437.
4. Reyrat, J. M., Berthet, F. X., and Gicquel, B. (1995) The urease locus of *Mycobacterium tuberculosis* and its utilization for the demonstration of allelic exchange in *Mycobacterium bovis* bacillus Calmette-Guérin. *Proc. Natl. Acad. Sci. USA* **92,** 8768–8772.
5. Azad, A. K., Sirakova, T. D., Rogers, L. M., and Kolattukudy, P. E. (1996) Targeted replacement of the mycocerosic acid synthase gene in *Mycobacterium bovis* BCG produces a mutant that lacks mycosides. *Proc. Natl. Acad. Sci. USA* **93,** 4787–4792.
6. Balasubramanian, V., Pavelka, M. S., Bardarov, S. S., Martin, J., Weisbrod, T. R., McAdam, R. A., Bloom, B. R., and Jacobs, Jr., W. R. (1996) Allelic exchange in *Mycobacterium tuberculosis* with long linear recombination substrates. *J. Bacteriol.* **178,** 273–279.
7. Aldovini, A., Husson, R. N., and Young, R. A. (1993) The *uraA* locus and homologous recombination in *Mycobacterium bovis* BCG. *J. Bacteriol.* **175,** 7282–7289.
8. Hinds, J., Mahenthiralingam, E., Kempsell, K. E., Duncan, K., Stokes, R. W., Parish, T., and Stoker, N. G. (1999) Enhanced gene replacement in mycobacteria. *Microbiology* **145,** 519–527.
9. Parish, T., Gordhan, B. G., McAdam, R. A., Duncan, K., Mizrahi, V., and Stoker, N. G. (1999) Production of mutants in amino acid biosynthesis genes of *Mycobacterium tuberculosis* by homologous recombination. *Microbiology* **145,** 3497–3503.
10. Guilhot, C., Jackson, M., and Gicquel, B. (1999) Mobile genetic elements and plasmids: tools for genetic studies, in *Mycobacteria: Molecular Biology and Virulence* (Ratledge, C. and Dale, J. W., eds.), Blackwell Science, Oxford, UK, pp. 17–37.
11. McAdam, R., Weisbrod, T. R., Martin, J., Scudri, J. D., Brown, A., Cirillo, J. D., Bloom, B. R., and Jacobs, Jr., W. R. (1995) In vivo characteristics of leucine and methionine auxotrophic mutants of *Mycobacterium bovis* BCG generated by transposon mutagenesis. *Infect. Immun.* **63,** 1004–1012.

12. Guilhot, C., Otal, I., Van Rompaey, I., Martin, C., and Gicquel, B. (1994) Efficient transposition in mycobacteria: construction of *M. smegmatis* insertional mutant libraries. *J. Bacteriol.* **176,** 535–539.
13. Sander, P., Meier, A., and Böttger, E. C. (1995) *rpsL+*: a dominant selectable marker for gene replacement in mycobacteria. *Mol. Microbiol.* **16,** 991–1000.
14. Norman, E., Dellagostin, O. A., McFadden, J., and Dale, J. W. (1995) Gene replacement by homologous recombination in *Mycobacterium bovis* BCG. *Mol. Microbiol.* **16,** 755–760.
15. Pelicic, V., Reyrat, J. M., and Gicquel, B. (1996) Generation of unmarked directed mutations in mycobacteria, using sucrose counter-selectable suicide vectors. *Mol. Microbiol.* **20,** 919–925.
16. Pelicic, V., Reyrat, J. M., and Gicquel, B. (1996) Positive selection of allelic exchange mutants in *Mycobacterium bovis* BCG. *FEMS Microbiol. Lett.* **144,** 161–166.
17. Pelicic, V., Jackson, M., Reyrat, J. M., Jacobs, W. R., Gicquel, B., and Guilhot, C. (1997) Efficient allelic exchange and transposon mutagenesis in *Mycobacterium tuberculosis. Proc. Natl. Acad. Sci. USA* **94,** 10,955–10,960.
18. Azad, A. K., Sirakova, T. D., Fernandes, N. D., and Kolattukudy P. E. (1997) Gene knockout reveals a novel gene cluster for the synthesis of a class of cell wall lipids unique to pathogenic mycobacteria. *J. Biol. Chem.* **272(27),** 16,741–16,745.
19. Pelicic, V., Reyrat, J. M., and Gicquel, B. (1996) Expression of the *Bacillus subtilis sacB* gene confers sucrose sensitivity on mycobacteria. *J. Bacteriol.* **178,** 1197–1199.
20. Steinmetz, M., Le Coq, D., Djema, H. B., and Gay, P. (1983) Genetic analysis of *sacB*, the structural gene of a secreted enzyme levansucrase of *Bacillus subtilis* Marburg. *Mol. Gen. Genet.* **191,** 138–144.
21. Daffé, M. and Draper, P. (1998) The envelope layers of mycobacteria with reference to their pathogenicity. *Adv. Microb. Physiol.* **39,** 131–203.
22. Pavelka, M. S. and Jacobs, Jr., W. R. (1999) A comparison of the construction of unmarked deletion mutations in *Mycobacterium smegmatis*, *M. bovis* BCG and *M. tuberculosis* H37Rv by allelic exchange. *J. Bacteriol.* **181,** 4780–4789.
23. Pavelka, Jr., M. S. and Jacobs, Jr., W. R. (1996) Biosynthesis of diaminopimelate, the precursor of lysine and a component of peptidoglycan, is an essential function of *Mycobacterium smegmatis*. *J. Bacteriol.* **178,** 6496–6507.
24. Guilhot, C., Gicquel, B., and Martin, C. (1992) Temperature-sensitive mutants of the Mycobacterium plasmid pAL5000. *FEMS Microbiol. Lett.* **98,** 181–186.
25. Quandt, J. and Hynes, M. F. (1993) Versatile suicide vectors which allow direct selection for gene replacement in Gram-negative bacteria. *Gene* **127,** 15–21.
26. Sambrook, J., Fritsch, E. F., and Maniatis, T. (1989) *Molecular Cloning: A Laboratory Manual.* Cold Spring Harbor, New York.
27. Curcic, R., Dhandayuthapani, S., and Deretic, V. (1994) Gene expression in mycobacteria: transcriptional fusions based on *xylE* and analysis of the promoter region of the response regulator *mtrA* from *Mycobacterium tuberculosis*. *Mol. Microbiol.* **13,** 1057–1064.

28. Dhandayuthapani, S., Via, L. E., Thomas, C. A., Horowitz, P. M., Deretic, D., and Deretic, V. (1995) Green fluorescent protein as a marker for gene expression and cell biology of mycobacterial interactions with macrophages. *Mol. Microbiol.* **17,** 901–912.
29. Kremer, L., Baulard, A., Estaquier, J., Poulain-Godefroy, O., and Locht, C. (1995) Green fluorescent protein as a new expression marker in mycobacteria. *Mol. Microbiol.* **17,** 913–922.

6

Gene Replacement using Pretreated DNA

Bhavna G. Gordhan and Tanya Parish

1. Introduction

1.1. Homologous Recombination in Mycobacterium tuberculosis

Gene replacement by homologous recombination (HR) is an invaluable tool in understanding the physiology and the significance of specific genes in the virulence of *Mycobacterium tuberculosis*. It will also allow for the development of rationally attenuated strains as candidate vaccines to prevent the spread of tuberculosis. Classically, allelic replacement involves the introduction of nonreplicating DNA (suicide plasmids) carrying a mutated copy of the targeted gene, most often disrupted by an antibiotic resistance determinant, into the chromosome. A single recombination event (cross-over) between the two alleles will result in integration of the entire plasmid to generate a single cross-over (SCO) strain carrying both wild-type and mutated copies of the gene. If two recombination events occur, a double cross-over (DCO) is generated where the wild-type allele is replaced by the mutant allele. Strains with an SCO can also give rise to DCO strains when a second recombination event takes place (**Fig. 1**).

Although targeted gene inactivation by HR has been achieved for a number of genes in the fast growing, nonpathogenic *Mycobacterium smegmatis (1–5)*, it has been notoriously difficult to accomplish in slow-growing mycobacterial species such as *M. tuberculosis* and *Mycobacterium bovis* BCG *(6)*. Initial attempts to achieve gene replacement by various selection methods in the *M. tuberculosis* complex resulted mainly in products of random integration or illegitimate recombination at an unusually high frequency *(2,7)*. Although it has been suggested that illegitimate recombination might be useful to generate libraries of mutants *(2)*, this process renders the isolation of DCO homologous recombinants virtually impossible in the absence of a counter-selectable marker

From: *Methods in Molecular Medicine*, vol. 54: *Mycobacterium Tuberculosis Protocols*
Edited by: T. Parish and N. G. Stoker © Humana Press Inc., Totowa, NJ

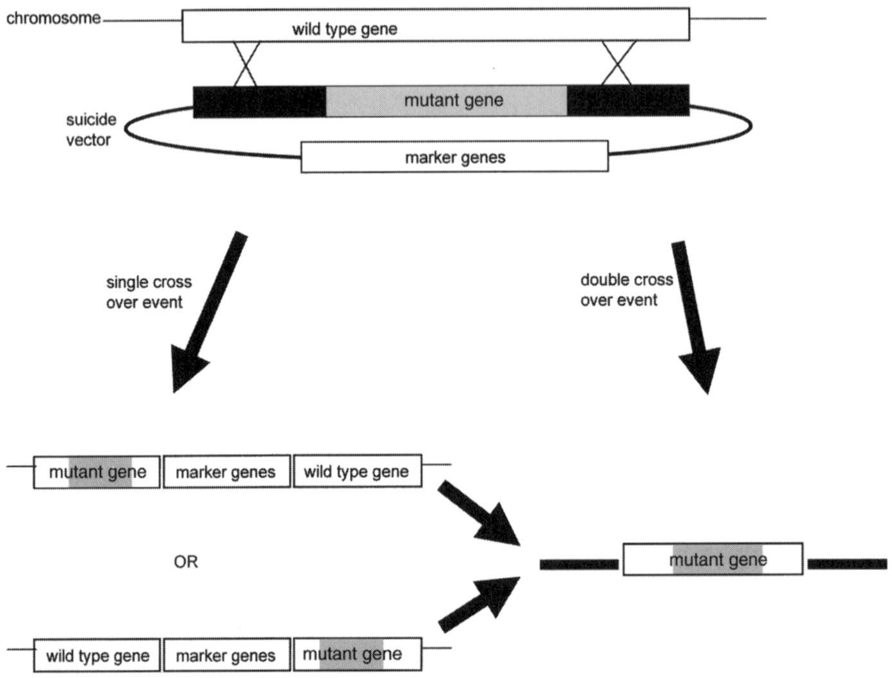

Fig. 1. Allelic replacement by homologous recombination. A nonreplicating (suicide) plasmid carrying a mutated version of the gene is introduced into the bacteria. Homologous recombination will lead to either single cross-overs, where a single recombination event has taken place or double cross-overs where two recombination events have occurred. SCOs will carry both wild-type and mutated alleles of the gene and any marker genes found on the plasmid, whereas DCOS will carry one copy of the gene and no marker genes.

or a mutant phenotype that is easy to discern ***(8–11)***. The basis of a counterselection strategy is that a marker gene in the vector renders the cell susceptible to the selective agent, and this marker is only incorporated into the chromosome in the event of an SCO or random integration, and not after a DCO has occurred. Therefore selection against a marker gene increases the proportion of DCO mutants. Several counter-selectable markers (*katG*, *rpsL*$^+$, *sacB*) have recently been described and used to facilitate allelic exchange in mycobacteria ***(6,12)*** (*see* Chapters 5 and 7).

Allelic replacement in *M. tuberculosis* was first demonstrated using a long linear substrate ***(13)***. The use of long linear fragments was thought to increase the probability of detecting targeted gene replacement, but the efficiency of isolating mutants has been much improved by the use of a counter-selectable strategy ***(14–16)***. Significant advances have recently been made in the development of suitable suicide and conditionally replicating vehicles for the delivery of inactivated genes into *M. tuberculosis* ***(17–19)***. A further increase in the efficiency of isolation of allelic replacement mutants has been achieved by combining the counter-selectable marker *sacB* with a temperature sensitive replicon for delivery ***(20)***. More recently, Hinds et al. ***(21)*** reported that single-stranded (ss) phagemid DNA, ultraviolet (UV) irradiation of double-stranded (ds) DNA and alkali denaturation of ds DNA enhanced HR. Application of this methodology led to successful allelic exchange at the *tlyA* locus in *M. tuberculosis* ***(21)***. This method has been further used to generate several auxotrophic mutants using the screenable marker gene *lacZ* ***(22)***. Now that efficient HR methods are available, analysis of mutants should give us vital information about mechanisms of pathogenicity. Although substantial progress has been made in the field of gene replacement in *M. tuberculosis*, there is still room for further major technical improvements. It will be useful to determine the effects of length of homology on recombination so that substrate construction can be standardized. Another interesting observation is that the frequency of allelic exchange is gene dependent (some genes are readily inactivated whereas others are refractory to the process), but the reason is unknown. There may also be a significant difference in the efficiency of the recombination process for replacement mutations vs insertion mutations of the targeted gene. The above are some of the questions that need to be addressed to optimize the process of HR in *M. tuberculosis*.

1.2. Structure and Function of M. tuberculosis recA

The RecA protein mediates HR in bacteria in addition to its roles in the repair of DNA damage, replication of chromosomal DNA, mutagenesis, induction of phage λ lysogens, and the regulation of the SOS response ***(23)***. Bacteria lacking the RecA protein are highly susceptible to DNA damaging agents and are recombination deficient. The *recA* gene of *M. tuberculosis* has been found to have a very unusual structure. The gene is interrupted by an in-frame open reading frame encoding an intein ***(24)*** that is removed by a novel mechanism of protein splicing to form mature and functionally active RecA ***(24–26)***. Until recently it was believed that the maturation requirement of RecA might conditionally limit the levels of functional RecA in *M. tuberculosis* ***(6,27)*** and hence limit HR. It has now been shown that the *M. tuberculosis recA* gene, with or without its intein, can complement a *M. smegmatis recA* deletion strain ***(28)***. This work revealed that both versions of the *M. tuberculosis recA* gene restored UV resistance to wild-type levels and most importantly, that the frequency of DCO HR events was identical regardless of whether the *recA* gene contained or lacked the intein. To rule out the possibility that the intein may nevertheless have an effect on recombination in *M. tuberculosis*, a similar experiment will have to be conducted in a *M. tuberculosis recA* mutant once such a mutant is isolated. This suggests that the intein coding sequence in the *recA* gene of *M. tuberculosis* is not a major factor leading to the low frequency of HR observed in *M. tuberculosis*.

1.3. Pretreatment of Donor DNA

Recently, it has been shown that HR in *M. tuberculosis* is enhanced by the use of ss DNA generated either by alkali denaturation or by the production of ss phagemid DNA, or alternatively by the use of UV-irradiated ds DNA ***(21)***. Introduction of pretreated donor DNA probably induces the expression of RecA and/or other proteins involved in DNA repair mechanisms, thus stimulating HR. Mutants of *M. tuberculosis* lacking a functional *tlyA* gene, which encodes a hemolysin, were isolated using either UV-irradiated DNA or ss phagemid DNA. No illegitimate recombination events were observed at this locus ***(21)***. Subsequently, the pretreatment of transforming DNA has allowed the construction of several auxotrophic strains of *M. tuberculosis* ***(22)***.

The principle effect of UV irradiation is the production of pyrimidine dimers, most commonly thymine dimers. Where two thymine residues are adjacent on the same DNA strand, UV-irradiation creates covalent links between them causing a distortion of the double helix at that point. Replication cannot proceed past these lesions and the damage has to be repaired in order for the cell to survive. Nucleotide excision repair by UvrABC produces a gapped duplex substrate, leading to the rapid formation of RecA filaments ***(29)*** which in turn stimulates HR.

Alkali treatment separates the two DNA strands (denaturation). In *Streptomyces coelicolor* A3(2) the number of transformants obtained by HR using ds circular DNA is greatly stimulated by denaturation of the donor DNA ***(30)***. Electroporation of *Mycobacterium intracellulare* with alkali-treated DNA similarly resulted in an increase in the number of DCO recombinants using an inactivated *19Ag* gene ***(21)***. Although both alkali treatment and UV-irradiation of donor DNA appear to stimulate HR in the slow-growing mycobacterial species, caution may be necessary when using UV-irradiated DNA, as there is the potential for the induction of point mutations in the recombined DNA. Although we have not assayed for this directly, our previous works suggests that such mutations would occur at a very low frequency, if at all ***(22)***. Little is known about the mutagenesis pathways which may be induced in response to DNA damage in *M. tuberculosis*. In *Escherichia coli*, the UmuDC proteins are involved in UV-induced mutagenesis, however, no *umuD* homolog has been found in the *M. tuberculosis* genome, thus this pathway may be missing.

1.4. Construction of Suicide Delivery Vectors

A prerequisite for a reliable HR system is the use of effective selection markers. Many different marker genes have been used in *M. tuberculosis*, both for positive and negative selection. There are only a few antibiotic resistance genes which may be used in *M. tuberculosis*, the most useful of these being hygromycin resistance (*hyg*). Kanamycin resistance (*kan*) has frequently been used, but the rate of spontaneous mutation to kanamycin is high. In experiments to isolate homologous recombinants, the rate of spontaneous mutation to kanamycin can be much higher than the rate of HR, making this marker of little use on its own. Therefore, it should be used in conjunction with other markers such as *hyg*. Other marker genes, such as *lacZ* and *xylE*, have been used as screening tools to confirm the presence of plasmid DNA; *lacZ*-containing cells are blue on plates containing 5-bromo-4-chloro-3-indolyl-β-D-galactopyranoside (X-gal) and *xylE*-containing cells turn yellow in the presence of catechol.

Negative selection markers such as *rpsL*$^+$ (*see* Chapter 7) conferring streptomycin sensitivity, *katG* ***(32)*** conferring isoniazid sensitivity and *sacB* conferring sucrose sensitivity (*see* Chapter 5) have all been successfully used. The disadvantage of both *rpsL*$^+$ and *katG* markers, is that antibiotic resistant strains of *M. tuberculosis* are required, whereas *sacB* works for all strains. In this chapter, we describe the use of *hyg*, *kan*, *lacZ*, and *sacB* marker genes. The strategy employed is a two-step strategy whereby SCOs are initially selected using *hyg* and *kan* markers, followed by screening and selection for those cells in which DCOs have occurred using *sacB* and *lacZ* markers (**Fig. 2**). The use of the two-step strategy allows the generation of both antibiotic resistance marked and unmarked (deletion) or point mutants ***(33)***.

Since we use different combinations of several marker genes in order to facilitate the two-step process for generating mutants and the subsequent need for multiple restriction enzymes sites, we have developed a simple cloning strategy based on two series of vectors (**Fig. 3** and **Table 1**).

The first series of plasmids (pNIL) is for cloning and manipulating the gene of interest (**Fig. 3A**). The plasmids consist of a simple cloning vector with an origin of replication for *Escherichia coli* (*oriE*), a kanamycin resistance gene (*kan*), and different multiple cloning sites (MCS) with a single *Pac*I restriction site.

The second series of plasmids (pGOAL) is used to generate and store a number of marker gene cassettes (**Fig. 3B** and **Table 1**). These plasmids contain *oriE*, an ampicillin resistance gene (*amp*), and different combinations of marker genes (*hyg*, *lacZ*, and *sacB*) flanked by two *Pac*I sites. Thus, the marker genes can be excised as a *Pac*I cassette and inserted into any of the pNIL series in a one-step cloning process (**Fig. 4**). The benefit of using *Pac*I sites is that none is present in the *M. tuberculosis* genome ***(34)*** or in the marker genes.

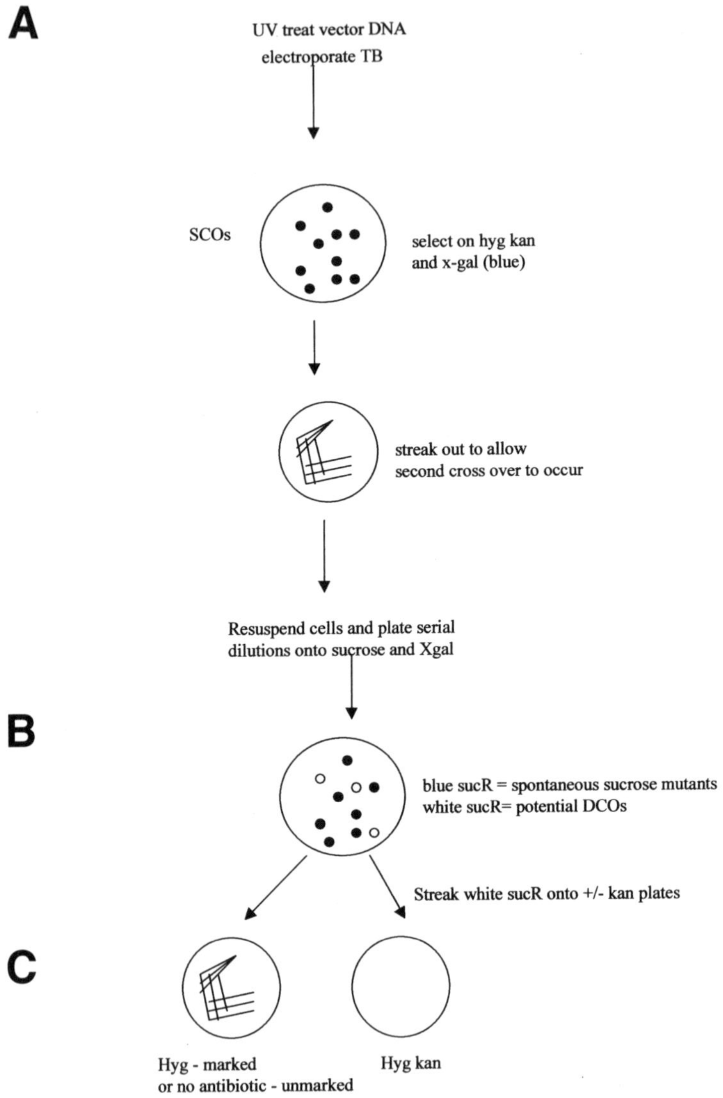

Fig. 2. Two-step strategy for generating *M. tuberculosis* mutants. **(A)** Pretreat suicide delivery vectors with UV light and electroporate *M. tuberculosis*. Select single cross-over transformants by plating onto hygromycin, kanamycin, and X-gal (colonies will be blue). Streak out a single transformant to allow the second cross-over to occur. Resuspend a loopful of cells in medium using 1 mm glass beads and vortexing and plate serial dilutions onto sucrose and X-gal plates. **(B)** Spontaneous sucrose resistant mutants will be blue, since they are single cross-overs and contain the *lacZ* gene, whereas double cross-overs will form white colonies, having lost all marker genes from the chromosome. **(C)** Streak out the white suc^R colonies onto plates with and without kanamycin to confirm the loss of all marker genes. before DNA preparation and Southern analysis on the kan^S colonies. For an unmarked mutation, no antibiotics are included in the plates in steps, for a *hyg* marked mutation hygromycin is included in the plates.

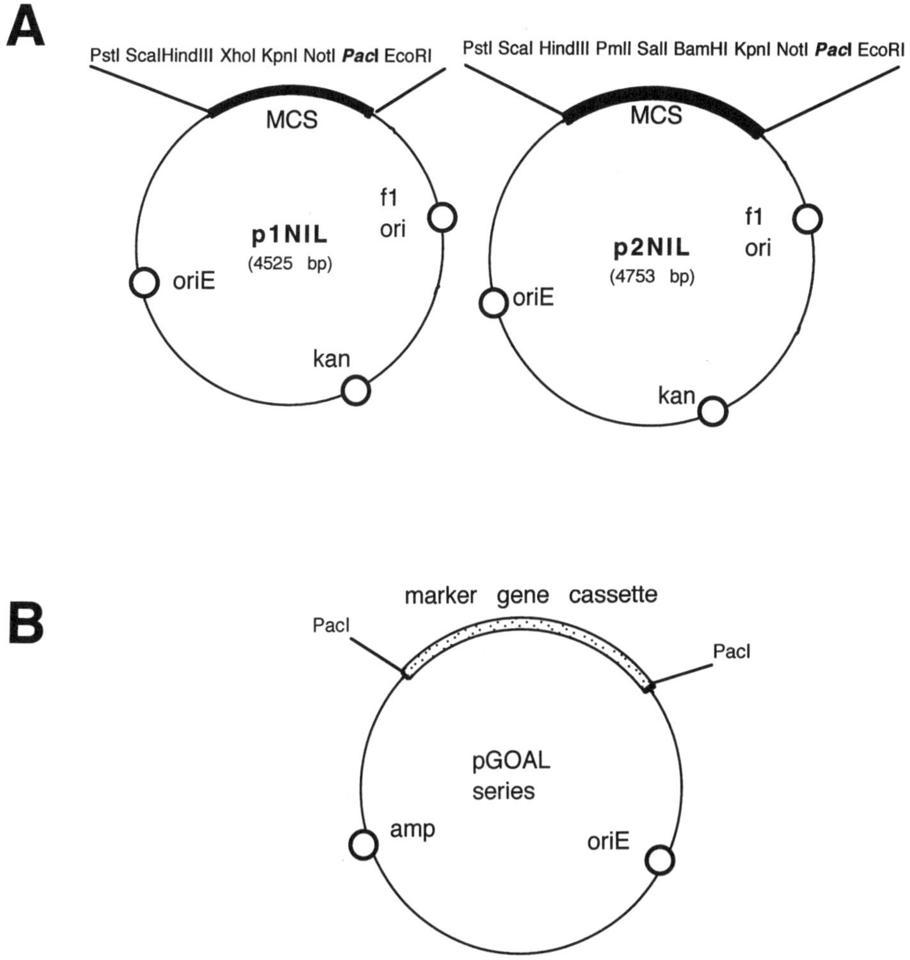

Fig. 3. General features of the **(A)** pNIL and **(B)** pGOAL vector series. pNIL vectors carry the *kan* gene for selection in both *E. coli* and mycobacteria, *oriE* for replication in *E. coli*, the f1 origin for generation of phagemid ssDNA if required, a small multiple cloning site and a single *Pac*I site. pGOAL vectors have different combinations of marker genes flanked by two *Pac*I sites, an *oriE* and *amp* for selection in *E. coli*. *kan* — kanamycin resistance gene; *amp* — ampicillin resistance gene; f1 ori — f1 origin; *oriE* — origin of replication in *E. coli*; MCS — multiple cloning site.

The protocols presented in this chapter deal with the construction of the suicide delivery vector using the rapid cloning method, two different treatment methods of donor DNA prior to electroporation into competent *M. tuberculosis* cells and the generation of mutants by a two-step process.

Table 1
Marker Gene Cassettes Available in the pGOAL Series

pGOAL number	Marker genes
14	*hsp60*p-*sacB*
15	hyg; *lacZ*[a]; *hsp60*p-*sacB*
17	Ag85p-*lacZ*; *hsp60*p-*sacB*
19	hyg; Ag85p-*lacZ*; *hsp60*p-*sacB*

[a]Not expressed in mycobacteria.

2. Materials

2.1. Construction of Suicide Delivery Vector

1. p1NIL and p2NIL cloning vectors (**Fig. 3A**).
2. Appropriate pGOAL vector (**Fig. 3B** and **Table 1**) (*see* **Notes 1** and **2**).

Vectors can be obtained from Neil Stoker, London School of Hygiene & Tropical Medicine on request.

2.2. Generation of Single Stranded DNA by Alkali Denaturation

1. 10 *M* NaOH: Dissolve 40 g of NaOH in 100 mL of water and autoclave.
2. 0.5 *M* ethylenediaminetetracetic acid (EDTA): Dissolve 18.6 g of EDTA in 70 mL of deionized water, pH to 8.0 with NaOH, make up to 100 mL and autoclave.
3. 0.2 m*M* EDTA/0.2 *M* NaOH solution: add 0.4 µL of 0.5 *M* EDTA and 20 mL of 10 *M* NaOH to 980 µL of sterile deionized water. Make fresh on day of use.
4. 3 *M* Sodium Acetate (NaOAc): Dissolve 40.8 g of NaOAc in 70 mL of deionized water, pH to 5.2 with acetic acid, make up to 100 mL and autoclave.
5. 70% ethanol: add 70 mL of 100% ethanol to 30 mL of deionized water.

2.3. Pretreatment of DNA with UV-Irradiation

1. Sterile 60 microwell plates with lids (NUNC, Roskilda, Denmark).
2. UV Stratalinker 1800 (Stratagene, La Jolla, CA).
3. Sterile distilled water.
4. 3 *M* sodium acetate (*see* **Subheading 2.2., step 4**).
5. 100% ethanol.
6. 70% ethanol (*see* **Subheading 2.2., step 5**).

2.4. Two-Step Strategy for Generating Mutants

1. Electroporation equipment (*see* **Note 3**).
2. 10% w/v Tween-80.
3. Middlebrook 7H9 liquid medium: dissolve 4.7 g of 7H9 powder (Difco Laboratories, Detroit, MI) in 900 mL of deionized water, add 5 mL of 10% Tween-80 and autoclave. Add 10% v/v OADC supplement (Difco) prior to use (*see* **Note 4**).

4. Middlebrook 7H10 solid medium: dissolve 19 g of 7H10 agar base (Difco) in 900 mL of deionized water, autoclave and cool to 50°C before adding 10% v/v oleic albumin dextrose catalase (OADC) supplement (*see* **Note 4**).
5. Sucrose stock solution: 50% w/v in water, autoclave. Use at a final concentration of 2% w/v.
6. Hygromycin B, obtained as stock solution. For selection use at 50–100 μg/mL.
7. Kanamycin sulfate: make up as 50 mg/mL stock solution, filter sterilize and store in aliquots at –20°C. For selection use at 10–20 μg/mL.
8. 5-bromo-4-chloro-3-indolyl-β-D-galactopyranoside (X-gal): make stock solution of 50 mg/mL in dimethyl sulphoxide and store at –20°C. Use at working concentration of 50 μg/mL.
9. 1 mm glass beads.

3. Methods

3.1. Construction of Suicide Delivery Vector

1. Clone the target gene into the appropriate pNIL vector depending on the restriction site required (*see* **Fig. 3**). Note that p2NIL has a *Pml*I site which generates blunt ends and can therefore be used for cloning PCR products directly.
2. Make the required mutation (*see* **Notes 5** and **6**). Check the construct by sequencing or restriction mapping.
3. Decide on the appropriate pGOAL *Pac*I marker gene cassette to use (*see* **Note 1**). Clone the *Pac*I cassette into the sole *Pac*I site of the vector containing the target mutant gene (*see* **Fig. 4** and **Note 7**).
4. Make a large scale preparation of delivery plasmid DNA (*see* **Note 8**).

3.2. Generation of Single Stranded DNA by Alkali Denaturation

1. Precipitate 2 μg of substrate DNA with 1/10 vol of NaOAc and 2.5 vol of 100% ethanol at 4°C for 20 min (*see* **Note 9**).
2. Centrifuge at 10,000*g* for 15 min and remove supernatant.
3. Dry the DNA pellet under vacuum and resuspend the pellet in 10 μL of sterile deionized water.
4. Add 3 μL of 0.2 m*M* EDTA/0.2 *M* NaOH to the DNA, mix and incubate at 37°C for 30 min.
5. Add 1.3 μL of 3 *M* NaOAc (1/10 vol) to the denatured DNA and precipitate the DNA with 2.5 vol of 100% ethanol at 4°C for 20 min.
6. Centrifuge at 10,000*g* for 15 min and remove supernatant.
7. Wash the DNA pellet twice with 70% ethanol (*see* **Note 10**)
8. Dry the pellet under vacuum and resuspend in 5 μL of sterile deionized water prior to electroporation (*see* **Notes 11** and **12**).

3.3. Pretreatment of DNA with UV-Irradiation

1. Precipitate 5 μg of substrate DNA as described under **Subheading 3.2., step 1** (*see* **Notes 9** and **12**).

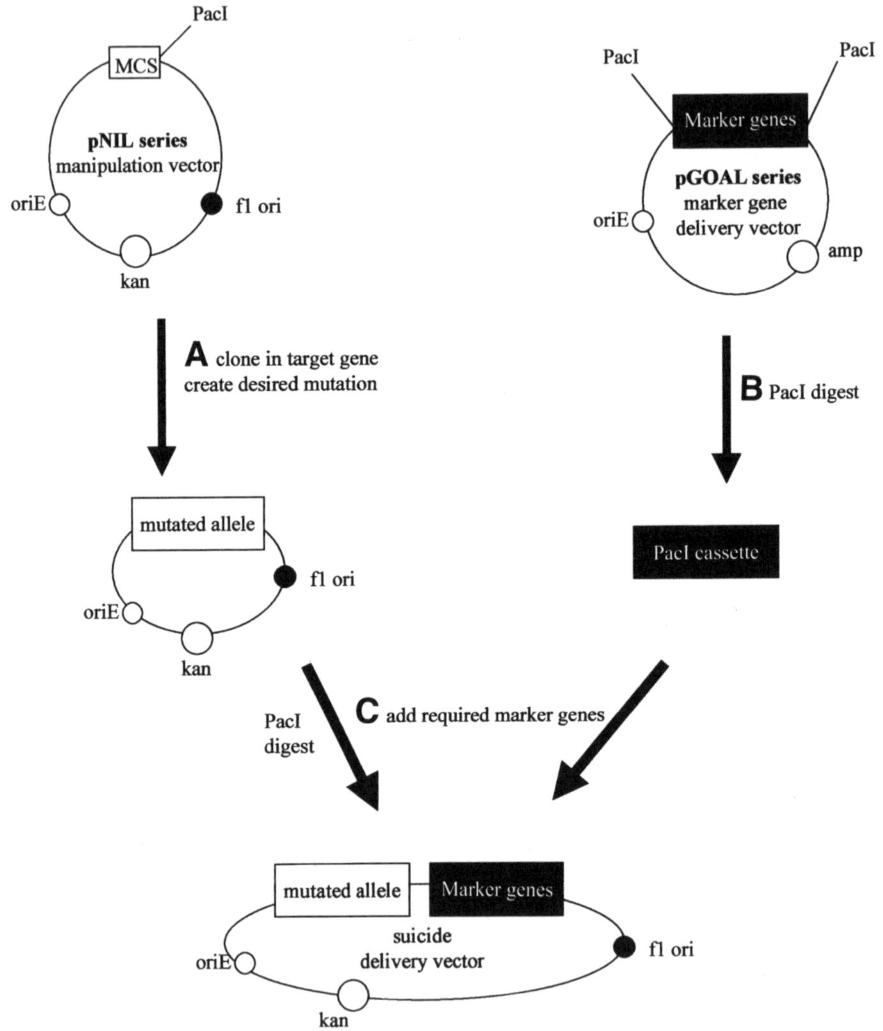

Fig. 4. Cloning strategy for generating suicide delivery vectors. **(A)** Clone the target gene into one of the pNIL vectors and generate the required mutation. **(B)** Excise the *Pac*I cassette containing the desired marker genes from the appropriate pGOAL vector and clone into the unique *Pac*I site of the pNIL-mutated-gene vector. This results in the final suicide delivery vector **(C)** containing an *oriE*, the kanamycin resistance gene (*kan*) and the f1 origin (f1 ori).

2. Wash the DNA pellet twice with 70% ethanol (*see* **Note 10**).
3. Dry the DNA pellet under vacuum and resuspend in 10 μL of sterile deionized water.
4. Place the DNA sample in a well of a sterile microwell plate (*see* **Note 13**).

5. Remove the cover of the microtiter plate and subject the DNA to 100 mJ cm^{-2} of UV energy (*see* **Note 14**).
6. Transfer the irradiated DNA into a microtube and store at –20°C until required.

3.4. Two-Step Strategy for Generating Mutants (see Figure 2)

1. Electroporate *M. tuberculosis* with the pretreated DNA from **Subheading 3.2.**, or **3.3.** (*see* **Note 15** and **16**).
2. Plate transformants onto 7H10 plates with hygromycin, kanamycin, and X-gal (*see* **Note 2**).
3. Seal plates with parafilm or in individual plastic bags and incubate at 37°C for 3–4 wk, until blue colonies appear. These are SCOs (*see* **Note 17**).
4. Streak two individual hygromycin resistant (hyg^R) kanamycin resistant (kan^R) transformants onto fresh 7H10 agar plates and incubate at 37°C for 2 wk (*see* **Notes 17** and **18**).
5. Scrape a loopful of cells from the plate and place into a universal containing approx 1 mL of 1 mm glass beads and 3 mL of 7H9/OADC/Tween.
6. Vortex vigorously until the majority of the cells are resuspended (*see* **Note 19**).
7. Let stand for 10 min to allow large clumps to settle.
8. Make serial dilutions and plate onto X-gal-containing plates with and without sucrose (and hygromycin where appropriate) (*see* **Notes 20** and **21**).
9. Seal plates and incubate at 37°C for 3–5 wk (*see* **Note 22**).
10. Count CFUs on each plate. Score blue and white colonies (*see* **Notes 20**, **23**, and **24**).
11. Streak (patch) approx 40 of the white sucrose resistant (suc^R) colonies onto plates with and without kanamycin and score for kanamycin sensitivity (kan^S) (*see* **Note 25**).
12. Prepare DNA from kan^S colonies and analyze by Southern blotting (*see* **Note 26**).

4. Notes

1. The pGOAL vector required will be dependent on the type of mutation being generated. For an unmarked mutation, pGOAL19 is the most appropriate, since it carries the *hyg* resistance gene, whereas for mutations marked internally with *hyg*, pGOAL17 will be more appropriate. Other combinations of markers are available, but we have found these two are the most useful in practice.
2. The use of two antibiotic resistance genes effectively abolishes the problem of obtaining spontaneous resistant colonies. Spontaneous kanamycin resistance occurs at a higher frequency than hygromycin resistance, thus *kan* should not be used on its own. Although, spontaneous hygromycin resistance occurs at a lower frequency, it can still be higher than the frequency of homologous recombination, so we do not recommend using hygromycin solely either.
3. We have used both the Bio-Rad Gene Pulser (Bio-Rad, Hemel Hempstead, Herts, UK) and the Flowgen Easyject (Lichfield, Staffordshire,UK). We recommend that electroporation efficiencies are optimized by the individual user depending on the equipment used.

4. Any of the commonly used media for mycobacteria may be used for growth of *M. tuberculosis*. However, it is important to allow for any supplement that the mutants may potentially require for growth.
5. There are two methods of generating a mutated allele. Either the gene can be cloned into the pNIL vector as one fragment and a subsequent deletion made, or two separate fragments containing the flanking DNA can be brought together to create a deletion. In either case the mutation can be marked by cloning the *hyg* gene into the deletion.
6. The minimum length of homology has not been determined, but it is likely that the frequency will fall progressively below 1 kb. We have used as little as 700 bp ***(22)***. We routinely use around 1 kb on either side of the mutation. In order to ensure that the second cross-over occurs with equal frequency to give wild-type and mutant alleles, the fragments on either side should be of approximately equal length.
7. The final vector should be checked using several different restriction enzymes, since the inclusion of the *sacB* gene can make plasmids unstable and cause deletions or rearrangements.
8. Both the UV-irradiation and alkali-treatment methods require an ultrapure, concentrated preparation of the plasmid (substrate) DNA. High yields of plasmid DNA can be obtained using the standard alkali lysis protocol ***(31)*** followed by purification of the DNA on a $CsCl_2$/ethidium bromide gradient or by phenol extractions. Due to the toxicity of these compounds these methods of purification are becoming redundant. Instead many commercial plasmid purification kits are now available that are safer and quicker.
9. An extra 1 µg of DNA should be precipitated to compensate for any loss that may occur during the precipitation and washing processes.
10. The DNA pellet is washed twice to remove all traces of salt. Excessive salts in the DNA sample causes arcing of the sample during the electroporation procedure with a consequent drop in transformation efficiency.
11. Alkali-denatured DNA in water will reanneal after a long period of time; however, it can be resuspended in sterile deionized water and stored at –20°C for short periods prior to electroporation.
12. DNA stored in water at –20°C for an extended period of time may undergo spontaneous hydrolysis causing nucleotides and salts to precipitate out. To prevent arcing, it is best to reprecipitate and wash the required amount of DNA prior to the electroporation procedure.
13. If more than one sample is to be irradiated, place them a few wells apart to prevent cross-contamination.
14. A setting of a 1000 on the energy scale on the UV Stratalinker 1800 delivers an output energy of 1000 µJ $cm^{-2} \times 100$ which is equivalent to 100 mJ cm^{-2}. Hinds et al. ***(21)*** tested the effect of 25, 100 and 300 mJ cm^{-2} of UV-irradiation on donor DNA using recombination assays. At 25 mJ cm^{-2} there was a slight increase in the number of recombinants whereas at 300 mJ cm^{-2} there was no net increase in the number of recombinants, since there was an increase in the rate of HR, but there was a sharp decrease in the number of transformants due to excessive DNA

damage. At 100 mJ cm^{-2} there was a marked increase in the number of HR transformants.

15. UV pretreatment is technically the least demanding and gives rise to the largest number of HR transformants. However, this may lead to the incorporation of additional point mutations in the introduced DNA. We have not routinely sequenced SCO strains, but the fact that we have isolated several hundreds of SCOs and not seen any loss of LacZ function suggests that the frequency of such an event is low. If this is a concern, the relevant DNA region in the mutants obtained should be sequenced to confirm that no extra mutations have been introduced. Alkali-denaturation is not expected to lead to any additional mutations and may be used as an alternative; using this method gives rise to fewer transformants and may necessitate the use of larger amounts of DNA. Since a two-step strategy is used, only one SCO transformant is required in order to generate a DCO, so the lower number of transformants should not be as large a problem. Another alternative is to use ss phagemid DNA. This has been shown to abolish illegitimate recombination as well. The main problem with this method is the generation of sufficient amount of single-stranded DNA, which can be technically challenging when using GC-rich DNA, such as *M. tuberculosis* DNA.
16. The electroporation efficiency of the cells should be assessed using a replicating vector. It is important to get an efficiency of at least 10^5 per μg of DNA, since the frequency of HR may be as low as 10^{-5}. Lower efficiencies may result in no HR transformants being obtained. However, since a two-step strategy is employed, only one SCO transformant is required in order to obtain a DCO mutant.
17. These transformants are SCO recombinants. Where a single recombination event occurs, the whole delivery vector will be integrated into the chromosome, so all marker genes will be present. Thus SCOs will be hyg^R kan^R and blue on X-gal plates. The SCO genotype can be confirmed by Southern blotting or PCR; in practice all the transformants we have analyzed so far have been SCOs, so this is not strictly necessary. If Southern blotting is not carried out, two transformants should be selected for the next stage.
18. This step allows the second cross-over to occur. X-gal should not be included in the plates, since this makes the cells even more sticky than usual and difficult to resuspend in liquid media. For an unmarked mutation, no antibiotics should be included in the plates. For *hyg* marked mutations, hygromycin should be included in the plates.
19. At this stage, it is not possible to make a completely homogeneous suspension of bacteria. The large clumps should be left to settle out, leaving a cell suspension which should be slightly cloudy. The majority of cells will not be in clumps, although a few may remain; this does not pose a problem, since mixed colonies derived from more than one cell will inevitably contain at least one SCO cell which will show up as kan^R in the subsequent step (and be discarded).
20. In practice, serial dilutions from 10^0 to 10^{-2} should be plated. Further dilutions are unnecessary, since there will be no colonies on the sucrose plates. The plates without sucrose are there to confirm that the SCO is sucrose-sensitive — a reduc-

tion of approx 10^{-4} to 10^{-5} CFUs should be seen on the sucrose plates. Exact colony counts are not required.

21. For an unmarked mutation, plate dilutions onto 7H10 plates plus X-gal, and 7H10 plus X-gal, and sucrose plates. For a *hyg*-marked mutation, plate onto 7H10 plus hygromycin and X-gal, and 7H10 plus hygromycin, X-gal, and sucrose.
22. Colonies will appear after 3 wk and can be screened for kanamycin sensitivity at this stage. However, it is important to note that if the mutant has a reduced growth rate, the mutant DCO colonies may not appear until later. Therefore, it is important to keep the plates for at least 5 wk.
23. The colonies on the sucrose plates are either spontaneous sucrose-resistant (suc^R) mutants (still SCOs) or DCOs. The rate of spontaneous sucrose resistance ranges from 10^{-4} to 10^{-5}. Spontaneous suc^R colonies should be blue, since they still carry the *lacZ* gene, whereas any DCOs should be white, having lost the *lacZ* marker gene. The relative frequency of blue to white colonies will depend on the frequency of recombination, which is highly gene dependent. We have seen between 10–90% of colonies being DCOs (white suc^R).
24. Some colonies may appear as pale blue. This is due to the variability of *lacZ* expression between cells. The use of a mycobacterial promoter to express *lacZ* reduces this problem, but it may still occur. However, since these are SCOs, they are easily excluded from Southern analysis by the fact that they are kan^R in the patch tests.
25. We routinely streak at least 40 colonies, this gives us a sufficiently large number of potential mutants for subsequent DNA preparation. Eight colonies can be streaked onto one 90 mm agar plate. DCOs will be kan^S.
26. We routinely pick eight colonies (one plate) at a time for DNA preparation. For an unmarked mutation, DCOs can either have the wild-type allele restored, or the mutant allele. Again, the relative frequency of each will depend both on the gene itself and the length of homologous DNA on either side of the mutation in the delivery construct. For *hyg*-marked mutations, all hyg^R kan^S colonies should carry the mutant allele.

References

1. Husson, R. N., James, B. E., and Young, R. A. (1990) Gene replacement and expression of foreign DNA in mycobacteria. *J. Bacteriol.* **172,** 519–524.
2. Kalpana, G. V., Bloom, B. R., and Jacobs, Jr., W. R. (1991) Insertional mutagenesis and illegitimate recombination in mycobacteria. *Proc. Natl. Acad. Sci. USA* **88,** 5433–5473.
3. Gordhan, B. G., Andersen, S. J., De Meyer, A. R., and Mizrahi, V. (1996) Construction by homologous recombination and phenotypic characterization of a *polA* mutant of *Mycobacterium smegmatis*. *Gene* **178,** 125–130.
4. Quan, S. W., Venter, H., and Dabbs, E. R. (1997) Ribosylative inactivation of rifampin by *Mycobacterium smegmatis* is a principle contributor to its low susceptibility to this antibiotic. *Antimicrob. Agents Chemother.* **41,** 2456–2460.

5. Boshoff, H. I. M. and Mizrahi, V. (1998) Purification, gene cloning, targeted knockout, overexpression, and biochemical characterization of the major pyrazinamidase from *Mycobacterium smegmatis*. *J. Bacteriol.* **180,** 5809–5814.
6. McFadden, J. (1996) Recombination in mycobacteria. *Mol. Microbiol.* **21,** 205–211.
7. Aldovoni, A., Husson, R. N., and Young, R. A. (1993) The *uraA* locus and homologous recombination in *Mycobacterium bovis* BCG. *J. Bacteriol.* **175,** 7282–7289.
8. Pelicic, V., Reyrat, J. M., and Gicquel, B. (1996) Expression of the Bacillus subtilis *sacB* gene confers sucrose sensitivity on mycobacteria. *J. Bacteriol.* **178,** 1197–1199.
9. Pelicic, V., Reyrat, J. M., and Gicquel, B. (1996) Generation of unmarked directed mutations in mycobacteria, using sucrose counter-selectable suicide vectors. *Mol. Microbiol.* **20,** 191–925.
10. Sander, P., Meier, A., and Bottger, E. C. (1995) A dominant selectable marker for gene replacement in mycobacteria. *Mol. Microbiol.* **16,** 991–1000.
11. Knipfer, N., and Shrader, T. E. (1997) Inactivation of the 20S proteasome in *Mycobacterium smegmatis*. *Mol. Microbiol.* **25,** 375–383.
12. Reyrat, J. M., Pelicic, V., Gicquel, B., and Rappuoli, R. (1998) Counterselectable markers: untapped tools for bacterial genetics and pathogenesis. *Infect. Immunol.* **66,** 4011–4017.
13. Balasubramanian, V., Pavelka, Jr. M. S., Bardarov, S. S., Martin, J., Weisbrod, T. R., McAdam, R. A., Bloom, B. R., and Jacobs, Jr. W. R. (1996) Allelic exchange in *Mycobacterium tuberculosis* with long linear recombination substrates. *J. Bacteriol.* **178,** 273–279.
14. Pelicic, V., Reyrat, J. M., and Gicquel, B. (1996) Positive selection of allelic exchange mutants in *Mycobacterium bovis* BCG. *FEMS Microbiol. Lett.* **144,** 161–166.
15. Azad, A. K., Sirakova, T. D., Rogers, L. M., and Kolattukudy, P. E. (1996) Targeted gene replacement of the mycocerosic acid synthase gene in *Mycobacterium bovis* BCG produces a mutant that lacks mycosides. *Proc. Natl. Acad. Sci. USA* **93,** 4787–4792.
16. Azad, A. K., Siakova, T. D., Fernandes, N. D., and Kolattukudy, P. E. (1997) Gene knockout reveals a novel gene cluster for the synthesis of a class of cell wall lipids unique to pathogenic mycobacteria. *J. Biol. Chem.* **272,** 16,741–16,745.
17. Bardarov, S., Kriakov, J., Carriere, C., Yu, S. U., Vaamonde, C., McAdam, R. A., Bloom, B. R., Hatfull, G. F., and Jacobs, Jr. W. R. (1997) Conditionally replicating mycobacteriophages: a system for transposon delivery to *Mycobacterium tuberculosis*. *Proc. Natl. Acad. Sci. USA* **94,** 10,961–10,966.
18. Baulard, A., Kremer, L., and Locht, C., (1996) Efficient homologous recombination in fast growing and slow growing mycobacteria. *J. Bacteriol.* **178,** 3091–3098.
19. Stolt, P., and Stoker, N. G. (1996) Functional definitions of regions necessary for replication and incompatibility in the *Mycobacterium fortuitum* plasmid, pAL5000. *Microbiology* **142,** 2795–2802.
20. Pelicic, V., Jackson, M., Reyrat, J. M., Jacobs, Jr. W. R., Gicquel, B., and Guilhot, C. (1997) Efficient allelic exchange and transposon mutagenesis in *Mycobacterium tuberculosis*. *Proc. Natl. Acad. Sci. USA* **94,** 10,955–10,960.

21. Hinds, J., Mahenthiralingam, E., Kempsell, K. E., Duncan, K., Stokes, R. W., Parish, T., and Stoker, N. G. (1999) Enhanced gene replacement in mycobacteria. *Microbiology* **145,** 519–527.
22. Parish, T., Gordhan, B. G., McAdam, R. A., Duncan, K., Mizrahi, V., and Stoker, N. G. (1999) Production of mutants in amino acid biosynthesis genes of *Mycobacterium tuberculosis* by homologous recombination. *Microbiology* **145,** 3497–3503.
23. Kowalczykowski, S. C., Dixon, D. A., Eggleston, A. K., Lauder, S. D., and Rehrauer, W. M. (1994) Biochemistry of homologous recombination in *Escherichia coli. Microbiol. Rev.* **58,** 401–465.
24. Davis, E. O., Sedgwick, S. G., and Colston. M. J. (1991) Novel structure of the *recA* locus of *Mycobacterium tuberculosis* implies processing of the gene product. *J. Bacteriol.* **173,** 5653–5662.
25. Davis, E. O., Jenner, P. J., Brooks, P. C., and Colston, M. J., and Sedgwick, S. G. (1992) Protein splicing in the maturation of *M. tuberculosis* recA protein: a mechanism for tolerating a novel class of intervening sequence. *Cell* **71,** 20 1–210.
26. Kumar, R. A., Vase, M. B., Chandra, N. R., Vijayan, M., and Muniyappa, K. (1996) Functional characteristics of the precursor and spliced forms of RecA protein of *Mycobacterium tuberculosis. Biochemistry* **35,** 1793–1802.
27. Davis, E. O., Thangaraj, H. S., Brooks, P. C., and Colston, M. J. (1994) Evidence of selection for protein introns in the recA's of pathogenic mycobacteria. *EMBO J.* **13,** 699–703.
28. Papavinasasundaram, K. G., Colston, M. J., and Davis, E. O. (1998) Construction and complementation of a *recA* deletion mutant of *Mycobacterium smegmatis* reveals that the intein in *Mycobacterium tuberculosis recA* does not affect RecA function. *Mol. Microbiol.* **30,** 525–534.
29. Friedberg, E. C., Walker, G. C., and Siede, W. (1995) DNA repair and mutagenesis. Wahington, DC: American Society for Microbiology.
30. Oh, S.-H. and Chater, K. F. (1997) Denaturation of circular or linear DNA facilitates targeted integrative transformation of *Streptomyces coelicolor* A3(2): possible relevance to other organisms. *J. Bacteriol.* **179,** 122–127.
31. Sambrook, J., Fritsch, E. F., and Maniatis, T. (1989) *Molecular Cloning: A Laboratory Manual*, 2nd ed. Cold Spring Harbor Laboratory Press, Cold Spring Harbor, New York.
32. Norman, E., Dellagostin, O. A., McFadden, J., and Dale, J. W. (1995) Gene replacement by homologous recombination in *Mycobacterium bovis* BCG. *Microbiology* **16,** 755–760.
33. Parish, T., and Stoker, N. G. (2000) Use of a flexible cassette method to generate a double unmarked *Mycobacterium tuberculosis tlyA plcABC* mutant by gene replacement. *Microbiology* **146,** 1969–1975.
34. Cole, S. T., Brosch, R., Parkhill, J., et al. (1998) Deciphering the biology of *Mycobacterium tuberculosis* from the complete genome sequence. *Nature* **393,** 537–544.

7

Gene Replacement in *Mycobacterium tuberculosis* and *Mycobacterium bovis* BCG Using *rpsL*⁺ as a Dominant Negative Selectable Marker

Peter Sander, Burkhard Springer, and Erik C. Böttger

1. Introduction

Much progress has been made in mycobacterial research in general and in mycobacterial genetics in particular during the past 10 yr. The complete genome sequences of two isolates of *Mycobacterium tuberculosis*, the widely distributed laboratory strain *M. tuberculosis* H37Rv *(1)* and a clinical isolate CDC1551 (http://www.tigr.org), have recently been determined, thus providing a complete blueprint of the genetic make-up of this pathogen.

How can we read this blueprint? Different approaches are possible to characterize the function of a gene. In general, heterologous expression of a particular gene in a different host, e.g., in *Escherichia coli* or in *Mycobacterium smegmatis* — a widely used surrogate strain in mycobacterial genetics — might help to characterize its function. However, from these experiments a gene can only be partially characterized. To fully understand the function of a gene or its contribution to a particular phenotype, it is necessary to investigate it functionally in its genetic background, especially when the gene is presumed to represent a regulatory gene or a virulence factor.

Isogenic mutants are widely used in bacterial genetics and are a powerful tool to investigate cause-effect relationships. Rather than selecting for mutants arising by chance, targeted gene inactivation allows the generation of a specific mutant, irrespective of whether the gene itself confers a recognizable phenotype. This is especially important for the investigation of phenotypes, which are based on genetic redundancy. Transposon mutagenesis allows the simultaneous isolation of many different mutants and recently this technique has been adapted to *M. tuberculosis* *(2–4)*. However, the distribution of IS-elements in the genome of *M. tuberculosis*

From: *Methods in Molecular Medicine*, vol. 54: *Mycobacterium Tuberculosis Protocols*
Edited by: T. Parish and N. G. Stoker © Humana Press Inc., Totowa, NJ

suggests that transposition might not be completely random and that it may prove difficult to target genes which are small in size *(5)*.

Generation of allelic replacement mutants is an important alternative to transposon mutagenesis. Here we describe a technique which allows the generation of allelic exchange mutants by the combination of a positive selectable marker (conferring kanamycin or hygromycin resistance) with a dominant negative selectable marker, *rpsL*+, the first negative selectable marker used in mycobacterial genetics ***(6)***. The *rpsL*+ allele is dominant under merodiploid conditions rendering a streptomycin-resistant strain whose resistance is caused by a mutation in *rpsL*, sensitive toward this compound *(7)*. When incorporated into a suicide vector outside the target gene, the *rpsL*+ gene facilitates the isolation of allelic replacement mutants. In contrast to transposon mutagenesis, targeted gene inactivation by allelic exchange requires a functional RecA-dependent recombination system. Despite the unusual structure of the *M. tuberculosis* RecA ***(8)*** and early reports that illegitimate recombination appears to be the predominant mechanism of integration of exogenous nucleic acids in *M. tuberculosis* complex ***(9)***, it has recently been demonstrated that the *M. tuberculosis* RecA is fully functional with respect to DNA repair mechanisms and homologous recombination ***(10,11)***.

More recent results obtained in our own as well as in other laboratories (*see* Chapters 9 and 10) strongly suggest that when difficulties are encountered with respect to the generation of mutants by allelic exchange, this is most likely resulting from some pecularities of the target gene itself (*see* **Note 1**). Here we describe the adaption of a technique, which has previously been used successfully in *M. smegmatis* ***(6,10,12,13)***, to generate allelic exchange mutants in *M. tuberculosis* and *Mycobacterium bovis* BCG. As transformation efficiencies are a critical issue (*see* **Note 2**), the original procedure has been modified by incorporating successive steps of positive and negative selections instead of a one-step double selection (*see* **Fig. 1**). The unfavourable ratio of single cross-over transformants to double cross-over (= allelic replacement) transformants in *M. tuberculosis* ***(14)*** clearly shows the advantage of a genetic system which uses a counter selectable marker to facilitate the isolation of knock-out mutants. A different strategy in mycobacterial genetics which uses negative selection markers for allelic exchange based on *sacB* conferring sucrose sensitivity and a replicative vector with a thermosensitive origin ***(15)*** is described in Chapter 9.

2. Materials

2.1. Bacterial Strains and Vectors

1. *E. coli* strains suitable for recombinant genetic work (e.g., *E. coli* XL1-Blue or DH5α (Stratagene Ltd, Cambridge, UK).

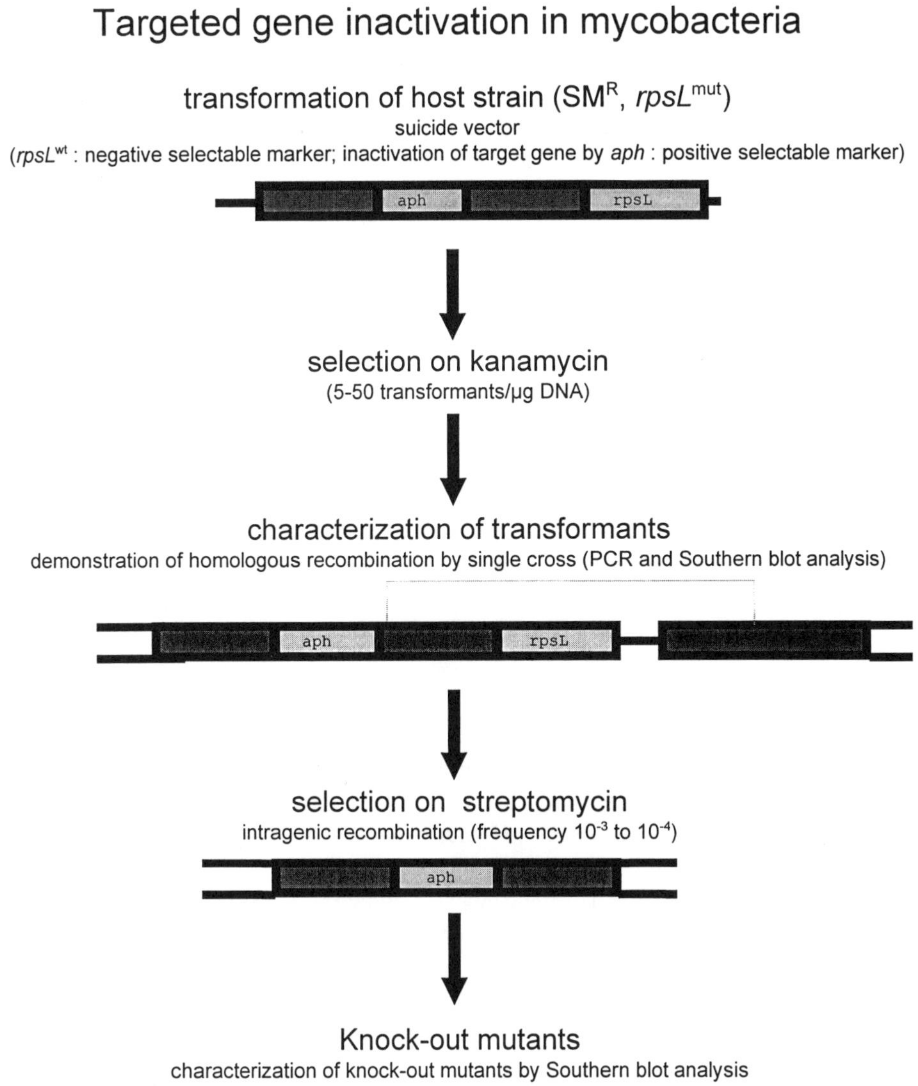

Fig. 1. Strategy to generate allelic exchange mutants of *M. tuberculosis* and *M. bovis* BCG by use of the *rpsL* wild-type allele as counter-selectable marker.

2. *M. tuberculosis* strains, e.g., H37Rv (ATCC) or *M. bovis* BCG Pasteur; from these strains streptomycin-resistant derivatives have been generated and are available from the authors upon request (*see* **Notes 3** and **4**).
3. *E. coli* cloning vector that does not replicate in mycobacteria and can therefore be used as a suicide vector for gene replacement (e.g., pUC-derivatives, like pBluescript SKII-).

4. Positive selection markers, e.g., *aph* from Tn*5* or Tn*903* conferring kanamycin resistance or hygromycin resistance cassette from plasmid pIJ963 ***(16)***.
5. *M. tuberculosis rpsL*$^+$ wild-type allele coding for ribosomal protein S12. The *rpsL*$^+$ gene is available from the authors on request as plasmid ptrpA–1-*rpsL* ***(6)***.
6. Replicative plasmids, e.g., pMV261 or integrative plasmid e.g pMV361 ***(17)***.
7. Integrative plasmid pMV361-*rpsL*$^+$ is also available from the authors.
8. For genetic manipulation of *M. tuberculosis*, a biosafety P3 facility is mandatory.
9. Laminar flow cabinet (mandatory for the work with *M. tuberculosis*) will also help to avoid contamination of the plates.
10. Centrifuges: microfuge and laboratory centrifuge.
11. Roller incubator set at 37°C.
12. Electroporator and 2-mm electroporation cuvets, e.g., BioRad Gene Pulser (BioRad, Hemel Hempstead, Hertfordshire, UK).
13. Middlebrook 7H9 broth (Difco, West Molsey, Surrey, UK): dissolve in deionized water at 4.7 g/900 mL, add Tween-80 to 0.05% final concentration and autoclave.
14. Middlebrook 7H10 agar (Difco): dissolve in deionized water at 18 g/900 mL, and autoclave.
15. Middlebrook OADC supplement (Difco): add 100 mL to 900 mL of 7H9 broth or 7H10 agar before use.
16. Roller bottles and apparatus.
17. 2 *M* glycine, sterilize by autoclaving.
18. 10% v/v glycerol, sterilize by autoclaving.
19. Antibiotic stock solutions: kanamycin 50 mg/mL; streptomycin 100 mg/mL: (filter-sterilize and store at –20°C). Use streptomycin and kanamycin at a final concentration of 100 µg/mL and 25 µg/mL, respectively.
20. Hygromycin B 50 mg/mL (Boehringer, Mannheim, Germany): store at 4°C. Use hygromycin at final concentration of 50 µg/mL.
21. 0.9% w/v NaCl.

3. Methods

3.1. Cloning Procedures

1. Isolate the target gene. For example, by screening of a genomic library, isolation from an ordered library or PCR-mediated DNA amplification.
2. Clone the fragment into an *E. coli* cloning vector (*see* **Note 5**).
3. Interrupt the open-reading frame of the target gene by deletion of a part of the coding region and insertion of one of the positive selectable marker genes (*aph* — conferring kanamycin resistance or *hyg* — conferring hygromycin resistance).
4. Clone the counter-selectable marker (*rpsL*$^+$) into the vector flanking the inactivated target gene.
5. Isolate sufficient amount of plasmid DNA for transformation of mycobacteria (> 10 µg) and resuspend in TE buffer.

3.2. *Transformation of* M. tuberculosis

1. Streak the streptomycin-resistant strain (*see* **Notes 3** and **4**) onto 7H10 agar plate (containing OADC) to obtain single colonies. Incubate at 37°C for approx 20 d.
2. Inoculate a single colony into 10 mL of 7H9 (containing OADC and Tween) in a tissue culture flask (200 mL). Incubate for 10–15 d at 37°C. Resuspend the settled cells once every day and measure growth by measuring optical density.
3. Inoculate 200 mL of 7H9 medium (containing OADC and Tween) in a roller bottle with 1 mL of the preculture and roll at 2 rpm until an optical density ($OD_{600\ nm}$) of approx 0.6 to 1.0 is achieved (approx 10–14 d).
4. Add 0.1 vol of 2 *M* glycine (final concentration of 1.5%) ***(18)***. Continue incubation at 37°C with rolling for an additional 20 to 24 h (*see* **Note 6**).
5. Collect cells by centrifugation for 30 min at 5000*g*. All following steps are performed at room temperature.
6. Resuspend the cells in an equal volume of 10% glycerol.
7. Repeat centrifugation and resuspend cells in approx 50 mL of 10% glycerol. Repeat twice more.
8. Collect cells by centrifugation and resuspend in approx 1/50th volume (4 to 5 mL) of 10% glycerol.
9. Take 400 µL competent cells and gently mix with up to 1 µg of supercoiled (sc) plasmid DNA. Set aside for 5 min. Include controls for competency of the cells by transformation of a replicative, e.g., pMV261 or integrative vector, e.g., pMV361 ***(17)*** as well as controls for the efficiency of counter selection by transformation of an integrative vector containing the *rpsL*+ gene, e.g., pMV361-*rpsL* ***(6)*** (*see* **Note 7**).
10. Electroporate with a single pulse using the following settings: 2.5 kV, 1000 Ohms, 25 µF.
11. Resuspend the cells immediately in 4 mL of 7H9 medium and incubate for 24 h at 37°C.
12. Plate 100–200 µL of the electroporated cells onto the appropriate antibiotic (kanamycin or hygromycin). In addition, concentrate the electroporated cells by centrifugation in a microfuge. Resuspend cells from 1 mL of the suspension in 50 µL 7H9 broth and plate onto 7H10 plus the appropriate antibiotic (kanamycin, hygromycin). In parallel, perform one-step double selection on plates containing the antibiotic used for positive selection plus streptomycin.
13. Seal the plates with parafilm and incubate the cells at 37°C for 28 d.
14. Expect 5–50 colonies on the plates used for single selection and 0–5 colonies on the plates used for double selection.
15. Pick single colonies and resuspend in 0.9% NaCl. Save an aliquot by freezing. Amplify the colony by streaking onto 7H10 agar containing an appropriate antibiotic. Incubate at 37°C for 20 d.
16. Isolate genomic DNA and perform PCR or Southern blot analysis for genetic characterization of the transformants (*see* **Note 8, Figs. 2** and **3**). At this stage, if no mutants are isolated, it will be necessary to carry out negative selection on single cross-over transformants.

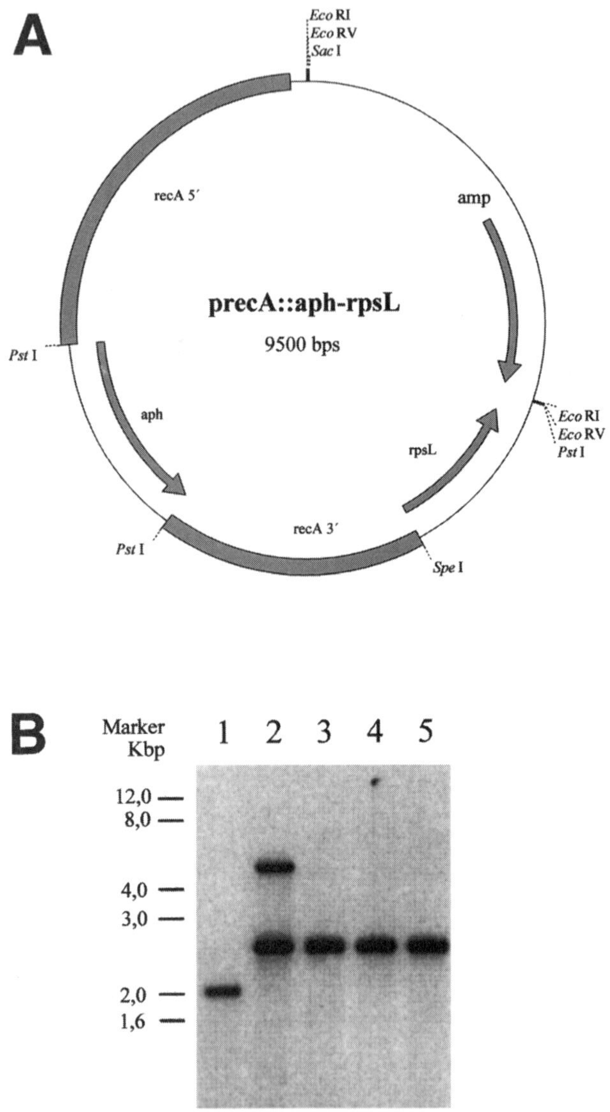

Fig. 2. Vector used to generate *M. bovis* BCG *recA* mutants and Southern blot analysis of recA mutants. **(A)** recA suicide vector with positive and negative selectable marker. aph: kanamycin resistance gene; *rpsL*: wild-type gene for ribosomal protein S12; amp: ampicillin resistance gene. **(B)** Southern blot analysis of *recA* mutants. lane 1: wild-type strain; lane 2: single cross-over recombinant, lanes 3–5: allelic exchange mutants obtained after selection of a single cross-over transformant on medium containing kanamycin plus streptomycin. The shift of the wild-type band (lane 2) and the presence of a second band indicates homologous single cross-over. The disappearance of the second band (lanes 3–5) indicates allelic exchange.

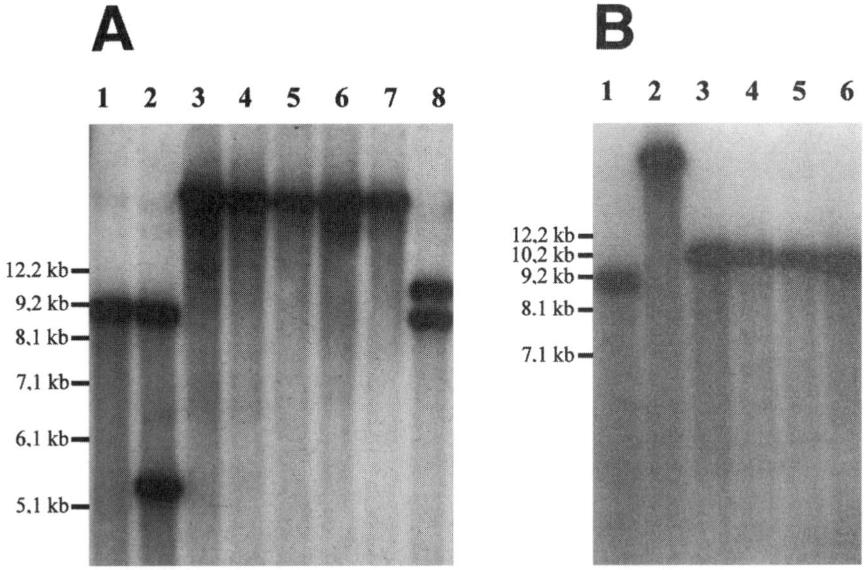

Fig. 3. Southern blot analysis of the *sigM* locus. **(A)** Southern blot analysis of *M. tuberculosis* strains obtained after transformation with a suicide vector targeting *sigM* and first positive selection. Lane 1: nontransformed wild-type, lanes 2 and 8: transformants resulting from illegitimate recombination, lanes 3–7: transformants resulting from homologous recombination by a single cross-over. Homologous recombination is indicated by a shift of the wild-type band (lanes 3–7). Illegitimate recombination is indicated by the presence of the wild-type band (unchanged) and the presence of an additional band (lanes 2 and 8). **(B)** Southern blot analysis of transformants obtained after selection of single cross-over transformants on medium containing kanamycin plus streptomycin. lane 1: wild-type, lane 2: single cross-over transformant, lanes 3–6: allelic exchange mutants obtained after subjecting the single cross-over transformant (lane 2) to counter selection. Allelic exchange is indicated by the shift of the band representing the homologous integration by a single cross-over recombination.

17. Inoculate transformants which have undergone a single cross-over into 5 mL of 7H9 medium and incubate at 37°C until an OD_{600} of approx 0.5 is reached.
18. Plate 100 µL of bacterial cells (10^{-2} to 10^{0} dilutions) directly onto 7H10-OADC plates containing the antibiotic used for positive selection plus streptomycin.
19. Calculate the efficiency of counterselection by plating 100 µL of serial dilutions (10^{-3} to 10^{-5}) onto a plate containing only the antibiotic used for positive selection (*see* **Note 9**). Incubate the plates at 37°C for 28 d.
20. Pick single colonies from the streptomycin plates and resuspend in 0.9% NaCl. Save an aliquot by freezing and amplify the remainder on plates containing the antibiotics used for positive selection. Incubate at 37°C for 20 d.

21. Isolate genomic DNA and perform PCR or Southern blot analysis (*see* **Figs. 2** and **3** and **Note 10**).

4. Notes

1. In our experiments (10 target genes) at least half of the primary transformants obtained after the first positive selection resulted from homologous integration by a single cross-over recombination.
2. Transformation efficiencies with replicative or integrative vectors (e.g., pMV261 or pMV361) in *M. tuberculosis*/*M. bovis* BCG (10^4/µg) are much lower than that in *M. smegmatis* (>10^6/µg). Transformation with suicide plasmids resulting in single cross-over recombinants are in the range of 10^{-3} or approx 1000 transformants per µg DNA for *M. smegmatis*. If the same ratio between replicating and suicide vectors is estimated when transforming *M. tuberculosis*, approx 10 transformants can be expected per µg DNA using a suicide vector. In *M. smegmatis*, the ratio of double cross-over to single cross-over transformants is in the range of 10^{-1}–10^{-2}. Due to the 100-fold lower transformation efficiencies in *M. tuberculosis* as compared to *M. smegmatis* the number of double cross-over transformants in a one-step selection procedure has to be estimated with 0.1 to 1 transformants per µg plasmid DNA when using a suicide vector. Our investigations have confirmed this calculation: all 400 clones obtained by transformation with suicide plasmids targeting different genes and selected on kanamycin or hygromycin, were generated by either a single cross-over event or illegitimate recombination. No knock-out mutants were observed when only positive selection was applied. Most clones obtained by direct selection on kanamycin plus streptomycin or hygromycin plus streptomycin (0–5 per plate; this number is in the range of no-DNA control transformation) are spontaneous antibiotic resistant mutants and only a few are allelic exchange mutants. Thus, the likelihood that single cross-over transformants have to be subjected to counter selection to achieve gene inactivation is high.
3. For the selection of streptomycin-resistant *M. tuberculosis* screen approx 5×10^{10} cells on medium containing 100 µg/mL streptomycin. Colony-purify resistant strains and determine genotype. In *M. tuberculosis*, the major mechanism of streptomycin resistance is the presence of mutations in *rpsL*; however, due to the presence of a single *rrn* operon, mutations in *rrs* can also cause streptomycin resistance ***(19,20)***. Therefore amplify the *rpsL* and *rrs* gene and determine sequence. The strategy described here only can be performed in a streptomycin-resistant strain where resistance is due to a mutation in *rpsL*.
4. Streptomycin resistance might be caused by different mutations in *rpsL*, by mutations in codon 43 or codon 88. Although all mutations confer high level of streptomycin resistance, the mutant alleles can be divided into restrictive and nonrestrictive classes. Investigations in *E. coli* have shown that ribosomes with restrictive RpsL proteins (i.e., RpsL43Lys→Asn, RpsL43Lys→Thr) are hyperaccurate and have decreased peptide elongation rates. This molecular effect in turn correlates with changes in exponential growth rate resulting in mutants which

grow more slowly than the wild-type strain ***(21–23)***. Investigations in *Salmonella* demonstrated that streptomycin-resistant mutants with restrictive mutations show reduced virulence, whereas wild-type virulence is observed in mutants carrying nonrestrictive mutations (RpsL43Lys→Arg) ***(24)***. Streptomycin-resistant in vitro isolates of mycobacteria show an approximately equal distribution of restrictive and nonrestrictive mutations in RpsL codon 43. In striking contrast, streptomycin-resistant clinical isolates of *M. tuberculosis* exclusively show a nonrestrictive mutation in *rpsL* codon 43 ***(25)***. This selection most probably reflects the necessity for nonattenuated strains. For genetic manipulation, only a strain which carries a nonrestrictive *rpsL* mutation (RpsL43Lys→Arg) should be used ***(25)***. These strains are available upon request from the authors' laboratory.

5. Construction of vectors: The frequency of homologous recombination in some species depends on the length of the cloned fragment. For homologous recombination in *M. tuberculosis*/*M. bovis* BCG approx 1500–2000 base pairs (bp) on each side of the positive selection marker have been shown to be sufficient. However, this is not the minimum length required for recombination as 750 bp has been demonstrated as sufficient for recombination in *M. tuberculosis* ***(26)***.
6. To achieve adequate transformation efficiencies, fresh competent cells should be prepared. Treatment of the cells with glycine prior to harvesting the cells increases transformation efficiencies.
7. Transformation efficiencies of pMV361-*rpsL* on plates containing kanamycin should be similar to those obtained with plasmid pMV361 and be in the range of 10^4/µg plasmid DNA. However, whereas the number of transformants obtained with plasmid pMV361 is not affected by the presence of streptomycin, the number of colonies obtained on kanamycin plus streptomycin should be zero when plasmid pMV361-*rpsL* is used.
8. To demonstrate integration by single cross-over or gene replacement, respectively, Southern blot analysis should be performed. In general, restriction enzymes for digestion of genomic DNA have to be chosen which result in different fragments when genomic DNAs from wild-type cells, single cross-over recombinants or allelic exchange recombinants are hybridized to a corresponding probe (*see* **Figs. 2** and **3**).
9. Typically 100 µL of undiluted culture should give 10^7 cfu on plates containing the positive selectable marker and approx 10^3 colonies on plates containing the positive selectable marker plus streptomycin.
10. Loss of the negative selectable marker by intragenic recombination resulting in a double cross-over can be expected in the range of 10^{-3} to 10^{-5} ***(27,28)***. Investigating transformants which have regained streptomycin resistance after the counter selection by Southern blot analysis demonstrated that some did not undergo a second cross-over. PCR mediated amplification and subsequent sequence determination demonstrated that resistance was due to the acquisition of a *rpsL* mutation in the vector derived gene. In all cases investigated, the mutation observed was identical to the mutation in the chromosomal *rpsL* allele. The frequency and the type of mutation suggested that the plasmid derived *rpsL* allele had acquired

the mutation by homologous recombination with the chromosomal *rpsL* allele. As the frequency of homeologous recombination, i.e., recombination between similar but not almost identical sequences, is dramatically reduced ***(29)***, we are in the process of generating a second generation of suicide vectors carrying a *M. smegmatis rpsL*$^+$ gene ***(30)*** instead of a *M. tuberculosis rpsL*$^+$ gene.

Acknowledgments

This work was supported by grants from the Deutsche Forschungsgemeinschaft: Schwerpunktprogramm "Ökologie bakterieller Krankheitserreger" and BO 820/13–1. We are indebted to Jo Colston and K.G. Papavinasasundaram giving us the possibility to use the P3 facility of the National Institute for Medical Research, Mill Hill.

References

1. Cole, S. T., Brosch, R., Parkhill, J., Garnier, T., Churcher, C., Harris, D., et al. (1998) Deciphering the biology of *Mycobacterium tuberculosis* from the complete genome sequence. *Nature* **393,** 537–544.
2. Pelicic, V., Jackson, M., Reyrat, J. M., Jacobs, W. R., Gicquel, B., and Guilhot, C. (1997) Efficient allelic exchange and transposon mutagenesis in *Mycobacterium tuberculosis*. *Proc. Natl. Acad. Sci. USA* **94,** 10,955–10,960.
3. Camacho, L. R., Energueix, D., Perez, E., Gicquel, B., and Guilhot, C. (1999) Identification of a virulence gene cluster of *Mycobacterium tuberculosis* by signature-tagged transposon mutagenesis. *Mol. Microbiol.* **34,** 257–267.
4. Cox, J. S., Chen, B., McNeil, M., and Jacobs, W. R. (1999) Complex lipid determines tissue-specific replication of *Mycobacterium tuberculosis* in mice. *Nature* **402,** 79–83.
5. Gordon, S. V., Heym, B., Parkhill, J., Barrell, B., and Cole, S. T. (1999) New insertion sequences and novel repeated sequence in the genome of *Mycobacterium tuberculosis* H37 Rv. *Microbiology* **145,** 881–892.
6. Sander, P., Meier, A., and Böttger, E. C. (1995) *rpsL*$^+$: a dominant selectable marker for gene replacement in mycobacteria. *Mol. Microbiol.* **16,** 991–1000.
7. Lederberg, J. (1951) Streptomycin resistance: a genetically recessive mutation. *J. Bacteriol.* **61,** 549–550.
8. Davis, E. O., Jenner, P. J., Brooks, P. C., Colston, M. J., and Sedgwick, S. G. (1992) Protein splicing in the maturation of *M. tuberculosis* RecA protein: a mechanism for tolerating a novel class of intervening sequence. *Cell* **71,** 20 1–210.
9. Kalpana, G. V., Bloom, B. R., Jacobs, W. R. (1991) Insertional mutagenesis and illegitimate recombination in mycobacteria. *Proc. Natl. Acad. Sci. USA* **88,** 5433–5437.
10. Frischkorn, K., Sander, P., Scholz, M., Teschner, K., Prammananan, T., and Böttger, E. C. (1998) Investigation of mycobacterial *recA* function: protein introns in the RecA of pathogenic mycobacteria do not affect competency for homologous recombination. *Mol. Microbiol.* **29,** 1203–1214.

11. Papavinasasundaram, K. G., Colston, M. J., and Davis, E. O. (1998) Construction and complementation of a *recA* deletion mutant of *Mycobacterium smegmatis* reveals that the intein in *Mycobacterium tuberculosis recA* does not affect RecA function. *Mol. Microbiol.* **30,** 525–534.
12. Sander, P., Prammananan, T., and Böttger, E. C. (1996) Introducing mutations into a chromosomal rRNA gene using a genetically modified eubacterial host with a single rRNA operon. *Mol. Microbiol.* **22,** 841–848.
13. Sander, P., de Rossi, E., Böddinghaus, B., Cantoni, R., Branzoni, M., Böttger, E. C., Riccardi, G., and Takiff, H. Contribution of the multidrug efflux pump LfrA to innate mycobacterial drug resistance (submitted).
14. Yuan, Y., Crane, D. D., Simpson, R. M., Zhu, Y., Hickey, M. J., Sherman, D. R., and Barry, C. E. (1998) The 16-kDa alpha-crystallin (Acr) protein of *Mycobacterium tuberculosis* is required for growth in macrophages. *Proc. Natl. Acad. Sci. USA* **95,** 9578–9583.
15. Berthet, F. X., Lagranderie, M., Gounon, P., Laurent-Winter, C., Ensergueix, D., Chavarot, P., Thouron, F., Maranghi, E., Pelicic, V., Portnoi, D., Marchal, G., and Gicquel, B. (1998) Attenuation of virulence by disruption of the *Mycobacterium tuberculosis erp* gene. *Science* **282,** 759–762.
16. Lydiate, D. J., Ashby, A. M., Henderson, D. J., Kieser, H. M., and Hopwood, D. A. (1989) Physical and genetic characterization of chromosomal copies of the *Streptomyces coelicolor* mini-circle. *J. Gen. Microbiol.* **4,** 1911–1919.
17. Stover, C. K., de la Cruz, V. F., Fuerst, T. R., Burlein, J. E., Benson, L. A., Bennett, L. T., Bansal, G. P., Young, J. F., Lee, M. H., Hatfull, G. F., Snapper, S. B., Barletta, R. G., Jacobs, W. R., Bloom, B. R. (1991) New use of BCG for recombinant vaccines. *Nature* **351,** 456–460.
18. Ward, B. J. and Collins, D. (1996) Electroporation at elevated temperatures substantially improves transformation efficiency of slow growing mycobacteria. *FEMS Microbiol. Lett.* **145,** 101–105.
19. Finken, M., Kirschner, P., Meier, A., Wrede, A., and Böttger, E. C. (1993) Molecular basis of streptomycin resistance in *Mycobacterium tuberculosis*: alterations of the ribosomal protein S12 gene and point mutations within a functional 16S ribosomal RNA pseudoknot. *Mol. Microbiol.* **9,** 1239–1246
20. Sreevatsan, S., Pan, X., Stockbauer, K. E., Williams, D. L., Kreiswirth, B. N., Musser, J. M. (1996) Characterization of *rpsL* and *rrs* mutations in streptomycin-resistant *Mycobacterium tuberculosis* isolates from diverse geographic localities. *Antimicrob. Agents Chemother.* **40,** 1024–1026.
21. Tubulekas, I. and Hughes, D. (1993) Suppression of *rpsL* phenotypes by *tuf* mutations reveals a unique relationship between translation elongation and growth rate. *Mol. Microbiol.* **7,** 275–284.
22. Schrag, S. J. and Perrot, V. (1996) Reducing antibiotic resistance. *Nature* **381,** 120–121.
23. Björkmann, J., Samuelsson, P., Andersson, D. I., and Hughes, D. (1999) Novel ribosomal mutations affecting translational accuracy, antibiotic resistance and virulence of *Salmonella typhimurium*. *Mol. Microbiol.* **31,** 53–58.

24. Björkmann, J., Hughes, D., and Andersson, D. I. (1998) Virulence of antibiotic-resistant *Salmonella typhimurium. Proc. Natl. Acad. Sci. USA* **95,** 3949–3953.
25. Böttger, E. C., Springer, B., Pletschette, M., and Sander, P. (1998) Fitness of antibiotic-resistant microorganisms and compensatory mutations. *Nat. Med.* **4,** 1343–1344.
26. Parish, T. Gordhan, B. G., McAdam, R. A., Duncan, K., Mizrahi, V., and Stoker, N. G. (1999) Production of mutants in amino acid biosynthesis genes of *Mycobacterium tuberculosis* by homologous recombination. *Microbiology* **145,** 3497–3503.
27. Pavelka, M. S., and Jacobs, W. R. (1999) Comparison of the construction of unmarked deletion in *Mycobacterium smegmatis, Mycobacterium bovis* Bacillus Calmette-Guerin, and *Mycobacterium tuberculosis* H37Rv by allelic exchange. *J. Bacteriol.* **181,** 4780–4789
28. Prammananan, T., Sander, P., Springer, B., and Böttger, E. C. (1999) RecA-mediated gene conversion and aminoglycoside resistance in strains heterozygous for rRNA. *Antimicrob. Agents Chemother.* **43,** 447–453.
29. Matic, I., Rayssiguiert, C., and Radman, M. (1995) Interspecies gene exchange in bacteria: The role of SOS and mismatch repair systems in evolution of species. *Cell* **80,** 507–515.
30. Kenney, T. J. and Churchward, G. (1996) Genetic analysis of the *Mycobacterium smegmatis rpsL* promoter. *J. Bacteriol.* **61,** 549–550.

8

Transcription Start-Site Mapping

Farahnaz Movahedzadeh, Jorge A. Gonzalez-Y-Merchand, and Robert A. Cox

1. Introduction

The synthesis of proteins is an essential process in cell growth and cell proliferation. The DNA sequence of a gene is first copied (transcribed) into an RNA sequence that is translated into a particular amino acid sequence. One strand of the gene, the RNA-like strand (or sense strand) has a nucleotide sequence equivalent to that of the RNA transcript (mRNA) with thymine replacing uracil. The complementary strand is often termed the template strand (or antisense strand), reflecting its role in the transcription process. Transcription takes place starting from the 5'-end and proceeding toward the 3'-end of the RNA product. The transcription process is usually described in three stages, namely, initiation, chain elongation, and termination. This chapter focuses on the initiation of transcription.

Transcription is brought about by the enzyme DNA-dependent RNA polymerase (Rpo) in association with other protein factors. Each transcript has a defined starting point referred to below as the transcription starting point (TSP), which defines the 5'-end of the transcript. The first nucleotide to be transcribed is defined as +1, nucleotides downstream are designated +2, +3, +4, and so on, whereas nucleotides upstream are designated –1, –2, –3 etc.

The observation that gene transcripts have defined starting points reflects the presence of DNA sequences upstream from the TSP that promote Rpo binding. These promoter sequences contain motifs that are essential for transcription to take place *(1,2)*. Control of the initiation of transcription is an important strategy used by cells, including mycobacteria *(3)*, to regulate protein biosynthesis. Investigations of elements that control the expression of a particular gene begin with the identification of the 5'-end sequences of RNA transcripts.

From: *Methods in Molecular Medicine*, vol. 54: *Mycobacterium Tuberculosis Protocols*
Edited by: T. Parish and N. G. Stoker © Humana Press Inc., Totowa, NJ

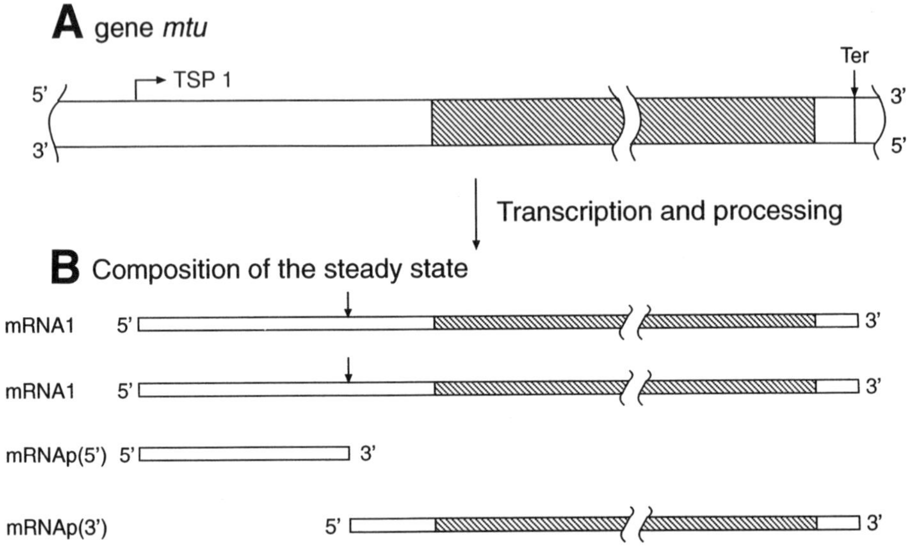

Fig. 1. Gene mtu and its transcripts. **(A)** The hypothetical gene *mtu*, in which transcription is controlled by a single promoter. The transcription starting point, TSP1, for mRNA1 relates to promoter P1. ter, denotes the site for termination of transcription. **(B)** Transcription of the gene leads to the formation of a steady-state between mRNA synthesis and degradation. ↓, Potential processing site. Cleavage at this site generates the products mRNAp (5') and mRNAp (3'). Intact mRNA1 transcripts are twice as abundant as processed transcripts.

Like other eubacteria, mycobacteria have a single Rpo core enzyme comprising four chains (two α, one β, and one β'), which is capable of forming several different holoenzymes (Eσ) through combination with sigma factors *(4–6)*. Each sigma factor recognizes a distinct class of promoter motifs. Sigma factors, which form part of the Rpo initiation complex, dissociate when Rpo switches into its elongation mode (for example, *see* **ref. *7***). Many, if not all, of the mycobacterial sigma factors have been identified. The best characterized promoter motifs are those recognized by the factor homologous to sigma 70 of *Escherichia coli*. The two elements, often referred to, as –10 (or Pribnow) and –35 boxes are hexamers centered around positions –10 and –35, respectively, from the TSP. The consensus sequences for the –10 and –35 boxes of *E. coli* $E\sigma^{70}$ promoters are 5' TATAAT 3' and 5' TTGAGA 3', respectively and they are usually separated by 16–18 base pairs (bp). Mycobacterial promoters with similar sequences have been identified (for review, *see* **ref. *6***).

The methods used to identify a TSP are mainly the primer extension procedure, and protection of a labeled RNA probe from RNAse treatment (RNAse protection analysis). The principles of these methods are described.

Primer extension and RNAse protection methods are illustrated by reference to a hypothetical gene *mtu* regulated by a single promoter (*see* **Fig. 1**) that generates a transcript with transcription starting point TSP1. The example chosen represents only one of a number of possibilities. For example, a gene may have tandem promoters or form part of an operon so that two or more genes are transcribed as a single unit, or another gene within the same operon may be transcribed not only as part of the operon but also under the direction of its own dedicated promoter ***(8)***. The degradation of mRNA is an important aspect of cell metabolism. Bacterial mRNA species are often short-lived ***(9,10)***. For example, the *hmp* gene of *Mycobacterium tuberculosis* was found to have a half-life of less than one minute ***(11)***. As a gene is transcribed, a steady state is established between the synthesis of transcripts and their degradation (mRNA turnover). The two analytical methods we describe reflect the steady-state concentrations of particular RNA components.

Both methods require knowledge of the nucleotide sequence of the gene and its upstream region. Each method is based on a bimolecular interaction between a nucleic acid probe and its target nucleotide sequence.

The identification of potential TSPs indicates the possible locations of promoter sequences. Functional evidence is then needed to confirm that the sequences identified function as promoters. Appropriate experiments include a study of the effects of site-directed mutagenesis on promoter activity.

1.1. Primer Extension

The method for primer extension ***(12–14)*** is illustrated in **Fig. 2**. A target sequence is identified near to the proposed 5'-end of a transcript. An oligonucleotide primer designed to interact with the target is synthesized. Once a complex is formed between the target and primer, the primer is extended by means of reverse transcriptase (RNA-dependent DNA polymerase), which incorporates deoxyribonucleotide triphosphates into DNA. The product is DNA, which is complementary to the RNA template. DNA synthesis stops when the 5'-end of the template strand is reached. The reaction is usually carried out at a temperature within the range 37°C–45°C although reactions have been carried out at 50°C ***(15)***. Primer extension using a ^{32}P-labeled primer has been found to be capable of detecting an RNA species, which accounts for 50–500 pg (0.00 1%–0.01%) of a 10–50 µg sample of total RNA ***(16)***.

1.1.1. The Primer Binding Site

The genome of mycobacteria is G+C-rich; with an overall G+C content of approx 67%. Individual gene sequences will contain regions that differ significantly from the average value. The stability of RNA secondary structures is

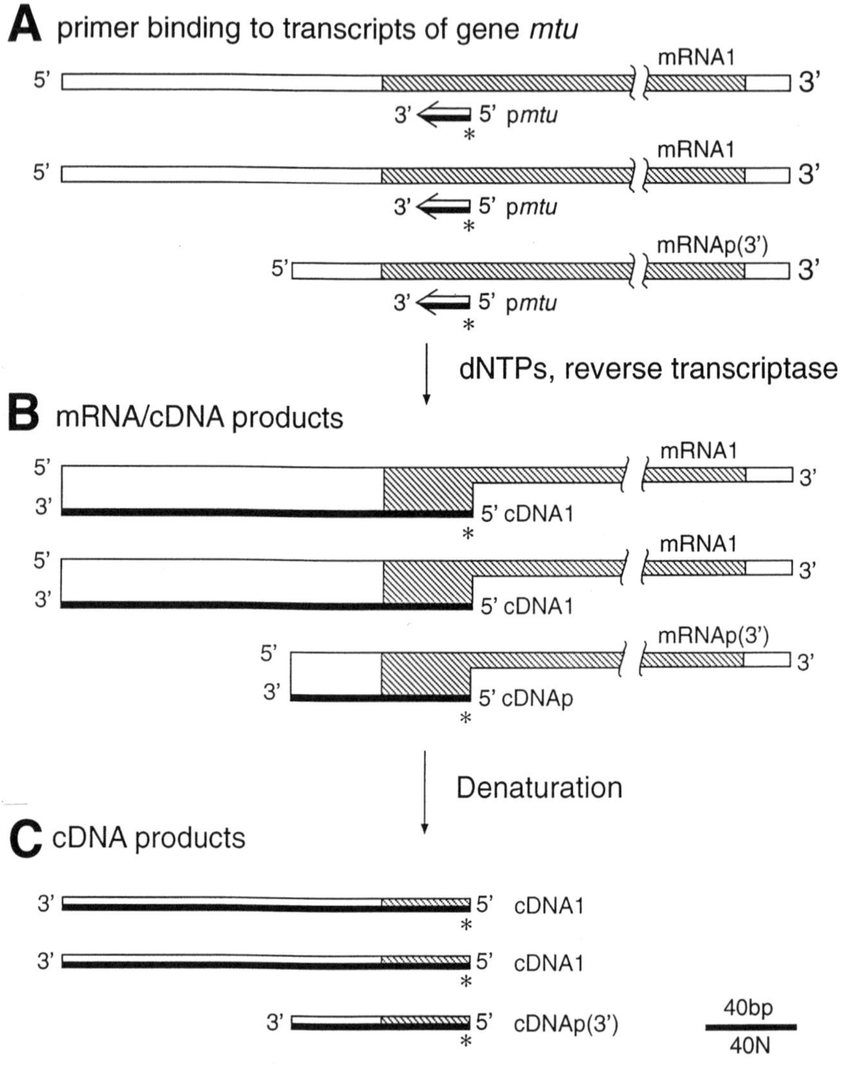

Fig. 2. Illustration of the primer extension method. The primer extension procedure is illustrated by reference to transcripts of the hypothetical gene *mtu* (*see* **Fig. 1B**). Intact mRNA1 transcripts are twice as abundant as processed transcripts. **(A)** Primer binding to transcripts of gene *mtu*. The composition of the steady state established between transcription and processing is the same as that illustrated in **Fig. 1B**. The asterisk denotes that the primer is tagged at the 5'-end. **(B)** Synthesis of mRNA-cDNA product. The enzyme reverse transcriptase is used to incorporate dNTPs into cDNA by extending the bound primer, using mRNA as template. **(C)** Products after denaturation. The final steps are the separation of products by denaturing polyacrylamide gel electrophoresis and their visualization by an appropriate method. Please note that the cleavage product mRNAp(3') is detected. bp, base pairs; N, nucleotides.

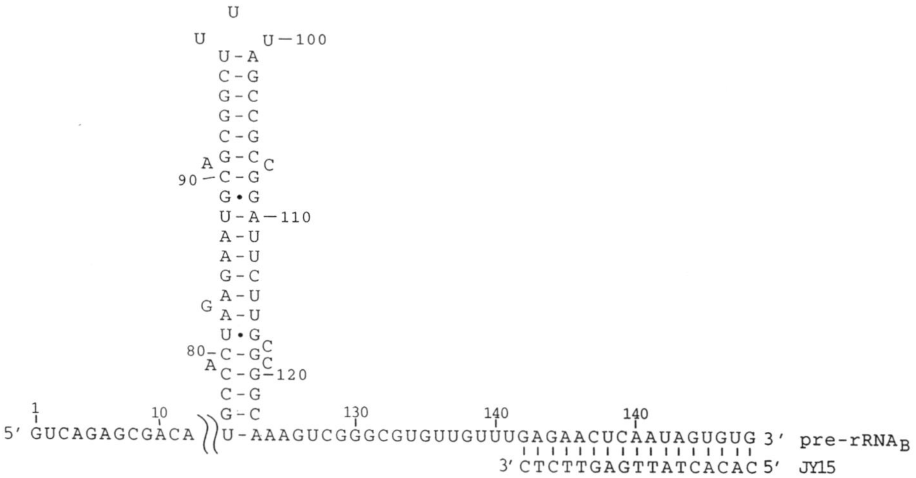

Fig. 3. Effects of G+C rich motifs and RNA secondary structure on primer extension. The 5'-end of a precursor-rRNA transcript was correctly identified using the primer JY15 illustrated. Thus, the G+C rich motifs (*see* text) located within the stem/Loop did not impede the progress of reverse transcriptase. No product was obtained using the primer 5' CAAGAATCCGCCGGCTAAAAGC 3' aimed at positions 95–116, presumably because the stability of the stem/loop structure prevents the primer from binding to its target.

affected by G+C content because G–C bp are more stable than A–U bp. It is likely that RNA transcripts form intramolecular secondary structures that are likely to be stable under the usual conditions of reverse transcription.

Our experience ***(17)*** suggests that G+C content of transcripts will not impede reverse transcription after initiation has taken place. For example, reverse transcriptase was found to read through the sequence 5' CGGCGCG 3' and its neighbors 5' GGCCGCCC 3' and 5' CGGCGACG 3' (*see* **Fig. 3**). However, the increased stability of RNA secondary structures could influence the primer extension reaction by preventing the primer from hybridizing with its target sequence. In other words, the primer may be prevented from binding to its target sequence by a competing RNA/RNA interaction that results from an intramolecular secondary structure stabilized by G+C rich motifs (*see* **Fig. 3**). Such intramolecular interactions are independent of RNA concentration and so proceed much faster than competing bimolecular primer/RNA interactions. Thus, the interaction between a primer and its target should be stronger than the interaction between the target and another RNA sequence. The length of the primer should be minimal to avoid inappropriate primer extension products arising from the primer binding imperfectly to nontarget sites. For these reasons primers are usually 16–24 nucleotides in length, depending on the nucleotide composition of the target and should ideally be located within 100–200 nucleotides of the 5'-end of the RNA species.

1.1.2. The Annealing Step

The purpose of this heating step is to make target RNA sequences available to the primer by "melting" local secondary structure and thereby facilitating the formation of a target/primer complex. The condition mentioned above, that the target/primer complex is required to be more stable than local RNA/RNA interactions at the temperature of the reverse transcriptase reaction, still applies. In other words, annealing helps to reveal potential binding sites without influencing the relative stability of the target/primer complex under the conditions of primer extension.

1.1.3. Product Size

For optimum results the size of a product should be within the range 60–200 nucleotides. The identity of the 5' terminal residue may then be revealed by comparison with homologous DNA fragments generated by sequencing reactions initiated by the primers used in the reverse transcription reaction. Products within the specified size range are least likely to be affected by the adverse effects of degradation of the RNA fraction during the course of the experiment, which may not only reduce the yield of the desired products but may also increase the apparent yield of RNA processing products. Such effects could lead to a false view of the composition of the steady state.

1.1.4. Identification of Primer Extension Products

Using a primer tagged at its 5'-end conveniently identifies the products of the primer extension reaction. Both radioactive and fluorescent labels have been used. The intensity of the end-labeled product is directly proportional to the number of molecules in a particular size fraction and is independent of molecular size. This property is valuable when several products are obtained. In this case the relative concentrations of the tagged products directly reflect the relative abundances of the target species.

1.2. Principle of the RNAse Protection Procedure

The 5'-end(s) of transcripts of a particular gene may be mapped by means of the RNAse protection assay *(18,19)*, as illustrated in **Fig. 4**. A transcript is a single-stranded RNA species and is therefore susceptible to hydrolysis by RNAses such as RNAse T1 and RNAse A. Protection against hydrolysis by the above mentioned RNAses is much increased by the formation of an RNA double helix. Thus, the method requires the synthesis of a tagged RNA sequence

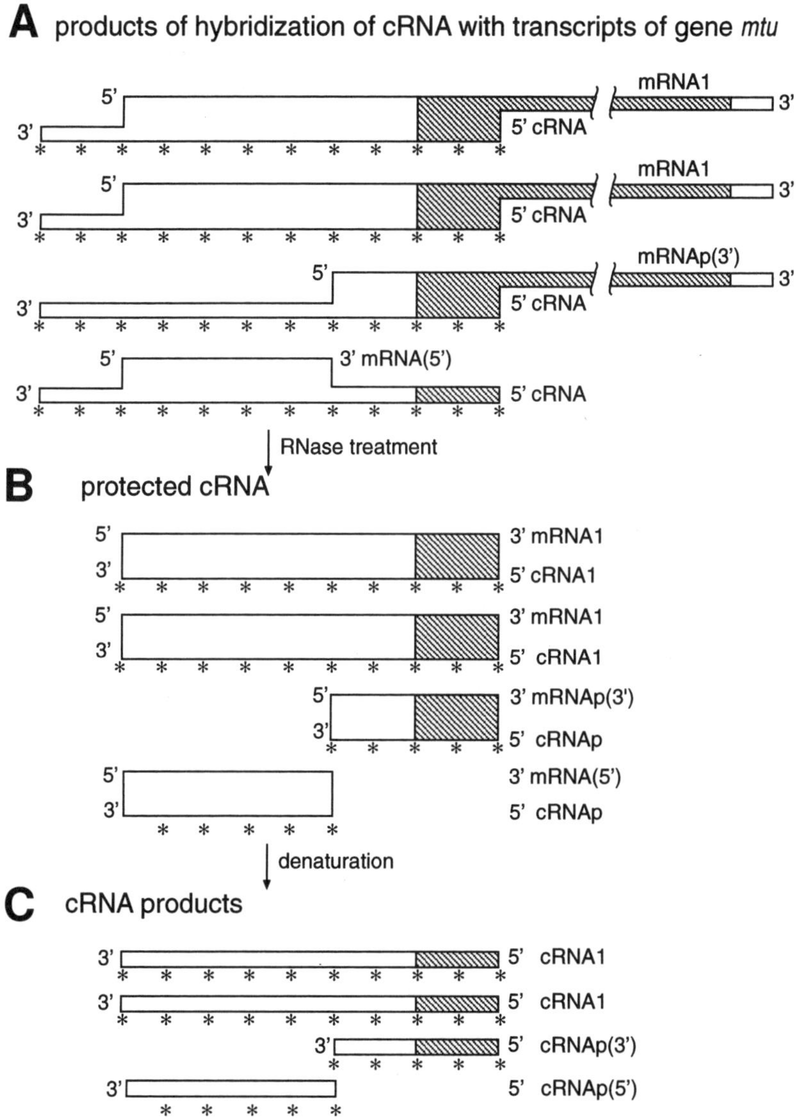

Fig. 4. Illustration of the RNAse protection method. **(A)** Transcripts (cRNA) of minigene-rpo1 have sequences complementary to transcripts of gene *mtu* namely mRNA1 and mRNAp, as defined in **Fig. 1**. which also shows that, in the steady-state mRNA1 is twice as abundant as the cleavage products mRNAp (5') and mRNA p(3'). Incubation of the total RNA fraction with tagged cRNA leads to the formation of RNA/RNA double-strands. **(B)** RNAse treatment removes overlapping single-stranded sequences. Probe sequences within the RNA double helix are protected from RNAse action and remain intact. **(C)** Component strands of the trimmed RNA double helix separate during denaturation. The final steps in the procedure are the separation of the products by electrophoresis and their visualization by an appropriate method. The scale shown in **(A)** also applies to **(B)** and **(C)**.

that is complementary to part of the target RNA species. The tagged probe is designed to extend beyond the 5'-end of the target sequence(s). Hence, products are easily recognized by their sizes, preferably in the range of 60–200 nucleotides. The probe and target RNA are hybridized in solution. The reaction mixture is then treated with at least two RNAses to hydrolyze unreacted probe, and single-stranded (nonprotected) tails of products formed between the probe and its target. Although both components are present at low concentrations, the method is successful because of the very high specific radioactivity of the probe. The products are conveniently separated on a polyacrylamide denaturing gel calibrated with DNA sequencing reactions catalyzed by the appropriate primer.

The S1 nuclease protection assay ***(20)*** is similar in principle to the RNAse protection assay ***(21)***. However, a DNA strand replaces the RNA probe and unprotected DNA sequences are hydrolyzed by S1 nuclease. The RNAse protection assay has become more popular because of the ease with which RNA probes may be generated. For this reason, we describe only the RNAse protection assay.

1.2.1. Construction of RNA Probes

We have found the construction of minigenes (*see* **Fig. 5**) to be a simple and direct procedure ***(19)***. An appropriate DNA sequence not less than 60 bp and not more than about 300 bp is identified for amplification polymerase chain reaction (PCR). It is convenient if the target sequence is available in a recombinant plasmid. One primer (p2 in **Fig. 5**) includes the promoter sequence for a viral-DNA-dependent RNA polymerase (we found it convenient to use T7 polymerase). A minigene, which has a T7 promoter, may then be obtained by PCR amplification. In vitro transcription using the appropriate polymerase results in cRNA, that is, transcripts of the minigene that are complementary to mRNA sequences. The transcripts of the minigene are conveniently labeled by using a radiolabeled NTP, for example, [α-^{32}P]CTP. One amplification reaction provides enough DNA for a very large number of in vitro transcription reactions. An alternative procedure is to amplify the required sequence with standard primers, that is, primers that do not carry a promoter sequence. The amplified DNA is cloned into an appropriate plasmid such as the pGEM™ series (Promega), which contain a P6 and T7 promoter, or Bluescript™ (Stratagene), which contains T7 and T3 promoters. The plasmids are linearized by using a suitable restriction endonuclease. Enzymes that generate 5'- protruding or blunt ends are preferred in order to avoid nonspecific initiation of transcription from 3'- protruding ends. cRNA is synthesized by in vitro transcription. Careful control of the ratio of enzyme to promoter is needed to ensure that only one plasmid strand is transcribed.

The in vitro transcripts should be treated with DNAase to remove template DNA and full-length transcripts should be recovered after polyacrylamide gel electrophoresis for use as riboprobes.

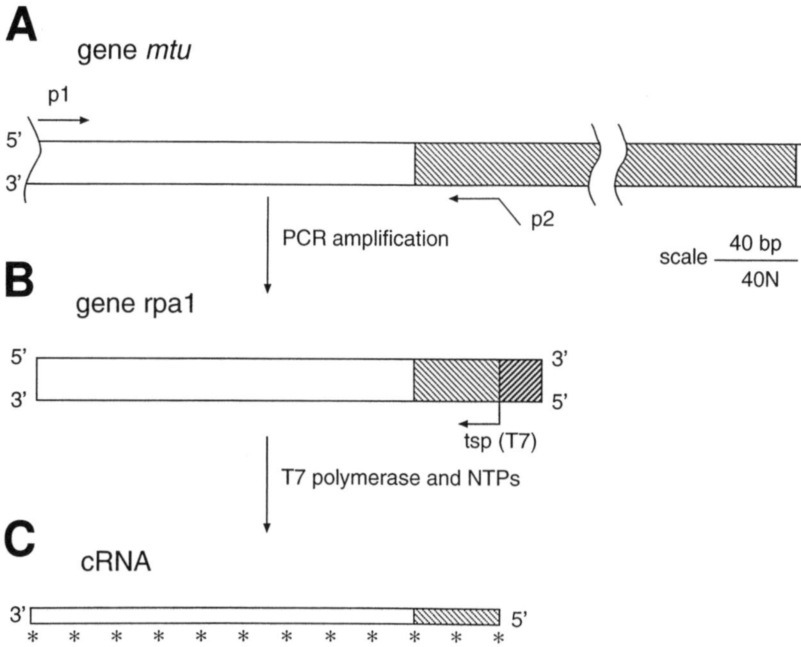

Fig. 5. A procedure for the construction and transcription of a minigene. **(A)** Construction of minigene rpo1. Part of the upstream region (180 bp) of the hypothetical gene *mtu* (*see* **Fig. 1**) is amplified by PCR using the deoxyribonucleotide primers p1 and p2. Primer p2 has the promoter sequence for a viral (e.g., T7) RNA polymerase at the 5'-end. The horizontal arrows show the binding sites for the primers; the angled part of the arrow labeled P2 denotes the T7 promoter sequence. Oblique shading indicates, coding region. **(B)** The product of PCR amplification is minigene rpo1 with a promoter specific for T7 RNA polymerase. **(C)** Transcripts of minigene rpo1 can be tagged, e.g., by using a radiolabeled NTP. Each asterisk denotes the incorporation of labeled nucleotides into RNA.

1.2.2. The Hybridization Reaction

The term hybridization is used to denote the formation of a duplex between an RNA probe and its target sequence. The underlying concepts were established when the processes of DNA denaturation and renaturation were investigated *(22)*. The concept of T_m was found to be valuable. A duplex nucleic acid was found to separate into its component strands over a narrow (10°C or less) temperature range. The mid-point of the transition, T_m, was found to depend on nucleotide composition (% G + C), ionic strength, and the presence of denaturing agents. Above a minimum size the T_m was not sensitive to the length of the duplex. Denaturation (strand separation) is independent of nucleic acid concentration. However the reverse reaction, renaturation (or hybridization, or duplex formation), is a bimolecular reaction and therefore depends on concentration. High salt concentrations (e.g., >0.5 *M* NaCl) favor duplex formation by screening the negatively charged phosphate residues of sugar phosphate backbone of nucleic acids, thereby reducing electrostatic repulsive forces between complementary strands. The temperature of the hybridization reaction is important, it cannot exceed the T_m of the product but should be adequate to "melt" intramolecular stem/loop structures that impede duplex formation. In the early days of the RNAse protection assay hybridization conditions were used which had been developed for the S1 nuclease assay. These conditions were designed to favor DNA/RNA hybridization and minimal competing DNA/DNA hybridization; considerations that do not apply to duplex formation between single stranded RNA species. Conditions described in ***(23)***, namely 90°C for 90 min in 25 m*M* PIPES, 1 *M* NaCl, 1 m*M* ethylenediaminetetracetic acid (EDTA), pH 6.8, are more appropriate to the RNAse protection assay and simplify the procedure.

1.3. Which Is the Better Method?

Each method has its strengths and its limitations. The strength of the primer extension method is that a tagged primer sequence lies at the 5' end of the product ensuring that the products obtained can be easily located within the sequence of interest; and the sizes of the products are readily obtained. Of course priming at sites closely related to the target can occur resulting in misleading information. Provided the primers are carefully selected, inappropriate reactions are uncommon. The use of end-labeled primers is valuable when more than one product is obtained because the relative concentrations of the tagged products are directly proportional to the relative concentrations of the target species (*see* **Fig. 2**). The main disadvantage of the method is that the primer selected may be prevented from binding to the target sequence by a competing RNA secondary structure (*see* **Fig. 3**). Raising the temperature of the primer extension reaction diminishes this effect (*see* **Subheading 1.1.**).

The RNA protection method is versatile. Hybridization of the tagged probe with its target sequence is unlikely to be prevented by RNA secondary structure. However, because the products are identified by size alone, the results may present ambiguities in their interpretation. This limitation in the method is illustrated in **Fig. 4**, when a single cleavage in the leader region of mRNA1 is the first step in RNA processing. This cleavage leads to two hypothetical fragments of different sizes, namely, mRNAp (5') and mRNAp (3'). The sizes of the products alone are not enough to lead to an unambiguous interpretation of the results. The method of choice is the one that is more likely to lead to an early identification of transcription start-sites. The use of both methods may be needed to achieve this end.

2. Materials (*see* Notes 1 and 2)

2.1. Isolation of RNA

1. Lysis buffer: 6 *M* guanidinium chloride, 10 m*M* EDTA, 1 m*M* 2-mercaptoethanol, 0.1% Tween-80.
2. 5X MOPS buffer: 0.1 *M* 3-(*N*-morpholino) propanesulfonic acid (MOPS), pH 7.0, (using 2 *M* NaOH), 40 m*M* sodium acetate, 5 m*M* EDTA, pH 8 (using 10 *M* NaOH).
3. Chloroform:butanol solution. 24:1 v/v.
4. Glass beads: 150–212 microns, acid-washed (Sigma, Poole, Dorset, UK).
5. Mini Bead-Beater device (Biospec Products, Bartlesville, OK) or Rybolyser device (Hybaid, Middlesex, UK) (*see* **Note 3**).
6. Refrigerated microfuge.
7. Ethanol.
8. 70% ethanol.

2.2. Primer Extension Procedure

1. Oligonucleotide primer specific for target gene (*see* **Note 4**)
2. 10X kinase buffer: 500 m*M* Tris-HCl, pH 7.5, 100 m*M* $MgCl_2$, 50 m*M* dithiothreitol (DTT), 1 m*M* spermidine.
3. [γ-^{32}p]ATP (at 3000 Ci/mmol, 10 mCi/mL).
4. T4 polynucleotide kinase (PNK): 8–10 U/µL
5. 2X primer extension buffer: 100 m*M* Tris-HCl, pH 8.3, 100 m*M* KCl, 20 m*M* $MgCl_2$, 20 m*M* DTT, 2 m*M* of each dNTPs, 1 m*M* spermidine.
6. Loading buffer: 98% formamide, 10 m*M* EDTA, 0.1% xylene cyanol, and 0.1% bromophenol blue.
7. 3 *M* sodium acetate, pH to 5.2 with glacial acetic acid and autoclave.
8. 40 m*M* sodium pyrophosphate.
9. Avian myeloblastosis virus (AMV) reverse transcriptase (Promega, Southampton, UK).
10. Phenol reagent: mixture of phenol:chloroform:isoamylalchohol (25:24:1).
11. TE buffer: 10 m*M* Tris-HCl, pH 7.5, 1 m*M* EDTA, pH 8.0.

2.3. RNAse Protection

2.3.1. Construction of Minigenes

1. TE buffer: 10 m*M* Tris-HCl, pH 7.5, 1 m*M* EDTA, pH 8.0.
2. *Taq* polymerase, 1 U/µL (Perkin-Elmer, Cheshire, UK). A 10X *Taq* polymerase buffer is supplied with the enzyme.

3. 1.25 m*M* dNTPs solution.
4. 10X TBE agarose gel-electrophoresis buffer: 890 m*M* Tris-HCl, pH 7.5, 890 m*M* boric acid, 25 m*M* EDTA.
5. QIAquick Gel extraction kit (QIAGEN, Sussex, UK): used to purify the PCR amplified DNA fragment.

2.3.2. Transcription of Minigenes (see **Note 5**)

1. 5X transcription buffer: 40 m*M* Tris-HCl, pH 7.5, 6 m*M* $MgCl_2$, 2 m*M* spermidine, 10 m*M* NaCl.
2. T7 RNA polymerase (Promega): 20 U/μL.
3. RNAsin ribonuclease inhibitor.
4. RNAse-free DNAse, RQ1 DNAase (Promega), 1 U/μL.
5. 2.5 m*M* ATP, GTP and UTP mixture.
6. 100 μ*M* CTP solution.
7. [α-^{32}P]cytidine 5'-[α-^{32}P]triphosphate (CTP): 50 μCi/μL, specific activity of 400 Ci/mmol.
8. Loading buffer: 98% formamide, 10 m*M* EDTA, 0.1% xylene cyanol, 0.1% bromophenol blue.
9. 6% polyacrylamide-urea gel.
10. Elution buffer: 0.5 *M* ammonium acetate, 1 m*M* EDTA, and 0.2% (w/v) sodium dodecyl sulfate (SDS).
11. 40% (v/v) acrylamide-*bis* acrylamide (29:1) stock solution (Amresco, Anachem, Bedfordshire, UK).
12. 3 *M* sodium acetate.
13. 100% ethanol.

2.3.3. RNAse Protection Assay

1. 5X PIPES/EDTA/saline (PES) buffer: 125 m*M* piperazine-*N,N'*-*bis*[2-ethanesulfonic acid] (PIPES), pH 6.8, 5 *M* NaCl, 5 m*M* EDTA. To prepare the 5X PES buffer, start with a 250 m*M* stock solution of PIPES. To prepare 25 mL of this stock solution, add the appropriate amount of PIPES to 12 mL of water. The solid will not dissolve until titrated with 1 *M* NaOH (added dropwise). Once PIPES is completely dissolved, make up to 25 mL (the final solution should be transparent). To prepare 50 mL of 5X PES buffer, take 25 mL of PIPES stock solution, add solid NaCl (14.6 g) and EDTA to 5 m*M* and adjust final volume to 50 mL. Note that 5 *M* NaCl is close to saturation and sometimes the NaCl will not dissolve until the final volume of the 50 mL is reached.
2. Scintillation counter.
3. Digestion buffer: 10 m*M* Tris-HCl, pH 7.5, 5 m*M* EDTA, 200 m*M* sodium acetate.
4. RNAse cocktail (AMBION, Austin, TX): 1 mg/mL of RNAse A and 20,000 U/mL of RNAse T1.
5. Loading buffer: 98% formamide, 10 m*M* EDTA, 0.1% xylene cyanol, and 0.1% bromophenol blue.

6. Sequencing equipment.
7. Phenol reagent: mixture of phenol:chloroform:isoamylalchohol (25:24:1).

3. Methods

3.1. Isolation of RNA

1. Collect cells from culture (*see* **Note 6**), resuspend them in 1 mL of lysis buffer, and incubate at –20°C for 15 min.
2. Transfer the suspension to a 2 mL screw-cap microcentrifuge tube containing 1 mL of heat-sterilized glass beads.
3. Lyse mycobacterial cells as follows: use three pulses of 1 min at low speed, and then four pulses of 15 s at high speed in the Mini Bead-Beater. After each pulse cool the solution in an ice-bath (*see* **Note 7**).
4. Sediment cellular debris and beads by centrifugation at 9400*g* for 5 min. Transfer the cleared lysate (supernatant) to a fresh tube.
5. Wash the sedimented mixture of beads and bacteria with 300 µL of fresh lysis buffer. Subject to four pulses of 15 s at high speed in the Mini Bead-Beater. Repeat **step 4**. Combine the supernatants in a microfuge tube.
6. Extract proteins from the supernatant by adding 2 vol of chloroform:butanol solution. Centrifuge at 16,000*g* for 2 min. Collect the aqueous upper layer and repeat this step three more times.
7. Add 0.5 vol of 100% ethanol by a dropwise procedure (*see* **Note 8**). Incubate at –70°C for at least 1 h.
8. Centrifuge at 16,000*g* for 30 min. Wash pellet with 1 mL of 70% ethanol and centrifuge at 16,000*g* for 10 min. Remove ethanol and dry at 37°C for 10 min.
9. Resuspend the RNA pellet in an appropriate volume of 1X MOPS buffer. Measure the OD at 230, 260, and 280 nm to check RNA quality and concentration. The absorbance at 230 should be similar to the value of absorbance at 280 and the OD260/280 ratio should be 2.0. Aliquot into small volumes and keep at –70°C (*see* **Notes 9** and **10**).
10. Check the integrity of the RNA by electrophoresis through formaldehyde-containing gels *(24)*. For subsequent analysis, the sample needs to be treated with RNAse-free DNAse *(25)*.

3.2. Primer Extension

3.2.1. Labeling the Primer

1. Add 10 pmol of the specific primer (*see* **Notes 4** and **11**), 1 mL of 10X kinase buffer, 3 µL of [γ-^{32}P]ATP, 1 µL of T4 PNK and autoclaved distilled water to a final volume of 10 µL *(27)*.
2. Incubate at 37°C for 15 min.
3. Heat to 90°C for 5 min to inactivate the T4 polynucleotide kinase and spin briefly
4. Store labeled primers at –20°C.

3.2.2. Hybridization and Primer Extension

The end-labeled primer complementary to the target RNA is used to synthesize cDNA.

1. Add 0.1–1 pmol of labeled primer, up to 40 μg of total RNA, and 5 μL of the 2X primer extension buffer.
2. Add an equal amount of water to a "No RNA" control tube for each primer
3. Anneal the RNA and primer by heating at the desired temperature (*see* **Note 12**) for 30 min.
4. Incubate at room temperature for about 10 min. Add 5 μL of 2X primer extension buffer, 1.4 μL of 40 m*M* sodium pyrophosphate, 1 U of AMV reverse transcriptase and 1.6 μL of nuclease free distilled water (*see* **Notes 13** and **14**).
5. Incubate the reaction at 42°C for about 1 h.

3.2.3. Precipitation, Electrophoresis, and Visualization of Products

1. Extract the reaction with an equal volume of phenol:chloroform:isoamylalchohol.
2. Precipitate by adding 0.1 vol of 3 *M* sodium acetate pH 5.2 and 2.5 vol of ethanol, incubate at –20°C for a few hours or overnight and spin at 16,000*g* for 30 min at 4°C.
3. Wash the pellet with 70% ethanol, remove the supernatant, and dissolve the pellet in 5 μL of TE buffer.
4. Add 5 μL of loading dye and heat the samples at 90°C for 10 min (*see* **Note 15**).
5. Analyze 5 μL of the samples by electrophoresis through a 6–8% polyacrylamide-urea gel along with suitable marker or DNA sequencing ladder and visualize by autoradiography (*see* **Note 16**).

3.3. RNAse Protection Assay

3.3.1. Construction of Minigenes

In order to construct a minigene, we use a general approach, which generates the transcription templates by PCR amplification of a cloned gene.

1. Choose the particular DNA region that is going to be amplified (*see* **Note 17**).
2. Design the 3' primer with two regions — the 5' end should have the T7 promoter sequence and the 3' end should have the sequence that corresponds to the 3' end of the transcript (*see* **Note 18**).
3. Design the 5' primer, usually 17–18 nucleotide long, corresponding to the 5'end of the transcript.
4. Amplify by PCR and check that a DNA fragment of the expected size has been produced. Estimate the amount of DNA by comparison with standards.
5. Purify the DNA by the use of QIAquick gel extraction kit and resuspend the DNA in an appropriate amount of TE buffer to 0.1–0.2 μg/μL.

3.3.2. Transcription of Minigenes

1. Prepare the reaction mixture at room temperature (to avoid precipitation of DNA-spermidine complex) as follows: 4 μL of 5X transcription buffer, 2 μL of 100 m*M* DTT, 20 U of RNAsin ribonuclease inhibitor, 4 μL of 2.5 m*M* ATP, GTP, and UTP mixture, 2.4 μL of 100 μ*M* CTP, 1–2 μL of template DNA, 5 μL of [α-^{32}P]CTP and 1 μL of T7 RNA polymerase. Final volume 20 μL.

2. Incubate for 60 min at 37°C.
3. Degrade the DNA template with 1 µL of RNAse-free DNAase for 15 min at 37°C.
4. Stop the reaction by adding 20 µL of loading buffer.
5. Purify the labeled transcript (RNA probe) as follows: incubate the sample for 3 min at 90–100°C, and run the total volume (20 µL) on a 6% polyacrylamide-urea gel. If radiolabel is used, after electrophoresis cover the gel with plastic wrap and expose it to film for 30 s to 2 min at room temperature to locate the full transcript. After aligning the developed film on the gel, excise the band from the gel using a sterile razor blade. Re-expose the cut gel to check that the correct band has been removed.
6. Elute the RNA from the gel by incubating the gel slice in 400 µL of elution buffer overnight at 37°C. Transfer only the elution buffer to a fresh tube (leaving the gel slice behind). Add 100 µL of 3 *M* sodium acetate and 800 µL of 100% ethanol. Precipitate on dry ice for at least 30 min. Spin for 30 min at 16,000*g* at 4°C.
7. Resuspend the probe RNA in about 20 µL of nuclease-free water. Take 1 µL of the probe and measure its radioactivity for example by means of its Cerenkov radiation (*see* **Note 19**).
8. The RNA probe should be used within 3 d of preparation.

3.3.3. RNase Protection Assay

1. Add 1–4 × 10^5 cpm RNA probe and 1 µg of cellular RNA in a total volume of 20 µL (*see* **Note 20**).
2. Add 5 µL of 5X PES buffer, mix and incubate at 90°C for 70 min (*see* **Note 21**) *(23)*.
3. Add 400 µL of digestion buffer to each sample and mix.
4. Add 1 µL of RNAse cocktail. Spin and incubate at 37°C for 30 min (*see* **Notes 22** and **23**).
5. Stop the reaction by adding 400 µL of phenol-chloroform. Mix and spin at 16,000*g* for 5 min. Transfer aqueous layer to a fresh tube.
6. Add 1 mL of 100% ethanol. Spin and keep at –70°C for at least 1 h.
7. Centrifuge at 16,000*g* for 30 min at 4°C. Carefully remove supernatant, because the pellet may be fragile at this state. Wash with 70% ethanol and spin as before.
8. Briefly, centrifuge again to remove any remaining ethanol.
9. Add 4–5 µL of loading buffer. Boil for 2–3 min and load the sample on a 6% polyacrylamide-urea sequencing gel (*see* **Note 24**).
10. Dry the gels and autoradiograph.

4. Notes

1. RNA is transcribed as a single-strand, a form that is very sensitive to RNAse action. RNAses are widespread and tenacious contaminants and are often found on fingertips and tend to stick to glassware. For these reasons, extreme care should be taken to avoid RNAse contamination in all procedures involving RNA. Gloves must be worn at all times, changed frequently, and care taken to avoid contaminating them; whenever possible sterile plasticware should be used in place of

glassware; essential glassware and pipet tips should be autoclaved; all reagents should be kept separate for RNA work.

2. Water: deionized water that has been autoclaved is recommended for the preparation of all solutions and for use in all procedures, including washing equipment. Treatment with diethyl pyrocarbonate to inactivate RNAse is not essential. If high-quality deionized water is not available, then treatment with diethyl pyrocarbonate (DEPC) is recommended. DEPC water: 0.1% DEPC in deionized water, stir to dissolve for about 30 min, then autoclave. Please note that any traces of DEPC left after autoclaving could inactivate enzymes and DEPC is suspected to be a carcinogen and should be handled with care.
3. A very good yield of RNA may be obtained using either of the two devices. One advantage of the Rybolyser is the safe handling of pathogenic mycobacteria but one disadvantage is that it is much more expensive than the Mini Bead-Beater.
4. DNA primers: the length of a primer should be the minimum required to give a product, usually in the range 16–24 nucleotides depending on GC content. This precaution is necessary to avoid inappropriate (and therefore misleading) products arising from interactions between a primer and nontarget but closely related sequences. A primer should not form "foldback" secondary structure that is stable during the priming reaction. The presence of such structures during the course of the reaction will reduce priming efficiency. When two primers are used in the same reaction, they should have minimal capacity to interact to form a duplex.
5. Except **items 5**, **6**, and **7**, all buffers and reagents in this particular subheading can be purchased either as a separate item or as part of the Riboprobe kit (Promega).
6. The required metabolic state of the mycobacterial culture influences the volume of culture needed to obtain sufficient RNA. Briefly, the volume of the culture should be geared to the cell density. The amount of RNA per average cell depends on growth rate. For example, the average amount of RNA per cell of *M. tuberculosis* was found to be approx 13 pg during exponential growth and approx 7 pg in the stationary phase.
7. There are several RNA-extraction procedures described in the literature ***(26)*** (*see* Chapter 3). We describe a protocol that we have found to be reliable. We have successfully isolated RNA from a wide range of fast-growers and *M. tuberculosis* ***(17,14,19,13,14)***. It is important to keep RNA samples on ice at all times to minimize any nuclease action. Once cells are resuspended in the lysis buffer, RNA will be protected from nucleases; however, we strongly recommend that samples should be kept on ice. All the centrifugations should be done at 4°C.
8. As this is a differential precipitation, the recommended amount of 100% ethanol should be used, otherwise a higher proportion of DNA will precipitate together with RNA.
9. We suggest that the purified RNA be dissolved in a very small volume (20–30 μL) of 1X MOPS buffer. In our experience, the approximate yield is 300–400 μg of RNA per 500 mL of culture.
10. Once the RNA concentration is measured, prepare appropriate aliquots according to the particular concentration of RNA needed for each experiment. Since

storage at –20°C is less reliable, storage at –70°C is recommended. Avoid thawing and freezing RNA samples, to prevent degradation.

11. Bring the final concentration of your primer to 0.1–0.2 pmol/µL by adding nuclease-free water or use directly from a 1 pmol/µL stock.
12. In most cases 45°C–65°C provides satisfactory results. The optimum temperature for annealing depends on the length of the primer and the GC content of the RNA. Preferably, determine the optimum temperature by means of a series of pilot experiments ***(28)***.
13. Prewarm sodium pyrophosphate, primer extension buffer, and nuclease-free water to room temperature or 37°C, since sodium pyrophosphate may precipitate in solutions that are cooler than room temperature.
14. For more than one reaction, prepare a master RT mix and add 9 µL to each reaction.
15. Caution: loading dye contains formamide, which is a teratogen.
16. Occasionally, a cluster of two or three products differing in lengths by a single nucleotide is found. Explanations for this effect include the possibility that the start of transcription takes place at more than one site (± one nucleotide) and that termination of reverse transcription takes place at or near the 5'-end of mRNA, that is, the 5'-terminal nucleotide or, to a lesser extent, at the penultimate 5'-terminal nucleotide.
17. It is convenient to design the size of the RNA to be bigger than the expected hybrid (probe RNA+ cellular RNA). We recommend that this difference in size should be around 100–150 nucleotides.
18. We have successfully used, in addition to the specific primer sequence, a 24 nucleotide T7 promoter sequence (5' AAT TCT AAT ACG ACT CAC TAT AGG 3'). It is important to make sure that, the T7 promoter sequence is located at the 5' end of the DNA template strand; note that the hybridization reaction will be carried out between cellular RNA (the target sequence) and its complement, the in vitro transcribed RNA (the probe).
19. The concentration of the RNA probe is difficult to measure. We usually measure Cerenkov radiation, which is emitted without the addition of scintillation fluid ***(29)***. Resuspend the probe in a very small volume (10–20 µL) of water; place 1 µL in the bottom of a microfuge tube, put this in an empty scintillation vial, and measure the radioactivity in a scintillation counter; it is usually in the range of $1–4 \times 10^5$ cpm/µL. Keep a sample (1 µL) of RNA probe at –70°C for use as the probe control at the end of this procedure.
20. Although we have obtained good results using 1 µg of cellular RNA, the results can be improved by using up to 40 µg of RNA for rare mRNA species. However, note that if the ratio of probe RNA/cellular RNA is very high, the background will increase. Therefore keep this ratio as close as possible to the suggested value.
21. Alternatively hybridization can be carried out in formamide buffer (80% deionized formamide, 1 m*M* EDTA, 40 m*M* PIPES, pH 6.4, 0.2 *M* sodium acetate) overnight at 50°C ***(24)***. Use the probe RNA and cellular RNA at similar concentrations as described. The final volume is not limited because the RNA is precipi-

tated using 0.1 vol of 3 *M* sodium acetate and 2.5 vol of 100% ethanol. Mix and incubate at –70°C for at least 1 h. Centrifuge at 16,000*g* at 4°C and wash with 1 mL of 70% ethanol. Allow the pellet to dry at 37°C for 5–10 min. The tubes may be monitored with a Geiger counter to avoid pellet loss. Resuspend pellet in 20 µL of formamide buffer. Mix by vortexing and spin. Add 12 µL of mineral oil (to avoid sample evaporation during incubation). Incubate at 80°C for 5 min and immediately incubate at 50°C overnight. After hybridization, transfer sample to a fresh tube. Care should be taken to avoid contamination from oil layer.

22. It is important to include a parallel negative control (with the same amount of probe RNA and cellular RNA) and keep it on ice to prevent hybridization, but treat with RNAses. This control will reveal if the concentration of RNAses and the length of incubation time are enough to degrade the equivalent amount of single-stranded RNA.
23. RNAses are inactivated by RNAse inhibitors; therefore the latter should be used with great care and if possible be avoided.
24. The gels can be calibrated by use of either *Hae*III-digested φX 174 DNA molecular size markers or the products of a known sequencing reaction; for example, the products obtained using the 3' primer (p2 in **Fig. 5**) without the T7 sequence and the target DNA sequence. Include a diluted (up to 1:10) sample of the purified RNA probe. Load sufficient probe to give a clear signal of similar intensity to the samples; too large a signal may mask regions of neighboring tracks.

Acknowledgments

Farahnaz Movahedzadeh is funded by the Wellcome Trust project grant 051880/Z/97/2. J.A.G-Y-M received financial support from COFAA and EDD, IPN, Mexico. This work was funded by grants from CONACYT, No. 27576-M, Mexico and from the European commission Research and Development program, contract ERBIC–18CT 9720253.

References

1. Fassler, J. S. and Gussin, G. N. (1996) Promoters and basal transcription machinery in eubacteria and eukaryotes: concepts, definitions and analogies. *Methods Enzymol.* **273,** 3–29.
2. Knaus, R. and Bujard, H. (1990) Principles governing the activity of *E. coli* promoters, in *Nucleic Acids and Molecular Biology* (Eckstein, F. and Lilley, D. M. J., eds.) Springer-Verlag, Heidelberg, pp. 110–122.
3. Mangan, J. A. and Butcher, P. D. (1998) Analysis of mycobacterial differential gene expression by RAP-PCR, in *Methods in Molecular Biology*, vol. 101, *Mycobacteria Protocols* (Parish, T. and Stoker, N. G., eds.), Humana, Totowa, NJ, pp. 307–322.
4. Bashyam, M. D., Kanshal, D., Dasgapta, S. K., and Tyagi, A. K. (1996) A study of the mycobacterial transcriptional apparatus: identification of novel features in promoter elements. *J. Bacteriol.* **178,** 4847–4853.

5. Smith, I., Dussanget, O., Rodriguez, G. M., Timm, J., Gomez, M., et al. (1998) Extra and intracellular expression of *Mycobacterium tuberculosis* genes. *Tuberc. Lung Dis.* **79,** 91–97.
6. Timm, J., Gomez, M., and Smith, I. (1999) Gene expression and regulation, in *Mycobacteria: Molecular Biology and Virulence* (Ratledge, C. and Dale, J., eds.), Blackwell Science, Oxford, pp. 59–92.
7. Krummel, B. and Chamberlin, M. J. (1989) RNA chain initiation by *Escherichia coli* RNA polymerase. Structural transitions of the enzyme in early ternary complexes. *Biochemistry* **28,** 7829–7842.
8. Zengel, J. M. and Lindahl, L. (1990) Mapping of two promoters for elongation factor Tu within the structural gene for elongation factor G. *Nucleic Acids Res.* **12,** 2181–2192.
9. Coburn, G. A. and Mackie, G. A. (1999) Degradation of mRNA in *Escherichia coli*: an old problem with some new twists. *Prog. Nucleic Acids Res. Molec. Biol.* **62,** 55–108.
10. Petersen, C. (1993) Translation and mRNA stability in bacteria: a complex relationship, in *Control of Messenger RNA Stability* (Belasco, J. S. and Brannerman, G., eds.), Academic, London.
11. Hu, Y., Butcher, P. D., Mangan, J. A., Rajandream, M.-A., Coates, A. R. M. (1999) The *hmp* gene of *M. tuberculosis* has a half life of less than one min. *J. Bacteriol.* **181,** 3486–3493.
12. Verma, A., Kringer, A. K., and Tyagi, J. S. (1994) Functional analysis of transcription of the *Mycobacterium tuberculosis* 16S rDNA-encoding gene. *Gene* **148,** 113–118.
13. Movahedzadeh, F., Colston, M. J., and Davis, E. O. (1997) Characterization of *Mycobacterium tuberculosis* LexA: recognition of a Cheo (*Bacillus*-type SOS) box. *Microbiology* **143,** 929–936.
14. Gonzalez-y-Merchand, J. A., Garcia, M. J., Gonzalez-Rico, S., Colston, M. J., and Cox, R. A. (1997) Strategies used by pathogenic and non-pathogenic mycobacteria to synthesize rRNA *J. Bacteriol.* **179,** 6949–6958.
15. Yamada, M., Izu, H., Nitta, T., Kurihara, K. abd Sakurai, T. I. (1998) High-temperature, non-radioactive primer extension assay for determination of a transcription initiation site. *Biotechniques* **25,** 72–78.
16. Triezenberg, S. J. (1987) Primer extension, in *Current Protocols in Molecular Biology*, vol. 1, Section 4.8.4. (Ausubel, F. M., Brent, M., Kingston, R. E., Moore, D. D., Seidman, J. G., Smith, J. A., and Struhl, K., eds.), John Wiley and Sons, New York.
17. Gonzalez-y-Merchand, J. A., Colston, M. J., and Cox, R. A. (1996) The rRNA operons of *Mycobacterium smegmatis* and *Mycobacterium tuberculosis*: comparison of promoter elements and neighbouring upstream genes. *Microbiology* **142,** 667–674.
18. DeMaio, J., Zhang, Y., Ko, C., Young, D. B., and Bishai, W. R. (1996) A stationary-phase stress-response sigma factor from *Mycobacterium tuberculosis*. *Proc. Natl. Acad. Sci. USA* **93,** 2790–2794.
19. Gonzalez-y-Merchand, J. A., Colston, M. J., and Cox, R. A. (1999) Effects of growth conditions on expression of mycobacterial *mur A* and *tyrS* genes and contributions of their transcripts to precursor RNA synthesis. *J. Bacteriol.* **181,** 4617–4627.

20. Berk, A. J. and Sharp, R. A. (1977) Sizing and mapping of early adenovirus mRNAs by electrophoresis of S1-endonuclease-digested hybrids. *Cell* **12,** 721–732.
21. Zinn, K., DiMaio, D., and Maniatis, T. (1983) Identification of two distinct regulatory regions adjacent to the human β-interferon gene. *Cell* **34,** 865–879.
22. Marmur, J., Rownd, R., and Schildkraut, C. L. (1963) Denaturation and renaturation of deoxyribonucleic acid. *Progr. Nucleic Acids Res.* **1,** 231–300.
23. Mironov, V. N., Van Montagu, M., and Inzé, D. (1995) High throughput RNase protection assay. *Nucleic Acids Res.* **23,** 3359–3360.
24. Sambrook, J., Fritsch, E. F., and Maniatis, T. (1989) *Molecular Cloning: A Laboratory Manual*, 2nd ed. Cold Spring Harbor Laboratory, Cold Spring Harbor, New York.
25. Mahenthiralingam, E. (1998) Extraction of RNA from Mycobacteria, in *Methods in Molecular Biology*, vol. 101, *Mycobacteria Protocols* (Parish, T. and Stoker, N. G., eds.), Humana, Totowa, NJ, pp. 65–75.
26. Mangan, J. A., Sole, K. M., Mitchison, D. A., and Butcher, P. D. (1997) An effective method of RNA extraction from bacteria refractory to disruption, including mycobacteria. *Nucleic Acids Res.* **25,** 675–676.
27. Promega, Technical Bulletin, "AMV Reverse Transcriptase primer extension system."
28. Walmsley, M., Leonard, M., Patient, R. (1998) Primer extension analysis of mRNA, in *Methods in Molecular Biology*, vol. 86, *RNA Isolation and Characterization Protocols* (Rapley, R. and Manning, L., eds.), Humana, Totowa, NJ, pp. 187–193.
29. Haviland, R. T. and Bieber, L. L. (1970) Scintillation counting of ^{32}P without added scintillator in aqueous solutions and organic solvents and on dry chromatographic media. *Anal. Biochem.* **33,** 323–334.

9

Fluorescence and Brightfield Cytology of Live *M. tuberculosis* Cells

Rory P. Cooney, Natalie J. Garton, and Michael R. Barer

1. Introduction

Although light microscopy fell out of favor as a research tool in prokaryotic biology in the 1980s, advances in the reagents available for cell labeling (staining) and in the user-friendliness of microscopes were underpinning a revolution in eukaryotic cell biology. The development of epifluorescence hardware, particularly confocal microscopy and low-light imaging systems, and computational deblurring and video enhancement methodologies, substantially extended the range of potential applications. These developments now enable us to detect weaker signals at higher levels of resolution than was previously possible. Finally the personal computer and related software developments have brought image analysis within affordable range for many laboratories and facilitate quantitation of cellular properties on an objective basis. We have sought to apply these advances across a range of prokaryotic applications and here we describe the methods we have applied to live *Mycobacterium tuberculosis* cells. Although we have principally been concerned with two applications, the determination of viability at the cellular level (*see* **Note 1**) and the nature and distribution of lipid domains, more general aspects of light microscopic cytological analyses are discussed below.

1.1. Applications of Light Microscopic (LM) Cytological Analyses

Light microscope images of bacteria can be used to determine cell morphology, to detect the presence or absence of specific cellular properties, and to quantify specific properties. In any analysis within these categories, it must be possible to prepare the bacteria for microscopy without altering the property to be determined, and to distribute the organisms so that individual cells can be

From: *Methods in Molecular Medicine*, vol. 54: *Mycobacterium Tuberculosis Protocols*
Edited by: T. Parish and N. G. Stoker © Humana Press Inc., Totowa, NJ

imaged. Confocal imaging systems offer the particular advantage that cells can be imaged within relatively thick specimens and signals separately assigned to cells occupying the same vertical (z) plane. The properties that can be determined, with the limitations discussed below are essentially those for which specific reagents are available or can be prepared. Thus specific immunological reagents and other affinity-based selective labels (e.g., lectins, oligonucleotides, and certain dyes) enable antigens and other specific cellular components (e.g., DNA) to be determined; cytochemical substrates allow enzyme activities to be detected; and physiological probes can be used to reveal such properties as integrity of the cell envelope and membrane energization. Finally the use of reporter genes, particularly *gfp*, can provide information about the expression of specific genes that is detectable at the single cell level.

1.2. Advantages and Limitations of LM Analyses

LM analyses offer special advantages for work with organisms that grow slowly or not at all, or in situations where analysis of small quantities of biomass is necessary. Around 10^7 *M. tuberculosis* cells are the minimum that can be studied with the methods described here, although there is no obvious reason why 100–1000 cells should not be amenable to analysis providing they can be accurately sampled and deposited at an easily located point on a microscope slide. Cytological analyses also provide opportunities to determine whether the specific property studied is heterogeneously distributed within a cell population, the cellular location of the property, and whether expression of the specific property is dependent on a spatial relationship.

Limitations of LM analysis relate to the equipment, processing, reagents, and safety. *M. tuberculosis* cells are often very small in culture, and cell profiles down to 0.5×2 μm are not unusual in our experience. The theoretical limit of resolution of light microscopy is 250–300 nm and this leaves little scope for point to point resolution of cellular structure in *M. tuberculosis* cells. However, fluorescence signals may be detectable from objects well below this diameter providing they are sufficiently intense. Ultrastructure is best explored by electron microscopy although the concerns that the necessary fixation procedures may substantially disturb the native organization are considerable. In contrast, because the signal yield from fluorescence labeling methods is relatively strong and detection methods are sensitive, they can often be applied to living cells and the disturbance of native structure and function is apparently minimal.

Processing and reagents provide limitations that relate to what can be done with the sample material to be studied (e.g., are the cells to be studied in pure culture, inside macrophages, or in tissue samples) and the nature of the analysis itself. In some ways, cytochemical methods may be seen as analyses in which each bacterial cell is both a test tube and a photometer cell. The technical challenge is in getting the reagents in and keeping the reaction products localized. Clearly these challenges increase with the complexity of the sample material to be analyzed, and we have discussed most of the central issues as they relate to mycobacteria and other bacteria elsewhere *(1,2)*. In spite of early pessimism about the degree to which cytochemical methods are applicable to bacteria *(3)*, our recent experience leads us to conclude that most areas of prokaryotic cell composition, biochemistry, and physiology are amenable to cytochemical analysis providing appropriate controls and standards are used and providing the incentive to develop the necessary reagents and procedures is strong enough *(1)*.

Finally, no procedure should be undertaken with an organism requiring level 3 biosafety containment without performance of a careful risk assessment. We have developed a chamber system in-house to make cell deposits suitable for microscopy *(4)*. However, the system itself imposes limitations regarding the range of cell numbers and sample types that can be processed, and workers wishing to develop our procedures for other applications may need to devise alternate means of sample processing.

1.3. Range of Appropriate Equipment for Microscopy and Image Processing and Analysis

It is possible to spend anything between a few thousand and a few hundred thousand US dollars on facilities to record and analyze the results of the methods described here. Even the simplest microscope equipped with a brightfield/phase contrast condenser, epifluorescence and a suitable oil immersion objective purchased from any of the major manufacturers can produce high quality images suitable for qualitative analysis. Compatibility between different manufacturers remains an important issue and you should make sure the microscope you buy will support the sort of imaging and control equipment you wish to add. If a good conventional camera system is available or desired, images taken on photographic film can be subjected to image analysis and it still remains difficult to beat this medium for the highest quality presentation images. However, photography of fluorescence images is technically demanding and does not compete with electronic imaging when the signals are weak.

The options for an electronic imaging and processing system are bewildering for the uninitiated. Quite powerful systems can be assembled for around $15,000 (excluding microscope), but the novice is probably better off getting a complete package (camera, camera mount, computer, camera control software, and image display, processing, and analysis software). Some systems also include motorized microscope stages and control software. This can be particularly useful for relocating objects, and can speed up the process of recording images after a sample has been scanned.

Optical sectioning of fluorescently labeled samples can be achieved by confocal imaging systems or by computational deconvolution of a z-series of digitized images. This approach may be necessary to study bacteria within cells or within relatively thick tissue samples, in order to obtain clear images from a single focal plane and exclude signals from other (out of focus) planes. Three-dimensional reconstructions of objects can be achieved with such systems. If thin sections or deposited monolayers of bacteria are to be studied, there is little advantage in a confocal system. Computational deblurring systems can be applied to single images and, in the elite systems, can achieve remarkable levels of apparent resolution (approx 100 nm) when applied to z-series.

Information about microscope imaging systems can be obtained from the major microscope manufacturers, local suppliers, volume 122 of the *Methods in Molecular Biology* series ***(5)*** and from many web pages (e.g., www.videomicroscopy.com — provides listings for many manufacturers; examples not listed include: www.improvision.co.uk; www.demon.co.uk/ffaltd/; www.datx.com; www.photonic-science.ltd.uk; www.synoptics.co.uk; www.optimas.com).

2. Materials

2.1. Preparation of Bacteria

2.1.1. Preparation of Bacterial Inoculum

1. *M. tuberculosis* frozen (–70°C) stock in 1 mL aliquots.
2. Middlebrook 7H10 agar (Difco Laboratories, Detroit, MI) containing 0.5% (v/v) glycerol and 10% oleic acid-albumin-dextrose-catalase supplement (OADC; Difco). Prepare according to manufacturer's instructions.
3. Middlebrook 7H9 broth (Difco) containing 0.2% (v/v) glycerol, 0.05% (w/v) Tween-80, and 10% albumin-dextrose-catalase (ADC; Difco) supplement. Prepare according to manufacturer's instructions.
4. Sterile 250 mL baffled polycarbonate conical flask (BDH, Poole, Dorset, UK).
5. Disposable 10 µL inoculating loops, disposable L-shaped speaders (STC, Technical Services Consultants Ltd., UK).
6. Laboratory sealing film (Whatman, Maidstone, UK).
7. Sealable plastic bags.
8. Sterile Pyrex glass test tubes (20-by-125-mm screw necked tubes fitted with screw-cap with latex liners).
9. Sterile glass rods (5 mm diameter, 160 mm length) with smooth fused ends.
10. Colorimeter: Jenway PCO1 (Jenway Ltd., Dunmow, Essex, UK).
11. Disposable polystyrene spectrophotometer cuvets (Sigma, Poole, Dorset, UK).

2.1.2. Preparation of Immobilized Bacterial Populations

1. Acetone.
2. 3-Aminopropyltriethoxysilane (APS) solution: freshly prepare a 2% (v/v) solution of APS (Sigma) in acetone (*see* **Note 2**).

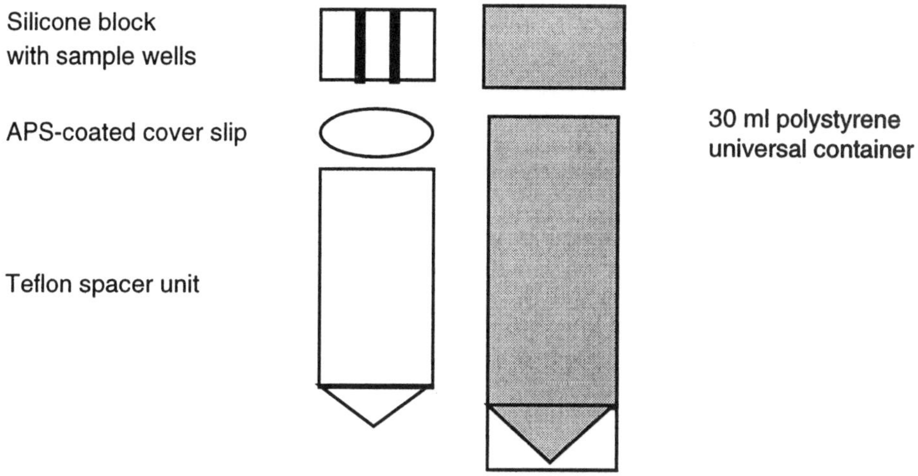

Fig. 1. Microchamber system used to deposit mycobacteria as monolayers on APS-coated cover slips *(4)*. The cover slip is placed between the spacer unit and silicone block in a 30 mL polystyrene universal container and held firmly in place by tightening the lid. The lid is predrilled with holes that are aligned over the sample wells.

3. 19 mm diameter circular cover slips, thickness no. 1 (BDH).
4. Shallow glass trough with lid.
5. Petroleum grease (Vaseline).
6. Microchamber system (*see* **Fig. 1**). This consists of a 30 mL polystyrene universal container, a Teflon spacer unit, and a silicone block with sampling wells. Teflon spacer units and silicone blocks were made to our specification by RAPRA Technology Ltd., Billingham, Cleveland, UK. Centrifuge with sealed centrifuge buckets designed to provide full aerosol containment.
7. Microscope slides.
8. Silicone fluid (Dow Corning 200/100 cs) (BDH).
9. Clear nail polish.

2.1.3. Exposure to Antibiotics

1. Antimycobacterial agents are purchased from Sigma and stored as recommended by the manufacturer. Prepare antimycobacterial drug stocks at 10 µg/mL in appropriate solvent. Sterilize by filtration, dispense into small aliquots, and store at –70°C for up to 12 mo.
2. Prepare working concentrations of antimycobacterial drugs in Middlebrook 7H9 broth from thoroughly thawed stocks. Working concentrations are prepared at 2X the required final drug concentration.
3. 0.22 µm disposable syringe filter units (Millipore, Watford, UK).

2.2. Rhodamine 123 (R123)/Propidium Iodide (PI) Labeling

2.2.1. Labeling of Bacterial Suspensions

1. Dimethyl sulfoxide (DMSO).
2. Phosphate-buffered saline (PBS), pH 7.3: 8.0 g NaCl, 0.2 g KCl, 1.15 g Na_2HPO_4, and 0.2 g KH_2PO_4 in 1 L of distilled water, adjust to pH 7.3 and sterilize by autoclaving.
3. Sterile distilled water (SDW).
4. R123 and PI (Sigma). Prepare stock solutions of 6.5 m*M* R123 and 7.5 m*M* PI in DMSO. Store at –20°C for up to 6 mo. Prepare working stock solutions of 50 μ*M* R123 and 150 μ*M* PI in PBS from completely thawed stocks on each day of use.
5. Carbonyl cyanide m-chlorophenyl hyrazone (CCCP) solution: 7.6 m*M* CCCP (Sigma) in ethanol.
6. Ethanol.
7. Screw-topped 1.5 mL centrifuge tube and/or 50 mm polystyrene Petri dishes (Bibby Sterilin Ltd.).
8. APS-coated cover slips (*see* **Subheading 3.1.2.**).
9. Microscope slides.
10. Silicone fluid (Dow Corning 200/100 cs).
11. Clear nail polish.

2.2.2. Microscopy

1. We routinely use a Nikon DIAPHOT-300 microscope (Nikon UK Limited, Surrey, UK) equipped with standard phase contrast and epifluorescence attachments. A 100 W high-pressure mercury-vapor lamp is used as a light source.
2. R123 fluorescence is viewed with an FITC specific filter block (excitation filter 420–490, barrier filter 530 ± 10, dichroic mirror 510) or a Nikon B–2A filter block (excitation filter 450–490, barrier filter 520, dichroic mirror 510). R123 and PI fluorescence are viewed simultaneously with a Nikon B–2E filter block (excitation filter 450–490, barrier filter 520–560, dichroic mirror 510).
3. Citifluor nonfluorescent immersion oil (Agar Scientific Limited, Essex, UK) is used with oil-immersion lenses for fluorescence microscopy to help prevent the fading of dyes.

2.2.3. Image Acquisition and Storage

1. Images are recorded using an integrating color charge-coupled device (CCD) camera (Model JVC KY-S55B, Foster Findlay and Associates, Newcastle upon Tyne, UK) linked to a Matrox Meteor frame grabber (Matrox Graphics Inc., Quebec, Canada; http://www.matrox.com) in a 90 MHz 35 MB RAM Pentium PC. Using this system RGB images are stored at 24-bit resolution (8 bits per color) in standard tagged image format as 768 × 576 square pixel *.TIF files.
2. Iomega Zip 100 drive and 100 MB Zip disks for image storage (Iomega Corporation, 1821 West Iomega Way, Roy, UT 84067, USA; http://www.iomega.com) (*see* **Note 3**).

2.2.4. Image Analysis

1. "Alpha" image analysis software (Adaptrix Limited, Gateshead, Tyne and Wear, UK).
2. Quattro Pro spreadsheet, statistical and graph-plotting computer program (Borland International Inc., Worldwide Headquarters, 100 Enterprise Way, Scotts Valley, CA 95066, USA; http://www.borland.com).

2.3. p-Iodonitrotetrazolium Violet (INT) Labeling

1. INT solution: prepare a fresh solution of 2 m*M* INT (Sigma) in SDW (*see* **Note 4**). Filter sterilize.
2. Sonic bath: Decon FS100b sonicator (BDH, Poole, Dorset, UK).
3. 0.22 μm disposable syringe filter units.
4. PBS, pH 7.3 (*see* **Subheading 2.2.1.**, **step 2**.).
5. Screw-topped 1.5 mL centrifuge tube.
6. APS-coated cover slips (*see* **Subheading 3.1.2.).**
7. Microscope slides.
8. Clear nail polish.

2.4. Gfp Expression

1. *M. tuberculosis* strain with required *gfp* construct *(11)*.
2. Middlebrook 7H10 agar, Middlebrook 7H9 broth (*see* **Subheading 2.1.1.**, **items 2** and **3**).
3. Kanamycin sulfate (Sigma): stock solution 10 mg/mL; filter-sterilize and store at –20°C.

2.5. Labeling of Lipid Domains

2.5.1. Preparation and Labeling of Liposomes

1. Glass tubes: 6 cm in depth and with a Quickfit ground glass joint, size B24.
2. Rotary evaporator.
3. Sonic bath: Decon FS100b sonicator (BDH, Poole, Dorset, UK)
4. Sonicator: MSE 150 W probe ultrasonic disintegrator (Sanyo Gallenkamp, Loughborough, Leicester, UK).
5. Sonic probe (19 mm in diameter, flat tip).
6. Dipalmitoyl L-α-phosphatidylcholine (DPPC) (Sigma).
7. Chloroform:methanol solution (2:1 v/v).
8. Fluorescent lipid probes from Molecular Probes (Cambridge Bioscience, Cambridge, UK) and Sigma. We have used the procedures described with dodecyl, hexadecyl and octadecyl aminofluorescein, BoDipy dodecanoate, and NBD stearate.
9. Nile red solution: 0.5 mg/mL Nile red (Sigma) in ethanol. Filter the solution and store with the exclusion of light at –20°C until required.

2.5.2. Microscopy

1. The set up described for R123/PI would suffice for most purposes (*see* **Subheading 2.2.2.**).
2. For higher resolution with weaker signals work we have used a Nikon Optiphot 2 microscope and a 16-bit digital Peltier cooled charge-coupled device (CCD) camera (Type KAF-0400, array 768H × 512V, pixel size 9 μm square, operating temperature 200K, Wright Instruments Ltd, Enfield, England) linked to a Viglen 486, 60 MHz microcomputer.
3. For deconvolution, we have used HazeBuster (VayTek Inc, Fairfield Imaging, England) to remove out of focus signals from fluorescent images.

3. Methods

3.1. Preparation of Bacteria for Microscopy

3.1.1. Preparation of Bacterial Suspensions

The preparation of *M. tuberculosis* cell suspensions for microscopy is problematic due to clumping. The method described here produces an evenly dispersed bacterial suspension of known cell density with a minimum of clumping.

1. Inoculate 50 mL of Middlebrook 7H9 broth in a 250-mL conical flask with 1 mL of frozen *M. tuberculosis* stock. Incubate for 6–7 d at 37°C with shaking at 180 rpm.
2. Inoculate predried Middlebrook 7H10 agar plates with 100 μL of this subculture and spread evenly over the surface using sterile spreaders. When the inoculum has dried, seal the Petri dishes with laboratory sealing film and incubate in closed plastic bags at 37°C for 6–7 d. By this time the culture has grown to a subconfluent lawn.
3. Transfer one loopful of mycobacterial growth to a sterile glass tube and gently homogenize with the rounded end of a sterile glass rod until a smooth paste is obtained. Add two 50 μL portions of Middlebrook 7H9 broth during homogenization so that an even suspension is produced; the volume is made up to 1 mL and thoroughly mixed.
4. A mycobacterial suspension prepared this way, and adjusted to an optical density (OD) of 0.2 at 580 nm (*see* **Note 5**) contains approx 1.0×10^8 cells/mL and produces between 5.0×10^7–1.0×10^8 colonies/mL.

3.1.2. Immobilization for Microscopy

Cells are immobilised as "monolayers" on APS-coated cover slips by centrifugation using a microchamber system developed in our laboratory ***(4)***. APS reacts with free hydroxyl groups on the glass surface. The resultant covalently-coated surface carries a positive charge at physiological pH to which mycobacteria strongly adhere.

1. Briefly clean cover slips by immersion in acetone and wipe clean with tissue.
2. Working in a chemical fume hood, lay the cover slips flat in a shallow glass dish and immerse the slides in freshly prepared 2% (v/v) APS solution. Smear the top of the dish with petroleum jelly and cover with a lid to prevent evaporation. Leave at room temperature between 16 and 24 h.
3. Remove the APS solution and immerse the cover slips in acetone to remove excess APS.
4. Remove the acetone and individually wash the cover slips by sequentially immersing them in two distilled water washes. Note that care must be taken to identify the upper (coated) surface. Clean gloves should be worn when handling the cover slips.
5. Drain the cover slips, gently blot with tissue paper, and leave at 37°C for 1 h to dry.
6. Mark the APS-coated face with permanent pen and store the cover slips for up to 1 mo in a clean, dry Petri dish.
7. Deposit mycobacterial suspensions onto APS-coated cover slips by centrifugation; aliquot 30 μL samples of bacterial suspension with a cell density of 10^6–10^8 mL^{-1} (these produce monolayers suitable for microscopy) onto the APS-coated cover slip. Place the spacer unit into the universal container then place a cover slip (APS coating outward) on top of the spacer. The silicone block is then secured in watertight contact with the cover slip (lipped surface downward) by screwing on the drilled universal cap and aligning the holes with the chambers made by the block (*see* **Fig. 1**). For pathogenic live mycobacteria, contain the complete microchamber in sealed centrifuge buckets. Centrifuge at 1000*g* for 5 min.
8. Remove the supernatant and dismantle the chamber assembly, taking care not to interfere with the deposited monolayers.
9. Further processing depends on the procedure. If cytochemical reactions were done prior to immobilization, dry the cover slips, mount (cell deposit face down) in an appropriate mountant, and seal in place with clear nail polish. Mark monolayer positions with permanent pen for easy location during microscopy. If the reactions are to be done with immobilized bacteria, transfer the cover slips to disposable polystyrene Petri dishes (50 mm diameter), which make useful "mini-staining trays."
10. Autoclave silicone blocks and packing units for reuse. Leave drilled universal caps and centrifuge pots overnight in 70% ethanol, and discard the 30 mL universals.

3.1.3. Exposure to Antibiotics

1. Prepare working stocks of antimycobacterial drugs at 2X the required final drug concentration.
2. Prepare *M. tuberculosis* cell suspension in Middlebrook 7H9 broth (*see* **Subheading 3.1.1.**).
3. Mix 5 mL of cell suspension and 5 mL of drug working stock in sterile test tubes.
4. Incubate at 37°C.
5. Mix thoroughly daily and sample for cytological studies.

3.2. Rhodamine 123/Propidium Iodide (R123/PI) Labeling — Cytoplasmic Membrane Energization and Cell Envelope Integrity (see Notes 6 and 7)

3.2.1. Labeling Prior to Immobilization

1. Add 1 µL aliquots of freshly prepared working stock R123 and PI solutions to 48 µL of *M. tuberculosis* cell suspension in a screw-topped 1.5 mL centrifuge tube. Final dye concentrations of 1 µ*M* and 3 µ*M*, respectively.
2. Mix thoroughly and incubate at 37°C for 15 min.
3. Pellet the cells by centrifugation at 10,000*g* for 2 min and discard the supernatant.
4. Wash the cells once with PBS, pellet by centrifugation, and resuspend thoroughly in 50 µL of SDW.
5. Deposit cells on APS-coated cover slips (*see* **Subheading 2.1.2.).**
6. Mount the cover slips in silicone fluid (*see* **Note 8**) on microscope slides and seal the edges with clear nail polish.
7. View cells using phase contrast and epifluorescence microscopy.

3.2.2. Labeling with Uncoupling Agent

In each experiment, samples of cells are labeled in the presence of the uncoupling agent CCCP to demonstrate that accumulation of R123 is dependent on cytoplasmic membrane potential. R123 labeling should be assessed as cytological activity only where labeling is shown to be uncoupler-sensitive (*see* **Note 9**).

1. Add 1 µL of freshly prepared CCCP stock solution to 49 µL of bacterial suspension in a 1.5 mL screw-topped centrifuge tube to give a final CCCP concentration of 150 µ*M* (*see* **Note 10**).
2. Mix thoroughly and incubate at 37°C for 15 min.
3. Label the CCCP-treated bacteria with R123/PI (*see* **Subheading 3.2.1.**).

3.2.3. Labeling After Immobilization

When large numbers of samples are being processed, it may be more convenient to immobilize the bacteria onto APS-coated cover slips before labeling. Background fluorescence tends to be slightly higher with this method.

1. Deposit 30 µL of each *M. tuberculosis* cell suspension onto APS-coated cover slips by centrifugation (*see* **Subheading 3.1.2.).**
2. Place the cover slips in polystyrene Petri dishes (50 mm) and immerse in 5 mL of PBS containing 1 µ*M* R123 and 3 µ*M* PI.
3. Incubate for 15 min.
4. Remove the labeling solution and gently wash the cover slips sequentially once with PBS and once with SDW.
5. Remove the SDW and leave the cover slips to dry.

6. Mount the cover slips in silicone fluid on microscope slides and seal the edges with clear nail polish.

3.2.4. Image Acquisition

1. View the preparation with a 100X oil immersion, phase contrast objective.
2. Acquire phase and fluorescence images from suitable fields of view to serve as the mask and data images.
3. R123 labeled cells fluoresce green and PI stained cells fluoresce red. These labels can be viewed simultaneously with Nikon B–2E filter block (excitation filter 450–490, barrier filter 520–560, dichroic mirror 510) (*see* **Note 11**).

3.2.5. Image Analysis

1. Analyze images using "Alpha" software as follows. An earlier version of this package and its use are described in Whiteley et al. *(2)*.
2. Use the phase contrast (mask) image to produce an outline of each cell; this and the contained pixels provide the mask defining the objects (cells) to be analyzed. The mask includes the morphometric data, and its superimposition on the fluorescence (data) image enables the signals therein to be quantified. Morphometric measurements obtained by image analysis include length, breadth, area, and perimeter of cells. Fluorometric measurements include integrated grey level (IGL) (sum of the 8 bit grey level intensity values for each of the objects pixels) and mean grey level (MGL) (IGL/number of pixels in object).
3. Save morphometric and intensity data to disc as comma-separated text files (*.prn files). Analyze comma-separated text files using spreadsheet, statistical, and graph-plotting computer programs. An example of analysis is shown in **Fig. 2**.

3.3. p-Iodonitrotetrazolium Violet (INT) Reduction — An Indicator of Cellular Oxidative Activity (see Note 12)

3.3.1. Labeling Procedure

1. Prepare cell suspensions of *M. tuberculosis* for INT labeling in sterile PBS, pH 7.3 (*see* **Subheading 3.1.1.**; *see* **Note 13**).
2. Add an equal volume of freshly prepared INT solution to the bacterial suspension in a 1.5 mL centrifuge tube, giving a final concentration of 1 m*M* INT (*see* **Note 14**).
3. Mix thoroughly and incubate at 37°C for 1 h (*see* **Note 15**). Samples with reduced INT become noticeably violet/purple.
4. Pellet the cells by centrifugation at 10,000*g* for 2 min, wash twice with PBS and deposit onto APS-coated cover slips (*see* **Subheading 3.1.2.**).
5. Mount the cover slips in PBS on microscope slides and seal the edges with clear nail polish.
6. View cells using phase contrast and brightfield microscopy.

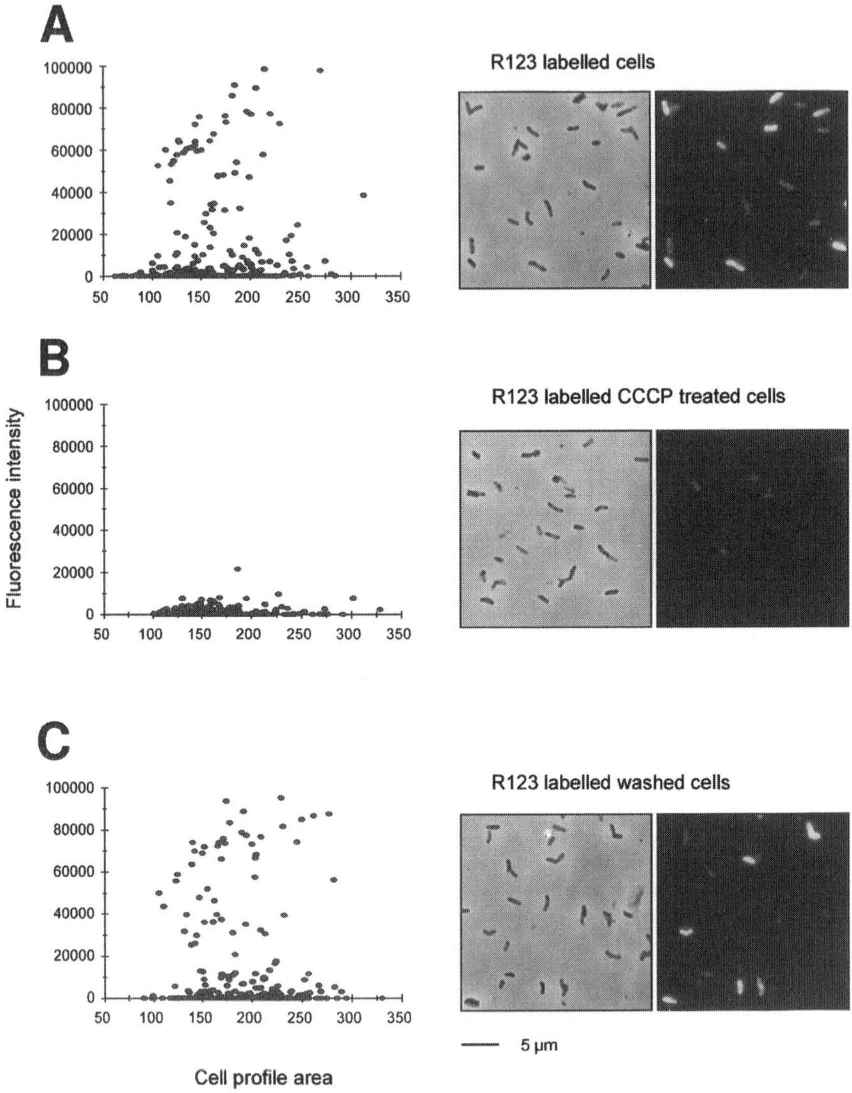

Fig. 2. Scatter plots showing uncoupler-sensitive accumulation of R123 by *M. tuberculosis* cells. Uncoupler sensitivity demonstrates that the R123 accumulation is due to membrane energization that can be short-circuited by CCCP and recovery after washing **(C)** show that the effect is reversible. We have found several treatments that produce cells that are insensitive to uncoupling. Both the mechanism of R123 labeling and its significance in these cells is uncertain. Bacteria were **(A)** labeled with 1 μ*M* R123, **(B)** treated with 150 μ*M* CCCP and labeled with R123, **(C)** treated with CCCP, washed in fresh broth, and labeled with R123. Phase contrast and fluorescence images of the same microscopic field of view are shown alongside results of image analysis of fluorescence intensity plotted against cell profile area. The scatter plots display cell signals according to size and fluorescence intensity and can help in the recognition of subpopulations.

3.3.2. Analysis of Results

1. Place the cover slip/slide on the microscope and view by phase contrast (100×). When a satisfactory field of view is obtained acquire and save an image of the cells.
2. Use this image to produce the mask (binary) image for subsequent analysis. The formazan deposits are best observed using brightfield illumination.
3. Focus on the same field of view, acquire and store the brightfield image. This is used as the data image.
4. Take densitiometric measurements from the brightfield (data) image and include integrated optical weight (IOW) (sum of the optical weights of each pixel of an object) and mean optical weight (MOW) (IOW/number of pixels in object) (*see* **Note 16**).

3.4. Gfp Expression (see Note 17)

1. For microscopy studies, harvest bacteria from agar or broth culture, wash with PBS, and deposit on APS-coated cover slips by centrifugation (*see* **Subheading 3.1.2.**).
2. Mount the cover slips in PBS on microscope slides and seal with clear nail polish.
3. View cells using phase contrast and epifluorescence microscopy with an FITC specific or Nikon B–2A filter combination (*see* **Subheading 2.2.2.**).
4. Results are analyzed as described for R123 (*see* **Subheading 3.2.5.**). Red signals are ignored.

3.5. Labeling of Lipid Domains (see Note 18)

3.5.1. Preparation and Storage of Liposomes

The procedure is adapted from that of New *(12)*. Dipalmitoyl L-α-phosphatidylcholine (DPPC) is used as the host lipid.

1. Weigh out accurately the desired amount of the fluorescent probe (routinely < 5 mg in our case) in a glass tube (6 cm in depth and with a Quickfit ground glass joint).
2. Add 40 mole equivalents of DPPC.
3. Dissolve in 5 mL of chloroform:methanol (2:1 v/v).
4. Dry the mixture *in vacuo* using a rotary evaporator (14 mmHg) for 3 h.
5. Add 5 mL of deionized water to the dry lipid mixture and place in a sonic bath. Sonicate continuously until all the lipid has been displaced from the sides of the tube.
6. Add a further 5 mL of deionized water to the tube and position it for sonication with the sonic probe. Thread a clean rubber sealing cap over the end of the probe to cover the tube which should be positioned so that the probe tip is 4 mm below the surface of the lipid suspension. In order to monitor the temperature during sonication, thread a thermocouple wire under the sealing cap and submerse in the lipid suspension, taking care it does not touch the probe.

7. Position an ice bath so that the contents of the tube are cooled during sonication.
8. Close the disintegrator cabinet and, with the power set at its lowest value, switch on the sonicator. Increase the power slowly until the amplitude of sonic radiation is 10 μm. Sonicate the mixture for 15 s at this amplitude and then switch off the power to allow the contents of the tube to cool to around 40°C (*see* **Note 19**). Repeat the sonication and cooling cycle until the mixture has had a total sonication time of 30 min.
9. Clean the probe by operating for 2 min in a large beaker of distilled water.
10. Dispense 1 mL aliquots of the liposome preparation into 1.5 mL centrifuge tubes and incubate these in a water bath at 50°C for 2 h to allow the "annealing" process to occur.
11. Centrifuge the liposome suspensions at 9000*g* for 1 min to pellet any metal particles shed from the probe. Remove the liposome supernatant and store with the exclusion of light at –20°C until required.

3.5.2. Labeling Mycobacteria with Liposome Suspensions

1. Dilute the stock liposome suspension 100-fold with deionized water and centrifuge for 10 min at 9,000*g* to pellet larger liposomes. Transfer the supernatant to a fresh microfuge tube. This is the working liposome suspension.
2. Prepare a mycobacterial suspension (OD_{580} = 0.2) in PBS (*see* **Subheading 3.1.1.**) and place 50 μL in a 1.5 mL centrifuge tube. Pellet the cells by centrifugation at 10,000*g* for 2 min.
3. Remove the supernatant and resuspend the pellet in 50 μL of the working liposome suspension.
4. Vortex the cell/liposome mixture briefly and incubate with the exclusion of light, at ambient temperature (approx 18–22°C) for 2 h.
5. Wash the cell/liposome mixture three times by alternate centrifugation and resuspension in 50 μL PBS.
6. Immobilize the labeled cells onto APS-coated cover slips (*see* **Subheading 3.1.2.**).
7. Mount the cover slips in PBS on microscope slides and seal the edges with clear nail polish.
8. Observe by phase contrast and epifluorescence microscopy with a Nikon B-2A filter combination (*see* **Subheading 2.2.2.**).

3.5.3. Staining Mycobacteria with Nile Red

1. Prepare a mycobacterial suspension (OD_{580} of 0.2) in PBS (*see* **Subheading 3.1.1.**) and place 50 μL in a 1.5 mL centrifuge tube.
2. Add 1 μL of Nile red stock solution. Vortex the mixture briefly, and incubate at 37°C for 10 min.
3. Wash the cells three times by alternate centrifugation and resuspension in 50 μL PBS.
4. Immobilize the labeled cells onto APS-coated cover slips (*see* **Subheading 3.1.2.**).

5. Mount the cover slips in PBS and seal the edges with clear nail polish.
6. Observe by phase contrast and epifluorescence microscopy with a Nikon G-2A filter combination (excitation filter 510–560, barrier filter 590, dichroic mirror 580).

3.5.4. Analysis of Results

Labeling with these methods produces either annular labeling, peripheral deposits apparently attached to the inner surface of the cell envelope, or internal deposits (inclusions). The pattern of labeling relates to the probe used and the physiological states of the organisms studied. These patterns can be recognized by direct observation in most cases. Where signals are weak, we have used the 16-bit cooled CCD camera (*see* **Subheading 2.5.2.**). We have also applied deconvolution algorithms according to the supplier's instructions to these images in order to display more detail *(2)*. Finally we have analyzed alkyl aminofluorescein and Nile red labeled images (*see* **Subheading 3.5.3.**) but have not found the results informative to date.

4. Notes

1. Although many publications implicitly or explicitly state that viability can be assayed at the cellular level by a variety of cytological methods, we consider that viability implies the capacity for replication and growth and have not found any method that can accurately predict these properties. In our view, direct demonstration of growth and replication by culture remains the only unambiguous operational definition of culturability applicable to bacteria. Although we have demonstrated R123 accumulation, INT reduction, and *gfp* expression in nonculturable *M. tuberculosis* cells on many occasions, we consider the viability of these cells to be indeterminate at present. Whereas these issues clearly have a bearing on the proposed dormancy states of *M. tuberculosis*, space precludes further discussion here and the reader is referred elsewhere ***(13–16)***.
2. Undiluted APS stock solution is stored at 4°C for a maximum of 1 mo as activity can fall rapidly with longer storage periods.
3. The 24-bit color images acquired using the camera/frame grabber described contain approx 1.3 MB of information. Iomega Zip disks (100 MB) prove a convenient and inexpensive means of storing these images without requiring computers with large memory. However, for long-term storage of large numbers of images, it is useful to have access to a CD writer.
4. INT is difficult to solubilize in water at 2 m*M* concentration; it is usually necessary to heat the mixture to 50°C followed by brief sonication to obtain a clear solution.
5. For safety reasons, cuvets containing *M. tuberculosis* cell suspensions are covered with laboratory sealing film and carefully sealed with tape. Alternatively, disposable polystyrene cuvets fitted with stoppers and sealed with tape may be used.

6. Although we originally developed the R123/PI and INT methods in order to determine viability at the cellular level, we now consider that definitive determinations at this level are not achievable by such indirect means and view these methods as indicators of physiological or biochemical activity. R123 is a cationic fluorescent dye originally used for selective labeling of mitochondria in living cells but has also proved to be an informative indicator of cellular activity in a wide range of bacteria including *M. smegmatis*, *M. bovis*, and *M. tuberculosis* ***(6–8)***. R123 is concentrated by cells with intact cytoplasmic membranes and membrane potential gradient. Membrane potential-dependent accumulation may be demonstrated by treatment with uncoupling agents which dissipate the electrochemical gradient ***(9)***.
7. We have used R123 labeling to assess the effect of antimycobacterial drugs on *M. tuberculosis*. The hydrophilic nucleic acid stain PI is included to identify cells with compromised cell envelopes. Although PI has a high affinity for DNA and RNA, its fluorescence yield is enhanced by binding to double-stranded DNA and intact cell envelopes exclude it.
8. Cells stained with R123 are mounted in silicone fluid to prevent leakage of accumulated dye; the dye quickly leaks from cells mounted in PBS resulting in poorly labeled cells and background fluorescence. We find that R123 labeled preparations mounted in silicone fluid may be stored for several days in the dark and do not fade significantly. Nonetheless, we prefer to view the cells and acquire images as soon as possible after staining.
9. We find that different tuberculocidal treatments, e.g., heat treatment (70°C for 30 min), 70% ethanol treatment, and 4% formaldehyde treatment, produce R123 labeled cells. However, this labeling is not sensitive to treatment with the uncoupler agent and therefore is not evidence of membrane potential. Nonspecific or energy independent labeling with R123 may be produced by binding of the dye to alternative cellular binding sites exposed/produced by the treatments.
10. Uncoupler sensitive accumulation of R123 by *M. tuberculosis* is demonstrated only where cells are treated with high concentrations of CCCP (150 μ*M*) and labeled with low concentrations of R123 (1 μ*M*). Higher concentrations of CCCP (10-fold higher than that normally used with nonmycobacterial species) may be necessary to produce uncoupling because of the additional barrier posed by the mycolic acid-containing layer of the mycobacterial cell envelope.
11. We use the red and green signals from our color camera to determine R123 and PI fluorescence, respectively; alternatively a monochrome camera could be used in combination with selective filter sets. The R123 emission spectrum extends into the red and this cross-talk between channels must be quantified with the specific set up used if PI signal quantitation is desired. Fluorescence from both dyes is relatively stable and fading does not occur quickly (i.e., there is little reduction in fluorescence intensity during observation). However, if fading is a problem, we recommend images are acquired with neutral density filters in the excitation path and extended integration times on the camera.

12. We have used the tetrazolium salt INT as a cytochemical indicator of oxidative metabolism in antibiotic-treated cultures of *M. tuberculosis*. INT is reduced intracellularly by physiologically active cells to an insoluble formazan deposit that is detected by light microscopy. Tetrazolium salts are redox indicators that are widely used to monitor oxidation reactions in biochemistry. As with R123, we developed the method as an indirect viability indicator but now consider the nomenclature inappropriate.
13. *M. tuberculosis* cell suspensions prepared in PBS produce larger INT formazan deposits than suspensions prepared in Middlebrook 7H9 broth.
14. Optimal reduction of INT by *M. tuberculosis* occurs at 1 m*M* INT. Higher concentrations of INT — such as those previously used in this laboratory with other bacteria, e.g., 10 m*M* with *Vibrio vulnificus* and *Pseudomonas putida* ***(17)*** and 5 m*M* with *Helicobacter pylori* ***(10)*** — are found to inhibit reduction.
15. INT formazan deposits increase in size with longer incubation times. We find that deposits formed after 1 h incubation are easily detectable by microscopy. With longer incubations, deposits become very large, producing swollen cells that may lyse.
16. Optical weight is a validated estimate of optical density and is determined per pixel. The IOW represents the sum of oxidative activity in a cell that produces reducing equivalents capable of reducing INT. This is determined by the availability of oxidizable substrates inside and outside the cells studied. A specific pattern of external substrate-accelerated tetrazolium reduction can be obtained from most bacteria we have studied ***(10)***. However, in limited studies we have found that INT reduction by *M. tuberculosis* is relatively uninfluenced by different exogenous substrate sources.
17. We have used *gfp* expression from the HSP60 promoter on pGFM11 ***(11)*** for our studies. We have examined the effects of antibiotics on levels of expression and have found the approach useful for studying cells that could not be labeled by the R123/PI or INT methods. The approach has much to offer for tracing cells in animal infections and, when coupled with fusions to specific promoters, to determine heterogeneity of expression within populations and location specific (e.g., intracellular) expression. *Gfp* is quite stable and the protein may take up to 4 h to become fluorescent. Thus, where relevant, careful consideration must be given to the likely timing of expression in relation to when the sample was taken.
18. Although a great deal is known about the lipid composition of *M. tuberculosis*, there remain considerable uncertainties about the distributions of the known lipid molecules within the cell. Moreover, it is not known whether cells in a population are heterogeneous with respect to these properties since such heterogeneity is not detected by chemical analysis. We have used labeling with lipophilic probes to address these issues ***(2)***. We describe a liposome-based and a direct labeling method. We have found that direct application of probes dissolved in chloroform or centrifugation of cells onto Langmuir-Blodget lipid films containing the probes does not produce technically satisfactory results although we feel the latter method is worthy of further consideration.

19. 40°C is the gel/fluid phase transition temperature (T_c) for DPPC. Below the T_c, breaking and resealing of vesicles does not occur efficiently, however, the temperature should not be allowed to rise above 60°C in order to prevent oxidative or thermal degradation of the lipid.

Acknowledgments

Plasmid pGFM11, GFP-expressing mycobacterial cloning vector, Kan^R $Strep^R$ (Kremer et al., 1995) was kindly provided by Dr. Camille Locht, Laboratoire de Microbiologie Génétique et Microbiologie, Institute Pasteur de Lille, F–59019 Lille Cedex, France. Work contributing to the methods described has been supported by the Medical Research Council and the Wellcome Trust.

References

1. Whiteley, A. S., Grewal, R., Hunt, A., and Barer, M. B. (1998) Determining biochemical and physiological phenotypes of bacteria by cytological assay, in *Digital Image Analysis of Microbes* (Wilkinson, M. H. F. and Schut, F., eds.), John Wiley and Sons, Chichester, pp. 281–307.
2. Christensen, H., Garton N. J., Horobin, R. W., Minnikin, D. E., and Barer, M. R. (1999) Lipid domains of mycobacteria studied with fluorescent molecular probes. *Mol. Microbiol.* **36,** 1561–1572.
3. Barer, M. R. (1991) New possibilities for bacterial cytochemistry: light microscopical demonstration of beta-galactosidase in unfixed immobilized bacteria. *Histochem. J.* **23,** 529–533.
4. Walker, D. R., Nwoguh, C. E., and Barer, M. R. (1994) A microchamber system for the rapid cytochemical demonstration of beta-galactosidase and other properties in pathogenic microbes. *Lett. Appl. Microbiol.* **18,** 102–104.
5. Paddock, S. W. (1999) Confocal microscopy methods and protocols, in *Methods in Molecular Biology*, vol. 122. Humana, Totawa, NJ, 446 pp.
6. Matsuyama, T. (1984) Staining of living bacteria with rhodamine-123. *FEMS Microbiol. Lett.* **21,** 153–157.
7. Resnick, M., Schuldiner, S., and Bercovier, H. (1985) Bacterial-membrane potential analyzed by spectrofluorocytometry. *Curr. Microbiol.* **12,** 183–185.
8. Bercovier, H., Resnick, M., Kornitzer, D., and Levy, L., (1987) Rapid method for testing drug-susceptibility of mycobacteria spp and gram-positive bacteria using rhodamine-123 and fluorescein diacetate. *J. Microbiol. Met.* **7,** 139–142.
9. Kaprelyants, A. S. and Kell, D. B. (1992) Rapid assessment of bacterial viability and vitality by rhodamine 123 and flow-cytometry. *J. Appl. Bacteriol.* **72,** 410–422.
10. Gribbon, L. T. and Barer, M. R. (1995) Oxidativemetabolism in nonculturable *Helicobacter pylori* and *Vibrio vulnificus* cells studied by substrate-enhanced tetrazolium reduction and digital image-processing. *Appl. Environ. Microbiol.* **61,** 3379–3384.

11. Kremer, L., Baulard, A., Estaquier, J., Poulaingodefroy, O., and Locht, C., (1995) Green fluorescent protein as a new expression marker in mycobacteria. *Mol. Microbiol.* **17,** 913–922.
12. New, R. R. C. (1990) Preparation of liposomes, in *Liposomes: A Practical Approach* (New, R. R. C., ed.), IRL, Oxford, pp. 33–103.
13. Nwoguh, C. E., Harwood, C. R., and Barer, M. R. (1995) Detection of induced beta-galactosidase activity in individual non-culturable cells of pathogenic bacteria by quantitative cytological assay. *Mol. Microbiol.* **17,** 545–554.
14. Barer, M. R. (1997) Viable but non-culturable and dormant bacteria: time to resolve an oxymoron and a misnomer? *J. Med. Microbiol.* **46,** 629–631.
15. Kell, D. B., Kaprelyants, A. S., Weichart, D. H., Harwood, C. R., and Barer, M. R. (1998) Viability and activity in readily culturable bacteria: a review and discussion of the practical issues. *Antonie Van Leeuwenhoek.* **73,** 169–187.
16. Barer, M. R. and Harwood, C. R. (1999) Bacterial viability and culturability. *Adv. Microb. Physiol.* **41,** in press.
17. Whiteley, A. S., O'Donnell, A. G., Macnaughton, S. J., and Barer, M. R. (1996) Cytochemical colocalization and quantitation of phenotypic and genotypic characteristics in individual bacterial cells. *Appl. Environ. Microbiol.* **62,** 1873–1879.

10

Phage Replication Technology for Diagnosis and Drug Susceptibility Testing

Ruth McNerney

1. Introduction

Of the world's infectious diseases, tuberculosis remains the leading cause of mortality and it has been estimated that of the eight million new cases that occur each year 95% are found in the less developed countries *(1,2)*. Diagnostic methods that involve culture of *Mycobacterium tuberculosis* are necessarily slow due to the protracted growth times required by these bacteria. Rapid molecular tests have been developed for both diagnosis *(3)* and drug resistance testing *(4)*. However, the high costs and requirement for specialized equipment prohibits the routine application of this technology in low-income countries, and there is an urgent need for sensitive, rapid tests that are affordable and appropriate for use in these areas of the world *(5)*.

The first bacteriophage found to infect the mycobacteria was isolated in 1947 *(6)* and over 250 mycobacteriophages (phages) have since been identified *(7)*. Although phages were utilized for typing isolates of tuberculosis *(8)*, they were not previously used in routine diagnosis. In recent years the potential of mycobacteriophages has been reexamined following the application of luciferase reporter phages to drug susceptibility testing in 1993 *(9,10)*. In 1965, Tokunaga and Sellers *(11)* had demonstrated that the antituberculosis drug streptomycin blocked phage replication in susceptible mycobacteria although not interrupting replication in a drug-resistant strain; similar effects were later shown with both kanamycin *(12)* and rifampicin *(13)*. In 1980, after investigating the inhibitory effects of seven drugs, David and colleagues *(14)* concluded that phages could be used to screen for antibacterial agents and that they might be used for testing the "difficult to grow" mycobacteria.

From: *Methods in Molecular Medicine*, vol. 54: *Mycobacterium Tuberculosis Protocols*
Edited by: T. Parish and N. G. Stoker © Humana Press Inc., Totowa, NJ

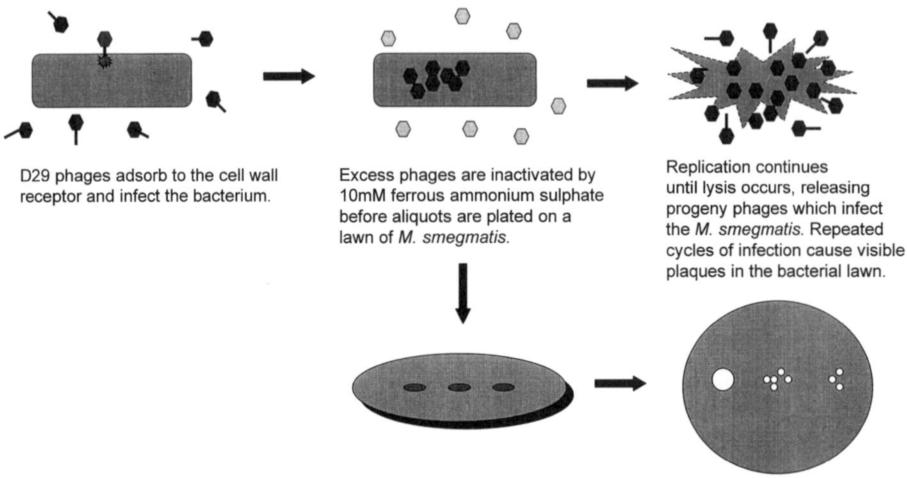

Fig. 1. Principles of phage replication assay.

David et al. ***(13–15)*** worked with mycobacteriophage D29, a lytic virus that infects a wide range of mycobacteria including *M. tuberculosis* and fast-growing saprophytic strains such as *Mycobacterium smegmatis*. Detection of progeny phages following infection was by plating onto a lawn of *M. smegmatis* bacteria where repeated cycles of infection and lysis caused clear areas known as plaques within the bacterial lawn. The plaques were visible after an overnight incubation at 37°C, and they were able to use *M. smegmatis* as the "universal indicator bacteria" for the rapid detection of D29 phages propagated in slow-growing strains of mycobacteria ***(15)***. When detecting progeny phages, it is desirable to remove those viruses that did not take part in infection but remain free in the culture media. Treatment with acid or sodium hydroxide may be used but reaction conditions have to be carefully controlled in order to prevent damage to host bacteria by these toxic reagents. The discovery that ferrous (iron II) salts inactivate D29 phages although not harming mycobacteria or those phages replicating inside them has enabled sensitive methods of detection to be developed (**Fig. 1**) ***(16)***. This simple technology has been applied both to drug susceptibility testing and to the detection of *M. tuberculosis* in clinical specimens.

Screening mycobacteria for susceptibility to those drugs that block phage replication, such as rifampicin or streptomycin, may be performed in less than 24 h. However, phages are only able to replicate in bacteria that are metabolically active, and slow-growing mycobacteria isolated on solid media require activation in broth before infection. Thus, when screening isolates of

M. tuberculosis grown on Lowenstein-Jensen (LJ), the bacteria are incubated in broth for at least 16 h before incubation with phages. A convenient microwell plate format has been adopted for rapid screening against rifampicin to reduce "hands on time" and enable the screening of large numbers of isolates ***(17)***. Drugs such as ethambutol and isoniazid do not block phage replication directly and are not active against bacteria at all stages of the cell cycle ***(14,18)***. When screening *M. tuberculosis* for resistance to these drugs, several days preincubation with the bacteria under test are necessary if accurate results are to be obtained ***(19)***. While the assay described here has been optimized for screening slow-growing species such as *M. tuberculosis*, D29 will infect a wide range of mycobacteria and the test can be adapted to screen fast-growing species. However, for accurate results, incubation times need to be adjusted due to the more rapid growth and cycle of infection of these organisms. When detecting mycobacteria in clinical specimens, such as sputum, pretreatment is required to decontaminate the sample and to separate the bacteria from mucous material or release intracellular organisms, thus permitting phage adsorption and infection to take place.

The simplicity and low-cost of this technology suggests it may be appropriate for transfer to laboratories in the less developed countries. Stocks of the phages and *M. smegmatis* indicator bacteria may be maintained "in-house" and indicator plates may be prepared in advance and stored at 4°C. The method requires no specialized equipment other than that utilized in the routine microbiology laboratory; however, stringent safety precautions should be observed when handling *M. tuberculosis* and all work with these organisms should be performed in a P3 microbiological safety facility. A commercial kit based on phage technology is marketed by Biotech Laboratories Ltd, Ipswich, UK.

2. Methods

2.1. Propagation of Mycobacteriophage D29

1. *Mycobacterium smegmatis* mc^2155 ***(20)*** (William R. Jacobs Jr., Howard Hughes Medical Institute, Albert Einstein College of Medicine, New York) or *M. smegmatis* 607 (American Type Culture Collection, Rockville, MD). Maintain stocks on solid medium.
2. Initial stocks of D29 ***(21)*** were obtained from Tanya Parish, London School of Hygiene & Tropical Medicine, London, UK. Phage stocks may be maintained in-house as described, prepared stocks of phages should remain viable for several months when stored at 4°C and for over 12 mo if lyophilized (*see* **Notes 1** and **2**).
3. Middlebrook 7H9 (Difco Laboratories, Detroit, MI). Middlebrook broth should be prepared according to the manufacturer's instructions and supplemented with 10% OADC (Difco Laboratories). For the culture of *M. tuberculosis*, add 0.2% glycerol. For infection by D29 add 1 m*M* calcium chloride. For agar plates, add 15 g/L Bacto agar prior to autoclaving. Storage is at room temperature, out of

direct sunlight. The detergent polyoxyethylenesorbitan (Tween) may not be included as it blocks adsorption of phages to the cell wall.

4. 0.45 µm filters (Whatman International Ltd, Maidstone, UK).

2.2. Production of Indicator Plates

1. Middlebrook 7H9 and *M. smegmatis* (*see* **Subheading 2.1., items 1** and **2**).
2. Luria-Bertani broth (LB) (Difco Laboratories) for the preparation of indicator plates and for testing susceptibilities to rifampicin and streptomycin. LB should be prepared according to the manufacturer's instructions (Difco) or can be prepared from its constituents: 10 g/L Tryptone, 5 g/L yeast extract, 10 g/L sodium chloride. For phage infection add 0.2% glucose and 1 m*M* calcium chloride (not required when preparing indicator plates).
3. Assay broth: LB broth containing 0.2% glucose and 1 m*M* calcium chloride.

2.3. Microwell Phage Replication Assay for Susceptibility to Rifampicin and Streptomycin

1. *M. smegmatis* SMR5 ***(22)***, a streptomycin-resistant strain (Peter Sander, Institut fur Medizinische Mikrobiologie, Hanover). *M. smegmatis* SMR5 should be maintained in 20 µg/mL streptomycin (*see* **Note 3**).
2. *M. tuberculosis* H37Rv (American Type Culture Collection, Rockville, MD). *M. tuberculosis* strains are maintained on LJ slopes (E & O Laboratories Ltd, Burnhouse, Scotland) (*see* **Note 4**).
3. Sterile flat bottom 96-well microtiter plates with lids (Greiner Labortechnik, Stonehouse, UK).
4. Disposable triple vented Petri dishes (Greiner Labortechnik).
5. Disposable 1 µL loops (Greiner Labortechnik).
6. Self-sealing polythene bags (Merck Ltd, Poole, UK).
7. 2.5 mm glass beads (Stratech Scientific Ltd, Luton, UK).
8. Ferrous ammonium sulfate hexadydrate (FAS) (Sigma-Aldrich Co. Ltd, Poole, UK). Solutions are not stable and should be prepared daily. Stock solutions of 100 m*M* are prepared in sterile water. Working stock solution of 30 m*M* is prepared in LB with 1 m*M* calcium chloride.
9. Antibiotic stock solutions. 10 mg/mL rifampicin in dimethyl formamide and 10 mg/mL streptomycin (Sigma-Aldrich Co. Ltd, Poole, UK). Store at –20°C for up to 6 mo. Dilute to the appropriate drug concentration in assay broth (**Subheading 2.2., step 3**). Prepare fresh on the day of use.
10. D29 phage (*see* **Subheading 2.1., step 2**).
11. *M. smegmatis* mc^2155 and *M. smegmatis* SMR5 indicator plates (*see* **Subheading 3.2.**)

2.4. Screening for Susceptibility to Isoniazid and Ethambutol

1. Antibiotic stock solutions: isoniazid (1 mg/mL) and ethambutol (2 mg/mL) in water (Sigma-Aldrich Co. Ltd). Store at –20°C for up to 6 mo. Dilute to the

appropriate drug concentration in assay broth (**Subheading 2.2., step 3**). Prepare fresh on the day of use.
2. Disposable triple vented Petri dishes (Greiner Labortechnik).
3. Disposable 1 µL loops (Greiner Labortechnik).
4. Self-sealing polythene bags (Merck Ltd, Poole, UK).
5. 2.5 mm glass beads (Stratech Scientific Ltd, Luton, UK).
6. 100 m*M* ferrous ammonium sulfate in sterile water.
7. Indicator plates (*see* **Subheading 3.2.**).

2.5. Detection of Mycobacteria in Sputum

1. Sodium hydroxide solution: 4% NaOH, 0.1 *M* trisodium citrate, 0.5% N-acetyl cysteine (Sigma-Aldrich Co. Ltd, Poole, UK).
2. 7H9 with OADC, glycerol and calcium chloride (*see* **Subheading 2.1., step 3**).
3. 50 m*M* ferrous ammonium sulfate (FAS).

3. Methods

3.1. Propagation of Mycobacteriophage D29 (see Note 5)

1. Mix Middlebrook 7H9 (with OADC and agar) and a 10% volume of stationary phase *M. smegmatis* mc^{2}155 culture and pour into a 90 mm Petri dish.
2. Inoculate by spreading 100 µL of D29 at approx 4×10^3 plaque-forming units (pfu)/mL in Middlebrook 7H9 broth with 1 m*M* calcium chloride.
3. Place in 37°C incubator and leave overnight.
4. Examine for bacterial growth; large numbers of plaques should be visible but lysis of the bacterial lawn should not be complete. If no bacterial lawn is visible, repeat plating with a more dilute suspension of phages.
5. Add 10 mL Middlebrook 7H9 with 10% OADC and 1 m*M* calcium chloride to the plate and return to 37°C incubator for a further overnight incubation.
6. Remove the broth and filter it through two sterile 0.45 µm filters to remove bacteria and debris. Aliquot and store at 4°C. Do not freeze and avoid exposure to UV light. 0.1% sodium azide may be added as a preservative (*see* **Note 6**).
7. To quantify the phage suspension, make 10-fold serial dilutions and spot 10 µL aliquots of each dilution onto a *M. smegmatis* indicator plate (*see* **Subheading 3.2.**). Use a fresh pipet tip for each dilution. Count the number of plaque forming units (pfu) visible after overnight incubation at 37°C. The phage stock should contain between 10^9 and 10^{10} pfu/mL.

3.2. Production of Indicator Plates

1. Seed 300 mL of Middlebrook 7H9/OADC broth in a 500 mL bottle with a single colony of *M. smegmatis*. Shake to mix and incubate at 37°C for 2 d until stationary phase is reached.
2. Store at 4°C until required (up to one month). Before using gently mix the suspension and leave to stand for a few minutes to allow any large clumps of bacteria to settle.

3. Prepare molten 1.5% bacto agar in LB broth and cool to approx 45°C before adding a 10–15% vol of *M. smegmatis* culture. Mix by inversion and pour into 90 mm Petri dishes (*see* **Notes 7** and **8**).
4. Store, sealed at 4°C for up to 2 wk. Prior to using, remove any surface liquid by drying in an incubator. Label plates with a marker pen.

3.3. Microwell Phage Replication Assay for Susceptibility to Rifampicin and Streptomycin

1. Prepare solutions of rifampicin or streptomycin at 0, 4, and 20 μg/mL (twice test concentration) in assay broth (*see* **Note 9**). Place 75 μL aliquots in the wells of a sterile microtiter plate.
2. Prepare *M. tuberculosis* cultured on LJ slope by transferring a 1 μL loopful to 2 mL assay broth in a bijou bottle with 4–8 glass beads (*see* **Note 4**). Vortex for 20 s to disperse the bacteria and leave to stand for 3 min to allow aerosols to settle.
3. Prepare a wild-type strain or *M. tuberculosis* H37Rv as a reference strain.
4. Place 75 μL of bacteria in each well containing the appropriate concentration of drug. Cover plate and seal in a plastic bag before incubating at 37°C for 24 h (*see* **Note 10**).
5. Prepare a suspension of phages at 10^8/mL in assay broth with drug at 0, 2, or 10 μg/mL and add 50 μL to the appropriate wells. Reseal plate and replace in 37°C incubator for 90 min.
6. Dry indicator plates and label with a marker pen.
7. To each well add 100 μL freshly prepared 30 m*M* FAS working stock. Mix by pipeting and place a 10 μL drop onto the surface of a *M. smegmatis* SMR5 indicator plate. Use a fresh pipet tip for each well. When the drops have been absorbed, plates may be sealed in plastic bags and placed in the incubator (*see* **Note 10**). Twelve samples (four strains) may be spotted on a single 90-mm plate, but care should be taken to ensure spots do not merge and contaminate each other
8. After overnight incubation record lysis (*see* **Notes 11–15**). Strains that produce plaques at concentrations of drug that inhibit plaque formation in the wild-type or reference strain are classed as resistant. If a strain fails to produce a high degree of lysis in the zero drug sample, then the result is invalid and the test should be repeated.

3.4. Screening for Susceptibility to Isoniazid and Ethambutol

1. Prepare solutions of isoniazid at 0, 0.4, and 10 μg/mL and ethambutol at 0, 16, and 30 μg/mL in assay broth. Place 1 mL in sterile bijou bottles.
2. Prepare *M. tuberculosis* from LJ slope by transferring a 1 μL loopful to 3.5 mL Middlebrook 7H9 supplemented with OADC, 0.2% glycerol and 1 m*M* calcium chloride with 4–8 glass beads (*see* **Note 4**). Vortex for 20 s to dissipate the bacteria and leave to stand for 3 min to allow aerosols to disperse.
3. Prepare a wild-type strain or *M. tuberculosis* H37Rv as a reference strain.
4. Place 1 mL of bacteria in each drug concentration and incubate at 37°C for 3 d.

5. Add 200 µL of a suspension of 3 × 10^8 D29 phages in Middlebrook 7H9 supplemented with 2 m*M* calcium chloride. Mix and incubate at 37°C for 90 min.
6. Prepare indicator plates.
7. Add 200 µL freshly prepared 100 m*M* FAS. Mix by vortexing.
8. Spot 10 µL aliquots on the surface of the indicator plate. When the drops have been absorbed plates may be sealed in plastic bags and placed in the incubator (*see* **Note 10**).
9. After overnight incubation record lysis (*see* **Notes 11–15**). Strains that produce plaques at concentrations of drug that inhibit plaque formation in the wild-type or reference strain are classed as resistant. If a strain fails to produce a high degree of lysis in the zero drug sample then the result is invalid and the test should be repeated.

3.5. Detection of Mycobacteria in Sputum

Detection of viable *M. tuberculosis* bacteria within clinical specimens such as sputum requires pretreatment to remove fast-growing organisms that could contaminate the test. Treatment is also required to separate the bacteria from mucous material and to release intracellular organisms, thus permitting phage adsorption and infection to take place (*see* **Note 1**).

1. Treat sputum specimen with an equal volume of sodium hydroxide solution for 15 min.
2. Dilute with 10 vol of sterile water and sediment by centrifugation at 3000*g* for 15 min.
3. Resuspend in 7H9 broth (with OADC, glycerol and calcium chloride) to twice the original volume and incubate at 37°C. To allow the mycobacteria to recuperate after the harsh decontamination treatment specimens should be cultured for at least 24 h prior to testing.
4. Control tubes containing no specimen and a tube containing 5 × 10^4 cfu *M. tuberculosis* H37Rv should be included with each batch processed.
5. Vortex samples and allow to stand for 3 min to allow aerosols to settle.
6. Add a 0.5 vol of D29 phages (10^8 pfu/mL) in Middlebrook 7H9 and 2 m*M* calcium chloride, mix and incubate at 37°C for 90 min.
7. Prepare molten 1.5% agar in LB broth, and cool to approx 50°C in a water bath.
8. Add 0.2 vol of 50 m*M* FAS and mix.
9. Place 1 mL of stationary phase *M. smegmatis* mc^2155 in a universal bottle, add 9 mL of molten LB agar and one 1 mL of sample. Mix by inversion and pour into a 90 mm Petri dish.
10. Allow to set before sealing in plastic bags and incubating at 37°C for 16 h.
11. Examine plates for lysis. The presence of plaques indicates the presence of viable mycobacteria in the original specimen. If no plaques are seen in the *M. tuberculosis* H37Rv positive control sample or plaques are observed in the negative control sample then discard results and retest with fresh reagents.

4. Notes

1. Mycobacteriophage D29 infects a wide range of mycobacteria and is not specific for *M. tuberculosis*. Speciation of mycobacteria should be undertaken by biochemical or molecular tests. It has been shown that p-nitro-alpha-acetylamino-beta-hydroxy propiophenone will inhibit phage replication in members of the *M. tuberculosis* complex but not in other mycobacteria and thus may be used to confirm the presence of *M. tuberculosis* complex bacteria ***(23)***.
2. Phages may be lyophilized with 0.1 vol of 0.75 *M* trehalose (Sigma-Aldrich, Poole, UK). Store at room temperature, avoid exposure to UV light. Rehydrate by adding sterile water to the original volume.
3. *M. smegmatis* mc^{2}155 or ATCC 607 may be used for propagation of phages. Either strain may be used as the indicator bacteria for testing susceptibility to rifampicin as they are naturally resistant to this drug. However, when testing susceptibility to streptomycin a resistant strain such as *M. smegmatis* SMR5 should be used as the indicator strain.
4. For susceptibility tests, it is recommended that cultures grown on LJ slopes for longer than 3 mo and those stored at 4°C be subcultured before testing.
5. In the event of contamination of work surfaces or instruments with phages, clean with bleach and 70% alcohol.
6. Sodium azide is toxic and may cause explosive mixtures in the presence of copper. Manufacturers' safety data sheets and local safety regulations should be consulted before handling this substance.
7. When preparing indicator plates, do not allow the molten agar to cool below 40°C as the *M. smegmatis* bacteria may not mix sufficiently to provide a uniform lawn. Alternatively, take care not to add bacteria while the agar is too hot. It is convenient to use a water bath at 45°C when handling large volumes.
8. When preparing indicator plates, use triple vented plastic Petri dishes in preference to glass. When using glass, always dry the indicator plates before using as they are prone to condensation.
9. The microwell assay may also be performed using Middlebook 7H9 broth with OADC and calcium chloride to replace the LB broth.
10. Plates are sealed in plastic bags to prevent drying by evaporation. To enhance safety, plates or tubes containing infectious material should be placed in sealed plastic boxes.
11. If growth of the *M. smegmatis* lawn on the indicator plates is not sufficient following overnight incubation, then leave at 37°C for longer. Use fresh *M. smegmatis* or increase the volume added when preparing the plates. Check that the bacteria are added when the molten agar is at 45°C.
12. If plaques are indistinct, check the viability of phage stocks and ensure calcium is included in the broth. Precipitation on the indicator plates following spotting may be caused by excess FAS or calcium chloride, less precipitation is observed when using LB broth than with Middlebrook 7H9. Yellow food coloring (Egg yellow 20 μL/mL, Supercook, Leeds, UK) may be added to the molten agar mix to facilitate identification of plaques.

13. If contamination with other microorganisms occurs, check the sterility of all reagents, and clean and decontaminate the working area.
14. If bacteria exposed to zero drug fail to produce plaques, then those bacteria are either dead, dormant, or not susceptible to infection by the phage. Retest with a fresh culture.
15. If plaques are produced from every sample, including negative controls of drug treated wild-type strains, then inactivation of exogenous phages was not effective. Repeat assay using fresh FAS.

Acknowledgments

We are grateful to Dr. Peter Sander, Institut fur Medizinische Mikrobiologie, Hanover, Germany for the gift of *M. smegmatis* SMR5 and William R. Jacobs, Jr., Howard Hughes Medical Institute, Albert Einstein College of Medicine, New York for the gift of *M. smegmatis* mc^2155. This study was funded by the Department for International Development, UK.

References

1. Dye, C., Scheele, S., Dolin, P., Pathania, V., and Raviglione, M. C. (1999) Global burden of tuberculosis. Estimated incidence, prevalence and mortality by country. *J. Amer. Med. Assoc.* **282,** 677–686.
2. Raviglione, M. C., Snider, D. E., Jr., and Kochi, A. (1995) Global epidemiology of tuberculosis. Morbidity and mortality of a worldwide epidemic. *J. Amer. Med. Assoc.* **273,** 220–226.
3. Sandin, R. L. (1996) Polymerase chain reaction and other amplification techniques in mycobacteriology. *Clin. Lab. Med.* **16,** 617–639.
4. Telenti, A. and Persing, D. H. (1996) Novel strategies for the detection of drug resistance in *Mycobacterium tuberculosis. Res. Microbiol.* **147,** 73–79.
5. McNerney, R. (1996) Diagnosis: present difficulties and prospects for the future. *Africa Health* **19,** 22–23.
6. Gardner, G. M. and Weiser, R. S. (1947) A bacteriophage for *Mycobacterium smegmatis. Proc. Soc. Exp. Biol. Med.* **66,** 205–206.
7. McNerney, R. (1999) TB: the return of the phage. A review of fifty years of mycobacteriophage research. *Int. J. Tuberc. Lung Dis.* **3,** 179–184.
8. Redmond, W. B. and Ward, D. M. (1966) Media and methods for phage-typing mycobacteria. *Bull. World Health Organ.* **35,** 563–568.
9. Jacobs, W. R., Jr., Barletta, R. G., Udani, R., Chan, J., Kalkut, G., Sosne, G., Kieser, T., Sarkis, G. J., Hatfull, G. F., and Bloom, B. R. (1993) Rapid assessment of drug susceptibilities of *Mycobacterium tuberculosis* by means of luciferase reporter phages. *Science* **260,** 819–822.
10. Riska, P. F. and Jacobs, W. R., Jr. (1998) The use of luciferase-reporter phage for antibiotic-susceptibility testing of mycobacteria, in *Methods in Molecular Biology*, vol. 101 (Parish, T. and Stoker, N. G., eds.) Humana, Totowa, NJ, pp. 431–455.
11. Tokunaga, T. and Sellers, M. I. (1965) Streptomycin induction of premature lysis of bacteriophage-infected mycobacteria. *J. Bacteriol.* **89,** 537–538.

12. Nakamura, R. M., Tokunaga, T., and Murohashi, T. (1967) Premature lysis of bacteriophage-infected mycobacteria induced by kanamycin. *Amer. Rev. Respir. Dis.* **96,** 542–544.
13. Jones, W. D., Jr. and David, H. L. (1971) Inhibition by rifampin of mycobacteriophage D29 replication in its drug-resistant host, *Mycobacterium smegmatis* ATCC 607. *Amer. Rev. Respir. Dis.* **103,** 618–624.
14. David, H. L., Clavel, S., Clement, F., and Moniz Pereira, J. (1980) Effects of antituberculosis and antileprosy drugs on mycobacteriophage D29 growth. *Antimicrob. Agents Chemother.* **18,** 357–359.
15. David, H. L., Clavel, S., and Clement, F. (1980) Adsorption and growth of the bacteriophage D29 in selected mycobacteria. *Ann. Virol.* **131,** 167–184.
16. McNerney, R., Wilson, S. M., Sidhu, A. M., Harley, V. S., al Suwaidi, Z., Nye, P. M., Parish, T., and Stoker, N. G. (1998) Inactivation of mycobacteriophage D29 using ferrous ammonium sulphate as a tool for the detection of viable *Mycobacterium smegmatis* and *M. tuberculosis*. *Res. Microbiol.* **149,** 487–495.
17. McNerney, R., Kiepiela, P., Bishop, K. S., Nye, P. M., and Stoker, N. G. (2000) Rapid screening of *Mycobacterium tuberculosis* for susceptibility to rifampicin and streptomycin. *Int. J. Tuberc. Lung Dis.* **4,** 69–75.
18. Phillips, L. M. and Sellers, M. I. (1970) Effects of ethambutol, actinomycin D and mitomycin C on the biosynthesis of D29-infected *Mycobacterium smegmatis*., in Host-virus relationships in Mycobacterium, nocardia and actinomyces (Juhasz, S. E. and Plummer, G., eds.), Charles C Thomas, Springfield, IL, pp. 80–102.
19. Wilson, S. M., al Suwaidi, Z., McNerney, R., Porter, J., and Drobniewski, F. (1997) Evaluation of a new rapid bacteriophage-based method for the drug susceptibility testing of *Mycobacterium tuberculosis*. *Nat. Med.* **3,** 465–468.
20. Snapper, S. B., Melton, R. E., Mustafa, S., Kieser, T., and Jacobs, W. R., Jr. (1990) Isolation and characterization of efficient plasmid transformation mutants of *Mycobacterium smegmatis*. *Mol. Microbiol.* **4,** 1911–1919.
21. Sander, P., Meier, A., and Bottger, E. C. (1995) rspL+: a dominant selectable marker for gene replacement in mycobacteria. *Mol. Microbiol.* **16,** 991–1000.
22. Froman, S., Will, D. W., and Bogen, E., (1954). Bacteriophage active against virulent *Mycobacterium tuberculosis*. I. Isolation and activity. *Am. J. Public Health* **44,** 1326.
23. Riska, P. F., Jacobs, W. R., Jr., Bloom, B. R., McKitrick, J., and Chan, J., (1997). Specific identification of *Mycobacterium tuberculosis* with the luciferase reporter mycobacteriophage: use of p-nitro-alpha-acetylamino-beta-hydroxy propiophenone. *J. Clin. Microbiol.* **35,** 3225.

11

Detection of Mutations in *Mycobacterium tuberculosis* by a Dot Blot Hybridization Strategy

Thomas C. Victor and Paul D. van Helden

1. Introduction

Genomic variation in any organism is of interest, because it may influence the phenotype of the organism. Special interest currently focuses on prokaryotic pathogens regarding mutations associated with resistance to therapeutic drugs, as well as those mutations involved in the evolution of the bacillus. The molecular basis of drug resistance in *Mycobacterium tuberculosis* to the front-line drugs is not mediated via plasmids, but is largely, if not entirely, owing to mutations in specific genes of *M. tuberculosis*. To date, 13 genes are known to be linked to resistance and many functional mutations have been described in these genes *(1,2)*. However, the *katG463* (Arg→Leu) and *gyrA95* (Thr→Ser) mutations have no apparent relationship to drug resistance, and the combination of these two polymorphisms has been used to place clinical isolates of the *M. tuberculosis* complex into three evolutionary distinct genotypic groups *(3)*.

Many strategies have been used to detect mutations in genes of interest, including DNA sequencing ***(1,4)***, dideoxy-fingerprinting ***(5,6)***, heteroduplex analysis ***(6)***, restriction fragment length polymorphism (RFLP) analysis ***(4,7)***, single-stranded conformational polymorphism (SSCP) analysis ***(4,8)***, and the use of probes for hybridization ***(9,10)***. Each system has inherent problems: for example, not all mutations result in the gain or loss of a restriction enzyme site, therefore limiting the use of RFLP analysis as a general method to screen for mutations. Other screening procedures that depend on DNA mobility shifts (e.g., PCR-SSCP) are often used, but are technically demanding and mutations are not always detected by these procedures. PCR amplification followed by DNA sequencing is a widely used technique for the identification of mutations, but is not readily available in routine laboratories. Furthermore, in countries

From: *Methods in Molecular Medicine*, vol. 54: *Mycobacterium Tuberculosis Protocols*
Edited by: T. Parish and N. G. Stoker © Humana Press Inc., Totowa, NJ

Table 1
Primers for PCR Amplification

Primer	Sequence 5'–3'	T_m	Fragment	Ref.
***katG* gene**				
RTB 59	TGGCCGCGGCGGTCGACATT			
RTB 36	TCGGGGTCGTTGACCTCCCA	66°C	804 bp	*11*
***inhA* gene**				
inhA 51	CGGGCAACAAGCTCGACGGG			
inhA 31	GGGTTCATGATCGGCAGGAG	64°C	169 bp	*4*
***inhA* promoter**				
inhA P5	CGCAGCCAGGGCCTCGCTG			
inhA P3	CTCCGGTAACCAGGACTGA	60°C	246 bp	*12*
***ahpC* intergenic**				
TB 90	CCGATGAGAGCGGTGAGCTG			
TB 91	ACCACTGCTTTGCCGCCACC	66°C	236 bp	*13*
***kasA* gene**				
kasA 51	ATTGAGTCGGAGAACCCCGA			
kasA 31	CCTTCCATATCGGTCCGACT	56°C	1389 bp	*14*
***rpoB* gene**				
TR 8	TGCACGTCGCGGACCTCCA			
TR 9	TCGCCGCGATCAAGGAGT	58°C	157 bp	*4*
***rpsL* gene**				
STR 52	GTCAAGACCGCGGCTCTGAA			
STR 34	TTCTTGACACCCTGCGTATC	60°C	272 bp	*4*
***rrs* gene**				
STR 53	TCACCATCGACGAAGCTCCG			
STR 31	CTAGACGCGTCCTGTGCATG	64°C	570 bp	*4*
***embB* gene**				
emb 151	CGGCATGCGCCGGCTGATTC			
emb 131	TCCACAGACTGGCGTCGCTG	65°C	260 bp	*14*
***pncA* gene**				
pncA 51	GCTGGTCATGTTCGCGATCG			
	CAGGAGCTGCAAACCAACTCG	64°C	673bp	*15*

most severely affected by tuberculosis, the clinical load would be too high for large-scale sequencing. Ideally, a simple technique that can detect mutations and that fulfills the criteria of accuracy, speed, and simplicity is required. A PCR-based dot-blot hybridization strategy to screen for mutations is described in this chapter. The examples that are given focus on the application of this technique to screen for mutations known to be associated with drug resistance in *M. tuberculosis*. However, the technique lends itself to the easy inclusion of any other locus and can also be used for other applications. The chapter is not aimed at describing techniques used to search for new or unknown mutations.

2. Materials

2.1. In Vitro Amplification

1. Primers (0.2 µ*M* per reaction) to amplify regions of the drug-resistant genes of *M. tuberculosis* (**Table 1**). These were designed according to published sequences (X68081, *kat*G; L05910, *rpo*B; L08011, *rps*L; U68480, *emb*B; U02492, *inh*A; U16243, *ahp*C; RV2245, *kas*A: X52917, *rrs*; U59967, *pnc*A) (*see* **Note 1**).
2. Genomic DNA (300 ng) isolated from clinical isolates and sputum or crude DNA templates prepared directly from cultures (*see* **Note 3**).
3. dNTP mixture: 2.5 m*M* of each dNTP, diluted in distilled water.
4. *Taq* DNA polymerase: 5 U/µL (Promega, Madison, WI).
5. 10X *Taq* Polymerase reaction buffer with magnesium chloride (10 m*M* stock) (Promega).
6. Mineral oil or paraffin wax.
7. Thermal cycler.
8. Variable-temperature heating block.
9. 12% polyacrylamide minigels.

2.2. Labeling of Oligonucleotides

1. Two heating blocks (set at 37°C and 65°C).
2. 160 pmol [^{32}P]-ATP (7000 Ci/mmol) (Amersham, Little Chalfont, Bucks, UK).
3. T4 polynucleotide kinase and 10X reaction buffer (Amersham).
4. Oligonucleotide stock solutions: 33 ng/µL. Wild-type and mutant-specific oligonucleotide probes to screen for the presence or absence of specific mutations in the drug-resistant genes of *M. tuberculosis* were designed according to published sequences. The names refer to the particular gene, the number indicates the codon (or position) involved, and wt or mu indicates wild-type or mutant sequence, respectively. Oligonucleotide sequences are given in **Table 2**.

2.3. Dot-Blot Hybridization

1. Dot-blot buffer: 0.4 *M* NaOH, 25 m*M* EDTA.
2. Heating block set at 95°C.
3. Hybond-N+ nylon membrane (Amersham).
4. Dot-blot apparatus and vacuum pump.
5. Oven set at 80°C.
6. Radioactive protective shields.
7. 5X SSPE: 50 m*M* sodium phosphate, pH 7.0, 0.9 *M* NaCl, 5 m*M* EDTA.
8. 10% sodium dodecyl sulfate (SDS) solution.
9. 5X Denhardt's: 0.1% w/v Ficoll, 0.1% w/v polyvinylpyrrolidone, 0.1% w/v bovine serum albumin.
10. Prehybridization solution: mix 7.2 mL of 5X SSPE with 0.4 mL of 5X Denhardt's and 0.4 mL of 10% SDS.

Table 2
Probes for Dot-Blot Hybridization

Probe	Sequence 5'–3'	T_m
katG315 wt	GATCACCAGCGGCATCGAGG	66°C
katG315 mu	GATCACCACCGGCATCGAGG	66°C
katG315 dmu	GCGATCACCACAGGCATCGA	64°C
katG463 mu	AGCCAGATCCTGGCATCGGG	66°C
katG463 wt	AGCCAGATCCGGGCATCGGG	68°C
katG275 wt	TTTCGGTAAGACCCATGGCG	62°C
katG409 wt	ACGAGTTCGCCAAGGCCT	58°C
inhp–34wt	CCGATTTCGGCCCGGCCG	64°C
inhp–10wt	CGGCGAGACGATAGGTTGTC	64°C
ahpC–40wt	GTGTGATATATCACCTTTGCCTG	66°C
ahpC–10wt	GGTTGCGACATTCCATCGTGCCGT	76°C
kasA 66wt	CCTCAAGGATCCGGTCGACA	64°C
kasA 269wt	GGTGCCGGTATCACCTCGGA	66°C
kasA 312wt	CAACGCGCACGGCACGGCGA	70°C
kasA 413wt	CGCTTGCCTTCGGGCGTTAC	66°C
rpoB531 wt	AGCGCCGACTGTCGGCGCTG	70°C
rpoB531 mu	AGCGCCGACTGTTGGCGCTG	68°C
rpoB533 wt	GTCGGCGCTGGGGCCG	64°C
rpoB526 wt	GGGTTGACCCACAAGCGC	60°C
rpoB516 wt	TTCATGGACCAGAACAACCG	50°C
rpsL43 wt	ACCACTCCGAAGAAGCCGAA	62°C
rpsL88 wt	CGGGTGAAGGACCTGCCT	60°C
rrs491 wt	AGAAGAAGCACCGGCCAA	56°C
rrs512/3 wt	ACGTGCCAGCAGCCGCG	60°C
rrs904 wt	GCTAAAACTCAAAGGAATTG	54°C
embB306 wt	CCTGGGCATGGCCCGAGTCG	70°C
pncA70 wt	GTAACCGGTGGCGCCGCGCT	70°C
pncA388 wt	GAGGTCGATGTGGTCGGTAT	62°C
pncA254 wt	CATCCCAGTCTGGACACGTC	64°C
pncA139 wt	TCGTGGCAACCAAGGACTTC	62°C

11. Wash solution: 2X SSPE, 0.1% SDS.
12. Hybridization oven and bottles.
13. Orbital shaker.
14. Darkroom facility, autoradiography cassettes and X-ray film.

2.4. Stripping of Blots

1. Hybridization oven.
2. Stripping solution: 4 *M* NaOH.

3. 20X SSC: dissolve 175.3 g NaCl and 88.2 g trisodium citrate in H_2O and adjust to a final volume of 1 L.
4. Neutralizing solution: 0.2 *M* Tris-HCl, pH 7.5, 0.1% SDS, 0.1X SSC.

3. Methods

3.1. PCR Amplification of the Target Drug Resistance Genes (see Note 3)

1. Add 5 µL (300 ng) of genomic DNA (or crude template) isolated from clinical isolates (*see* Chapter 2 and **Note 2**) in a reaction mixture consisting of 2.25 m*M* $MgCl_2$, 200 µ*M* dNTPs (dATP, dGTP, dCTP, and TTP), 0.2 µ*M* each of 5' primer and 3' primer (*see* **Notes 1** and **4**), and 1.5 U of *Taq* DNA Polymerase in a final volume of 100 µL (*see* **Note 5**).
2. Cycle reaction mixtures in a thermal cycler as follows: 93°C for 3 min; then 35 cycles of 93°C for 1 min, annealing at T_m (*see* **Table 1**) for 1 min and an extension step at 72°C for 2 min. Final extension at 72°C for 10 min (*see* **Note 6**).
3. Confirm amplified products by gel electrophoresis (*see* **Notes 7** and **8**).

3.2. Labeling of Oligonucleotide Probes

Incubate 10 µL (330 ng) of wild-type or mutant oligonucleotide for 1 h at 37°C in a 30 µL reaction mixture containing 160 pmol of [γ-^{32}P]-ATP, 1X reaction buffer and 20 U of T4 polynucleotide kinase *(16)* (*see* **Notes 9** and **10**).

3.3. Dot-Blot Hybridization

1. Mark the top left hand corner of a Hybond N+ Nitrocellulose membrane and mount onto dot-blot apparatus.
2. Add 200 µL of dot-blot buffer to each well and aspirate.
3. Mix 10 µL of PCR product (from **Subheading 3.1.**) with 190 µL of dot-blot buffer and denature at 95°C for 5 min.
4. Load 200 µL of the denatured samples onto the dot-blot apparatus and aspirate.
5. Wash wells with 200 µL dot-blot buffer and aspirate.
6. Repeat **steps 3–5** above, but using known mutant and wild-type PCR-amplified DNA controls for each membrane (*see* **Note 2**).
7. Bake membrane at 80°C for 2 h.
8. Prehybridize the membrane in 8 mL prehybridization solution at 10°C lower than the calculated T_m (T_m = 4[G+C] + 2[A+T]) (*see* **Notes 6** and **10**).
9. Add 5 µL of the labeled primer to the prehybridization mix and continue to hybridize at T_m = –10°C for 60 min.
10. After hybridization, wash the membrane twice for 30 min each in wash solution at room temp.
11. Wash the membrane in Wash solution at the T_m for 10 min (*see* **Notes 12** and **13**).
12. Expose the membrane to an X-ray film for 3–6 h.
13. **Figure 1** is a sample result obtained by the dot-blot hybridization strategy for one of the prominant mutations (codon 531) found in the *rpoB* gene from clinical isolates of *M. tuberculosis*. DNA (*n* = 18) from drug-resistant and susceptible

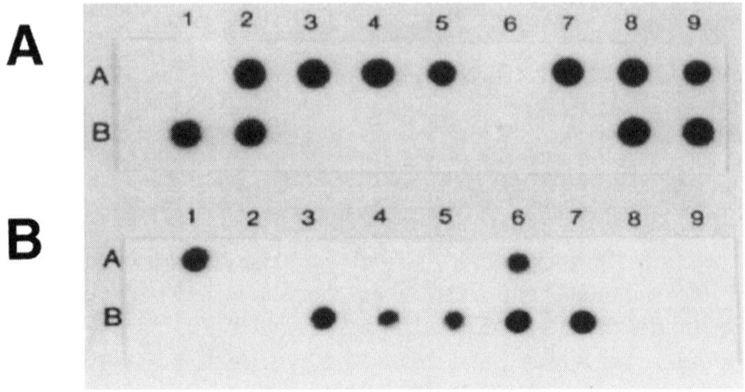

Fig. 1. Dot-blot hybridization. DNA (n = 18) from drug-resistant and susceptible isolates of *M. tuberculosis* were amplified with primers TR 8 and TR 9 and hybridized in a dot-blot format with radiolabeled probes rpoB531 wt (filter A) and rpoB531 mu (filter B; same as filter A, but stripped and reprobed with rpoB531 mu). Good discrimination was obtained for samples B7 and B8 which are known mutant (C-T) and wild-type for codon 531, respectively, as characterized previously ***(4)***. Amplified DNA from the control $H_{37}Rv$ was loaded in B9. (Reprinted from **ref. *14***.)

isolates of *M. tuberculosis* amplified with primers TR8 and TR9 and hybridized in the dot-blot format with radiolabeled probes rpoB531wt (filter A) and rpoB531 mu (filter B; same filter as A, but stripped and reprobed with rpoB531 mu.) Good discrimination was obtained for the control samples (B7 and B8 are known mutant [C-T] and wild-type for codon 531 respectively and amplified wild-type DNA from H37Rv was loaded in B9) and demonstrated that the different probes hybridize specifically to the amplified regions containing wild-type and mutant sequences respectively. The codon 531 mutation (C-T) in clinical isolate B6 was confirmed by sequence analysis and reflects the results obtained for the controls. Both wild-type and mutant probes clearly indicate which of the other clinical samples loaded onto the filter have a mutation at codon 531 (*see* **Notes 12–15**).

3.4. Preparation of Blots for Reuse (Stripping)

1. Incubate the membrane at 50°C in hybridization oven in 200 mL of stripping solution for 45 min. Shake occasionally.
2. Wash membrane at 42°C in 200 mL of neutralizing solution for 30 min.
3. Store membrane in sealed plastic bag.

4. Notes

1. As the predictive value of any test is dependent on prevalence, a mutational screening strategy should initially focus on the mutations most frequently diag-

Table 3
Genotype and Phenotype Resistance Data[a]

Isolate	Drug pattern (Phenotypic)	Mutations (Genotypic)
1	INH, RMP, SM, EMB	*katG315, katG463, rpoB531, rrs513, embB306*
2	INH, RMP SM	*katG315, rpoB531, rpsL43*
3	INH	*katG315*
4	INH, RMP, SM, EMB	*katG315, katG463, rpoB531, rrs513, embB306*
5	INH	*kasA269*
6	RMP	*rpoB531*
7	INH, RMP	*katG315, rpoB531*
8	INH, RMP, SM, EMB	*katG315, katG463, rpoB531, rrs513, embB306*
9	INH, RMP, SM	*katG315, rpoB531, rpsL43*
10	INH	*katG315*
11	INH, RMP, SM	*katG315, rpoB526, rpsL43*
12	S	—
13	S	—
14	S	—

[a]Phenotype (traditional culture-based drug susceptibilty testing) and genotype (mutation analysis by the PCR-based dot-blot hybridization procedure) results are examples from drug resistant and -susceptible clinical isolates originated from a high incidence community.

INH = isoniazid, RMP = rifampicin, SM = streptomycin, EMB = ethambutol, S = susceptible (reprinted from **ref.** ***14***)

nosed in the geographic area studied. Codons 315, 463 (*kat*G), 531, 526, 516 (*rpo*B), 43 (*rps*L), 491, 513 (*rrs*), and 306 (*emb*B) are frequently seen to be altered in clinical isolates from a number of studies ***(1,2,4,5,8,12–15,18)***. It would therefore be beneficial to focus the initial mutational screening strategy on these mutations. Probes and primers to be used in the PCR-based dot-blot hybridization strategy for ten genes associated with drug resistance are described in this chapter. Examples of the genotypic and phenotypic data obtained with drug-resistant and -susceptible isolates obtained from a high incidence community ***(14)*** are shown in **Table 3**.

2. It is important to include positive (mutant) and negative (wild-type) controls on each blot. These controls are molecularly well-characterized DNA samples with known mutations in the respective genes. More stringent final washes (increased temperature or lower salt concentration during final washes) can be done to obtain better discrimination between controls if necessary.
3. As with any PCR-based DNA amplification procedure, special care ***(17)*** must be taken to avoid false results due to amplicon contamination.

4. Although this chapter focuses on selected regions in some of the most important target genes, the flexibility of the dot-blot strategy ensures that additional loci can easily be incorporated into the screening strategy as described, e.g., the recently described *kas*A gene *(2)*.
5. This technique could be adapted to amplify and detect drug resistant mutations directly from sputum samples or microscopy stained slides. The high daily output possible with this strategy would enable the focus of drug resistance control strategies to include all smear-positive samples.
6. The annealing temperature for each primer set was calculated as follows: T_m = 4(G+C) + 2(A+T) and the optimal annealing temperature for each is given in **Table 1**.
7. The following experimental flow is recommended: PCR amplification → confirmation of amplification by gel electrophoresis → labeling of probe for region of interest → dot-blot hybridization → overexposure of first time autoradiography to ensure that samples were sufficiently blotted → final autoradiography.
8. Although it is important to confirm DNA amplification by gel electrophoresis, small differences in efficiency of amplification do not have a significant effect on the outcome of the hybridization results.
9. Purification of labeled oligonucleotides is not necessary.
10. The process to establish critical hybridization conditions is greatly enhanced by the use of radioactively labeled probes, since the membranes could easily be rewashed at higher stringency hybridization conditions. However, detection with nonradioactive labeled probes gives similar results. For nonradioactive detection, probes can be 3' end-labeled with digoxigenin (DIG) by terminal transferase (Roche Diagnostics, Germany) according to the specifications of the manufacturer. Hybridization should be carried out in 5X SSPE and the final wash and detection steps using anti-DIG alkaline phosphatase as described by the manufacturer.
11. The dot-blot hybridization strategy with wild-type probes can be used to detect drug resistant mutations since these do not hybridize to mutant loci encoding drug resistance *(15)*. The wild-type probe strategy however is unable to provide a precise understanding of the different mutations occurring at a specific codon. It is known that >99% of mutations within these loci confer resistance and therefore the absence of a hybridization signal has been interpreted to directly reflect drug resistance. These results are confirmed by phenotyping.
12. The application of specific mutant probes can be applied to identify or confirm the nature of this mutational event, although it may be argued that it would not be possible to identify cases where both the resistant and sensitive bacilli are present in the host. This may also be true for all other molecular methods. The dot-blot hybridization strategy with mutant probes can detect drug resistant alleles when they represent 1–2% of the overall population (results not shown). However, a review of the literature suggests that mixed infections in active tuberculosis cases are rare.
13. Efficiency of DNA amplification, hybridization time, buffer salt concentration, the temperature used in the final washing step, and the length of exposure to the

X-ray film are all conditions that can affect discrimination between positive and negative results. These conditions can be evaluated empirically with the aid of positive and negative controls for each locus. We found good discrimination for all the probes described after the filters were washed finally in 1.5X SSPE for 10 min at 74°C after hybridization.

14. The method is reproducible, not technically demanding and it takes about two normal working days to obtain results from the start of amplification (done in batches of 30–40 samples) to the final autoradiography step of the dot-blot hybridization (done in batches of up to 150 samples, including controls).

References

1. Musser, J. M. (1995) Antimicrobial agent resistance in mycobacteria: molecular genetic insights. *Clin. Microbiol. Rev.* **8,** 496–514.
2. Mdluli, K., Slayden, R. A., Zhu, Y., Ramaswamy, S., Pan, X., Mead, D., Crane, D. D., Musser, J. M., and Barry, C. E. (1998) Inhibition of a *Mycobacterium tuberculosis* β-ketoacyl ACP synthetase by isoniazid. *Science* **280,** 1607–1610.
3. Sreevatsan, S., Pan, X., Stockbauer, K. E., Cornell, N. D., Kreisworth, B. N., Whittam, T. C., and Musser, J. M. (1997) Restricted structural gene polymorphism in the *Mycobacterium tuberculosis* complex indicates evolutionarily recent global dissemination. *Proc. Natl. Acad. Sci. USA* **94,** 9869–9874.
4. Victor, T. C., Warren, R., Butt, J. L., Jordaan, A. M., Felix, J. V., Venter, A., Sirgel, F. A., Schaaf, H. S., Donald, P. R., Richardson, M., Cynamon, M. H., and van Helden, P. D. (1997) Genome and MIC stability in *Mycobacterium tuberculosis* and indications for continuation of use of isoniazid in multidrug-resistant tuberculosis. *J. Med. Microbiol.* **46,** 847–957.
5. Felmlee, T. A., Lin, Q., and Whelen, A. C. (1995) Genomic detection of *Mycobacterium tuberculosis* rifampicin resistance: comparison of single-strand conformation polymorphism and dideoxy fingerprinting. *J. Clin. Microbiol.* **33,** 1617–1623.
6. Williams, D. L., Wagnespack, C., Eisenach, K, Crawford, J. T., Portaels, F., Salfinger, M., Nolan, C. M., Abe, C., Sticht-Groh, V., and Gillis, T. P. (1994) Characterization of rifampicin resistance in pathogenic mycobacteria. *Antimicrob. Agents Chemother.* **38,** 2380–2386.
7. Wegenack, N. L., Uhl, J. R., St. Amand, A. L., Tomlinson, A. J., Benson, L. M, Naylor, S., Kline, B. C., Cockerill, F. R., III, and Rusnak, F. (1997) Recombinant *Mycobacterium tuberculosis* KatG (S315T) is a competent catalase peroxidose with reduced activity towards isoniazid. *J. Infect. Dis.* **176,** 722–727.
8. Telenti, A., Imboden, P., Marchesi, F., Lowri, D., Cole, S., Colston, M. J., Matter, L., Schopfer, K., and Bodmer, T. (1993) Detection of rifampicin-resistance mutations in *Mycobacterium tuberculosis. Lancet* **341,** 647–650.
9. De Beenhouwer, H., Lhiang, Z., Jannes, G., Mijs, W., Machtelinckx, L., Rossau, R., Traore, H., and Portaels, F. (1995) Rapid detection of rifampicin resistance in sputum and biopsy specimens from tuberculosis patients by PCR and line probe assay. *Tuberc. Lung Dis.* **76,** 425–430.

10. Rossau, R., Traore, H., De Beenhouwer, H., Mijs, W., Jannes, G., De Rijk, P., and Portaels, F. (1997) Evaluation of the INNO-LIPA Rif. TB assay, a reverse hybridization assay for the simultaneous detection of *Mycobacterium tuberculosis* complex and its resistance to rifampicin. *Antimicrob. Agents Chemother.* **41,** 2093–2098.
11. Pretorius, G. S., van Helden, P. D., Sirgel, F., Eisenach, K. D., and Victor, T. C. (1995) Mutations in *katG* gene sequences in isoniazid-resistant clinical isolates of *Mycobacterium tuberculosis* are rare. *Antimicrob. Agents Chemother.* **39,** 2276–2281.
12. Morris, S., Han Bai, G., Suffys, P., Portillo-Gomez, L., Fairchok, M., and Rouse, D. (1995) Molecular mechanisms of multiple drug resistance in clinical isolates of *Mycobacterium tuberculosis. J. Infect. Dis.* **171,** 954–960.
13. Telenti, A., Honoré, N., Bernasconi, C., March, J., Ortega, A., Heym, B., Takiff, H. E., and Cole, S. T. (1997) Genotype assessment of isoniazid and rifampicin resistance in *Mycobacterium tuberculosis*: a blind study at reference laboratory level. *J. Clin. Microbiol.* **35,** 719–723.
14. Victor, T. C., Jordaan, A. M., van Rie, A., van der Spuy, G. D., Richardson, M., van Helden, P. D., and Warren, R. (1999) Detection of mutations in drug resistance genes of *Mycobacterium tuberculosis* by a dot-blot hybridization strategy. *Tuberc. Lung Dis.* **79,** 343–348.
15. Hirano, K., Takahashi, M., Kazumi, Y, Fukasawa, Y., and Abe, C. (1998) Mutation in *pncA* is a major mechanism of pyrazinamide resistance in *Mycobacterium tuberculosis. Tuberc. Lung Dis.* **78,** 117–122.
16. Victor, T., du Toit, R., Jordaan, A. M., Bester, A. J., and van Helden, P. D. (1990) No evidence for point mutations on codons 12, 13 and 61 of the *ras* gene in a high-incidence area for esophageal and gastric cancers. *Cancer Res.* **50,** 4911–4914.
17. Dragon, E. A., Spadoro, J. P., and Madej, R. (1993) Quality control of polymerase chain reaction, in *Diagnostic Molecular Microbiology: Principles and Applications* (Persing, D. H., ed.) ASM Press, Washington, DC, pp. 160–168.
18. Van Rie, A., Warren, R. M., Beyers, N., Gie, R. P., Classen, C. N., Richardson, M., Sampson, S. L., Victor, T. C., and van Helden, P. D. (1999) Transmission of a multidrug-resistant *Mycobacterium tuberculosis* strain resembling "Strain W" among non-institutional, HIV seronegative patients. *J. Infect. Dis.* **180,** 1608–1615.

12

Restriction Fragment Length Polymorphism Typing of Mycobacteria

Dick van Soolingen, Petra E. W. de Haas, and Kristin Kremer

1. Introduction

In principle, restriction fragment length polymorphism (RFLP) typing can be applied to strains of all mycobacterial species for which suitable probes have been identified. International consensus has been achieved regarding the methodology of IS*6110* RFLP typing of *Mycobacterium tuberculosis* complex isolates *(1)* and IS*1245* RFLP typing of *Mycobacterium avium* strains *(2)*. This chapter describes the technical details of these standardized methods regarding the isolation of DNA, restriction enzymes, electrophoresis conditions, internal- and external-size markers, Southern blotting, and several probes used for hybridization. Furthermore, RFLP typing of isolates of some other mycobacterial species is described.

1.1. RFLP Typing of M. tuberculosis *Complex*

The discovery of transposable elements and other repetitive DNA elements in *M. tuberculosis* complex strains in the early 1990s has led to various DNA fingerprinting methods to differentiate strains belonging to the complex. Some of these methods are based on the amplification of repetitive DNA sequences using the polymerase chain reaction (PCR) *(3–7)*. Other methods visualize restriction fragments containing particular repetitive DNA elements like insertion sequence (IS) elements *(1,8–12)*. A comparison between PCR-based and RFLP typing methods revealed that IS*6110* RFLP typing is the most discriminative and reproducible typing method currently available *(13)*. Because IS*6110* RFLP typing has been internationally standardized with regard to the choice of restriction enzyme, probe, and size markers, interlaboratory comparison is enabled by computerization of DNA fingerprints. The accurate com-

From: *Methods in Molecular Medicine*, vol. 54: *Mycobacterium Tuberculosis Protocols*
Edited by: T. Parish and N. G. Stoker © Humana Press Inc., Totowa, NJ

parison of IS*6110* RFLP patterns by computer has been described in detail elsewhere ***(14)***. This standardization has led to new possibilities for studying the transmission of tuberculosis on different scales.

Initially, in the early 1990s, the use of IS*6110* RFLP typing for outbreak management of multidrug-resistant *M. tuberculosis* was reported frequently ***(15–18)***. In more recent years, population-based molecular epidemiological studies in San Francisco ***(19)***, New York ***(20)***, Denmark ***(21)***, Amsterdam ***(22)***, Zürich ***(23)***, and The Netherlands ***(24)*** have provided insight into risk factors for the transmission of tuberculosis. Recently, transmission of tuberculosis across country borders ***(25)*** and the spread of particular *M. tuberculosis* genotype families in different areas have been recognized ***(13,26,27)***. Some species within the *M. tuberculosis* complex can be identified using IS*6110* RFLP typing; e.g., the majority of *Mycobacterium bovis* strains contain only a few copies of IS*6110*, mostly including a hybridizing restriction fragment of 1.9 kb ***(8)***. *M. bovis* BCG strains contain either one or two copies of IS*6110* on *Pvu*II restriction fragments of 1.5 and 1.9 kb ***(28)***. The *Mycobacterium microti* strains typed so far also exhibit characteristic IS*6110* RFLPs not found among other *M. tuberculosis* complex strains ***(29)***.

In addition to IS*6110*, other genetic markers for typing of *M. tuberculosis* complex isolates have been described. Polymorphic GC rich sequence (PGRS)-based RFLP typing can be used as an additional typing method for *M. tuberculosis* complex strains containing less than five copies of IS*6110*, as the interpretation of the IS*6110* RFLP typing results of these strains has proven unreliable ***(8,9,30–32)***. The IS*1081* RFLP pattern of *M. bovis* BCG is, in combination with the two characteristic IS*6110* RFLP patterns, a reliable tool to recognize this attenuated *M. bovis* strain ***(11,33)***. The B9 probe ***(34)*** and the *pmb64* gene ***(35)*** can be used to distinguish between *M. bovis* BCG substrains. Furthermore, strains of the recently described *M. tuberculosis* complex species *Mycobacterium canettii* contain only a single IS*1081* copy, whereas strains of the other species in the complex contain between four and seven copies of this IS element ***(11,36)***. The *mtp40* sequence has also been shown to be associated with genetic polymorphism among *M. tuberculosis* strains ***(37,38)***, whereas this sequence is absent in most *M. bovis* strains ***(37–40)***. Other sequences like the direct repeat (DR) ***(8,9,31,41)***, the major polymorphic tandem repeat (MPTR) ***(42)***, the GTG repeat ***(12)***, IS*1547* ***(43)***, the IS-like element ***(44)***, and *katG* ***(45)*** can also be used to differentiate *M. tuberculosis* complex strains and these are usually applied to answer specific research issues.

The completion of the genome sequence of *M. tuberculosis* strain H37Rv has disclosed the presence of 25 additional IS elements, which are present in one to three copies ***(46,47)***. Furthermore, two prophages and a novel repetitive sequence, the REP13E12 family, which is present in seven copies, were identified ***(46)***.

1.2. RFLP Analysis of M. avium Complex

M. avium is one of the most frequently encountered species among non-*M. tuberculosis* complex strains isolated from humans. The epidemiology of *M. avium*-related infections is not clear. Possible reservoirs for *M. avium* infections in humans have been found in tap water ***(48)***, soil of potted plants ***(49)***, hard cheese ***(50)***, cigarettes ***(51)***, and animals like birds and pigs ***(52–54)***. Recently, the presence of the insertion sequence IS*1245* was found to be restricted to *M. avium*, *Mycobacterium silvaticum*, and *Mycobacterium paratuberculosis* ***(53,55)***. In both *M. paratuberculosis* isolates and *M. avium* isolates from birds, particular IS*1245* RFLP patterns were found of eleven and three bands, respectively ***(53)***. In contrast, highly polymorphic multibanded IS*1245* RFLP patterns were found among *M. avium* isolates from humans and pigs ***(53,56,57)***. Furthermore, a significant part of the IS*1245* DNA fingerprints of *M. avium* isolates from pigs shared a high degree of similarity with the human isolates ***(56,57)***. As the "bird-type" IS*1245* RFLP pattern was only rarely encountered among human isolates it was concluded that birds are not an important source of *M. avium* infections in humans in the Netherlands ***(53,57)***. Extensive RFLP typing studies of *M. avium* isolates from the above-mentioned and other reservoirs are needed to investigate their epidemiological relatedness with strains isolated from humans. This will also provide more insight in the taxonomy and evolutionary divergence within the *M. avium* complex.

Besides IS*1245*, other IS elements have been used for RFLP typing of the *M. avium* complex. IS*1311*, which is closely related to IS*1245*, has also shown a large degree of polymorphism among human and animal isolates ***(58)***. IS*901* enables differentiation of the bird-type IS*1245* RFLP pattern isolates, but is absent in most other *M. avium* complex strains ***(53)***. IS*902*, originally identified in *M. silvaticum*, has 98% similarity to IS*901* ***(59)***. IS*1110* is only rarely found in *M. avium* complex strains, but has been shown to hybridize at low stringency to an unidentified DNA sequence present in some strains ***(60,61)***. Finally, members of the closely related species *M. paratuberculosis* can be typed with IS*900*, which is exclusively present in strains of this species ***(61,62)***. However, the level of discrimination of IS*900* RFLP among *M. paratuberculosis* isolates is poor ***(63)***.

1.3. RFLP Analysis of Isolates from Other Mycobacterial Species

Other non-*M. tuberculosis* complex mycobacterial species that frequently occur in humans are *Mycobacterium gordonae*, *Mycobacterium kansasii*, and *Mycobacterium xenopi*. The PGRS ***(30)*** and the MPTR ***(42,64)*** sequences can be used as probes in RFLP typing to differentiate isolates of the species *M. gordonae* and *M. kansasii*. IS*1652* is only suitable for typing isolates of particular *M. kansasii* subspecies ***(64,65)***. IS*1512* ***(66)*** is associated with a high degree of genetic polymorphism in *M. gordonae*. An IS*1081*-related element (IS*1395*) has been found in *M. xenopi* and can be used as a probe in RFLP typing ***(67,68)***. In the emerging pathogen *Mycobacterium hemophilum*, a "multiple-copy-genetic-element" has been found, associated with a limited degree of genetic polymorphism ***(69)***.

2. Materials

2.1. Isolation of High-Molecular-Weight Genomic DNA from Mycobacteria

1. Solid medium: Löwenstein Jensen, or Löwenstein Jensen supplemented with pyruvate ***(70)*** (ICN Pharmaceuticals, Costa Mesa, CA).
2. Liquid medium: Middlebrook 7H9 ***(70)*** (Difco Laboratories, Detroit, MI).
3. 10X TE buffer: 100 m*M* Tris-HCl, pH 8.0, 10 m*M* EDTA in distilled water. Autoclave. Store at room temperature (RT) for up to 1 yr.
4. 1X TE buffer: add 1 vol of 10X TE buffer (*see* **Subheading 2.1., item 3**) to 9 vol of distilled water. Autoclave. Store at room temperature for up to 1 yr.
5. 10 mg/mL lysozyme in distilled water: Store in small aliquots at –20°C for up to 1 yr.
6. 10% sodium dodecyl sulfate (SDS): dissolve 10 g SDS in 100 mL distilled water by heating at 65°C for 20 min (*see* **Note 1**). Do not autoclave. Store at room temperature for up to 1 mo.
7. 10 mg/mL proteinase K in distilled water: Store in small aliquots at –20°C for up to 1 yr.
8. SDS/proteinase K solution: Prepare a fresh mix for all samples. Mix 70 µL of 10% SDS (*see* **Subheading 2.1., item 6**) and 5 µL of 10 mg/mL proteinase K (*see* **Subheading 2.1., item 7**) for each sample. Vortex briefly.
9. 5 *M* NaCl: dissolve 29.2 g of NaCl in 100 mL of distilled water. Autoclave. Store at room temperature for up to 1 yr.
10. CTAB/NaCl solution: Dissolve 4.1 g NaCl in 80 mL of distilled water. While stirring, add 10 g *N*-cetyl-*N*,*N*,*N*,-trimethyl ammonium bromide (CTAB). Heat the solution to 65°C to dissolve. Adjust the volume to 100 mL with distilled water. Store at room temperature for up to 6 mo.
11. Chloroform/isoamyl alcohol (24:1) (*see* **Note 2**): Mix 24 vol of chloroform with 1 vol of isoamyl alcohol. Store at room temperature for up to 1 yr.
12. Isopropanol. Store at room temperature for up to 1 yr.
13. 70% ethanol: Mix 7 vol of ethanol with 3 vol of distilled water. Store at –20°C.
14. Water baths set at 37°C, 65°C, 80°C.
15. Thermomixer (Thermomixer 5436, Eppendorf, Hamburg, Germany) (*see* **Note 3**).
16. Microcentrifuge.
17. Aspirator (*see* **Note 4**).

2.2. Quantification of the Extracted DNA

2.2.1. Ethidium Bromide Staining and UV Irradiation

1. Agarose.
2. 1X TBE: 89 m*M* Tris, 89 m*M* boric acid, and 2.5 m*M* EDTA in distilled water. Adjust the pH to 8.2. Autoclave. Store at room temperature for up to 1 yr.
3. 1000X ethidium bromide (500 µg/mL) (*see* **Note 5**). Add 3 mL of 10 mg/mL ethidium bromide (BDH Laboratory Supplies, Poole, Dorset, UK) to 57 mL of distilled water. Store at 4°C protected from light for up to 1 yr. Dilute this stock solution 1:1000 to achieve a working concentration of 0.5 µg/mL.
4. 5X DNA sample buffer: 50% (w/v) glycerol, 50 m*M* Tris-HCl, pH 7.5, 5 m*M* EDTA, 0.05% w/v bromophenol blue, 30 µg/mL RNase. To prepare this solution mix the following reagents:

Glycerol	50 g
1 *M* Tris-HCl, pH 7.5	5 mL
100 m*M* EDTA	5 mL
Bromophenol blue	0.05 g
10 mg/mL RNAse	300 µL

   Add distilled water to a final volume of 100 mL. Heat for 15 min in a 100°C water bath to dissolve. Store at 4°C for up to 1 yr.
5. 1X DNA sample buffer: Dilute 5X DNA sample buffer 1:5 in distilled water. Store at 4°C for up to 1 yr.
6. Microwave or water bath set at 100°C.
7. Water bath set at 70°C.
8. DNA electrophoresis equipment.
9. UV transilluminator.
10. Photo equipment.

2.2.2. GeneQuant Spectrophotometer

1. 1X TE (*see* **Subheading 2.1., item 4**).
2. GeneQuant spectrophotometer RNA/DNA calculator (GeneQuant II, Pharmacia Biotech Ltd., Cambridge, UK).
3. Quartz cuvet, light path 10 mm (Hellma GmbH & Co., Müllheim, Germany).
4. Aspirator (*see* **Note 4**).

2.3. Digestion of Chromosomal DNA by a Restriction Enzyme

1. External markers (*see* **Notes 6** and **7**, and **Table 1**): Depending on the RFLP typing method, DNA of one or more of the following mycobacterial reference strains should be used as external markers (these strains can be obtained upon request from the authors):

   M. tuberculosis Mt14323
   M. bovis BCG P3
   M. avium R13
   M. avium IWGMT49

Table 1
Requirements and Conditions for the Various RFLP Typing Methods[a]

Species	Restriction enzyme	External markers[c]	Internal marker[d]	Gel: Agarose (% ,w/v)	Gel: Size (length × width)	Electrophoresis: Marker[e]	Electrophoresis: Voltage (V)	Electrophoresis: Time (h)	Indicator band: size (kb)	Indicator band: cm from slots[f]	Probe	Nature of the probe	Refs.
M. tuberculosis complex	*Pvu*II	Mt14323	SDL/phi	0.8	16 × 20	lambda/phi	20	20	2.0	7.0	IS*6110*	PCR prod.	***1,10***
		P3	SDL/phi	0.8	16 × 20	lambda/phi	20	20	2.0	7.0	IS*1081*	PCR prod.	***11,33***
		Mt14323	SDL/phi	0.8	16 × 20	lambda/phi	20	20	2.0	7.0	B9	PCR prod.	***34***
		Mt 14323, P3	SDL/phi	0.8	16 × 20	lambda/phi	20	20	2.0	7.0	*mtp40*	PCR prod.	***37,38***
		Mt14323	SDL/phi	0.8	16 × 20	lambda/phi	20	20	2.0	7.0	*katG*	insert	***45***
	*Alu*I[b]	Mt14323	marker IV	0.7	24 × 20	marker IV	30	40	2.3	19.5	PGRS	oligol	***8,9,30***
		Mt14323	SDL/phi	1.5	16 × 20	lambda/phi	20	18	0.60	7.5	DR	oligo2	***8,9,41***
	*Hinf*I	Mt14323	SDL/phi	0.7	16 × 20	lambda/phi	20	18	2.0	7.0	$(GTG)_5$	oligo2	***12,13***
M. avium	*Pvu*II	IWGMT 49, R13	SDL/phi	0.7	24 × 20	lambda/phi	40	20	0.87	20	IS*1245*	PCR prod.	***2,53***
			SDL/phi	0.7	24 × 20	lambda/phi	40	20	0.87	20	IS*901*	PCR prod.	***53,73***
M. paratuberculosis	*Bste*II	ATCC 19698	marker X	0.8	24 × 20	marker IV	50	20	1.1	17	IS*900*	PCR prod.	***62,66***
M. kansasii	*Bste*II	MkG59	SDL/phi	0.8	16 × 20	lambda/phi	20	20	2.0	7.0	MPTR	oligo3	***42***
M. gordonae	*Bste*II	ATCC 19277	SDL/phi	0.8	16 × 20	lambda/phi	20	20	2.0	7.0	MPTR	oligo3	***42***

[a]Standardization has only been achieved for IS*6110* RFLP typing of *M. tuberculosis* complex and IS*1245* RFLP typing of *M. avium*, the conditions indicated for the other RFLP typing methods are recommendations.

[b]*Alu*I digests the internal marker, therefore the digestion mix needs to be heat-inactivated prior to adding the internal marker.

[c]See **Subheading 2.3.**, **item 1**.

[d]See **Subheading 2.4.**, **items 4–6**.

[e]See **Subheading 2.5.**, **items 3** and **4**.

[f]±0.3 cm.

M. paratuberculosis ATCC 19698
M. gordonae ATCC 19277
M. kansasii MkG59.

2. Restriction endonuclease (10 U/µL) and digestion buffer (Boehringer Mannheim): Depending on the RFLP typing method either *Pvu*II, *Alu*I, or *Bste*II should be used (*see* **Note 6** and **Table 1**).
3. Microcentrifuge.
4. Water bath or Thermomixer (*see* **Note 3** and **Subheading 2.1., item 15**).

2.4. Estimation of the DNA Concentration in the Samples After Digestion

1. Materials to perform gel electrophoresis, ethidium bromide staining, and UV irradiation.
2. Internal marker (*see* **Note 8**): Depending on the RFLP typing method, either SDL-Phi, marker IV, or marker X should be used as internal marker (*see* **Note 6** and **Table 1**).
3. Supercoiled DNA ladder-*Pvu*II (SDL-*Pvu*II) (*see* **Note 9**): The DNA must first be precipitated to remove inhibitory substances that will prevent cleavage by *Pvu*II. Precipitate 50 µL of supercoiled DNA ladder (200 ng/µL, Gibco-BRL, Life technologies, Paisy, UK) by adding 150 µL of 1X TE, 500 µL of absolute ethanol (do not use the last 250 mL of the 1 L bottle), and 25 µL of 5 *M* NaCl. Incubate at –20°C for 30 min and centrifuge for 15 min at 11,000*g*. Discard the supernatant, air dry the pellet, and redissolve the pellet in 58 µL of 0.1X TE. Add 5 µL *Pvu*II and 7 µL digestion buffer and incubate at 37°C for at least 2 h. Add 1 µL 5X DNA sample to 4 µL of the digested and 4 µL of the undigested supercoiled DNA ladder. Estimate the DNA concentration of the digested marker and verify that the DNA has been digested completely by agarose gel electrophoresis (*see* **Subheading 3.2.1.**).
4. Internal marker SDL-phi: Add the size markers to small volumes (1 mL) of 5X DNA sample buffer (*see* **Subheading 2.2.1., item 4**) to get a final concentration of: 3 ng/µL SDL-*Pvu*II (*see* **Subheading 2.4., item 3**) and 1 ng/µL PhiX174-*Hae*III (marker IX, Boehringer Mannheim). Store at –20°C for up to 1 yr. For direct use, store one aliquot at 4°C.
5. Internal marker IV: Add marker IV (Boehringer Mannheim) to small volumes (1 mL) of 5X DNA sample buffer (*see* **Subheading 2.2.1., item 4**) to get a final concentration of 4 ng/µL. Store at –20°C for up to 1 yr. For direct use, store one aliquot at 4°C.
6. Internal marker X: Add marker X (Boehringer Mannheim) to small volumes (1 mL) of 5X DNA sample buffer (*see* **Subheading 2.2.1., item 4**) to get a final concentration of 2 ng/µL. Store at –20°C for up to 1 yr. For direct use, store one aliquot at 4°C.

2.5. Electrophoresis

1. *See* **Subheading 2.2.1., items 1–10**.

2. Electrophoresis marker: Depending on the RFLP typing method, either lambda-phi or marker IV should be used as electrophoresis marker (*see* **Note 6** and **Table 1**).
3. Electrophoresis marker lambda-phi: To prepare a mixture of lambda-*Hin*dIII (40 ng/µL) and PhiX174-*Hae*III (50 ng/µL) in sample buffer, add the following reagents to a microcentrifuge tube:

   16 µL lambda-*Hin*dIII (Marker II, 500 ng/µL, Boehringer Mannheim)
   40 µL PhiX-*Hae*III (Marker IX, 250 ng/µL, Boehringer Mannheim)
   104 µL 1X TE buffer (*see* **Subheading 2.1., item 4**)
   40 µL 5X DNA sample buffer (*see* **Subheading 2.2.1., item 4**)

   Mix and store in small aliquots of 50 µL at –20°C for up to 1 yr. For direct use, store one aliquot at 4°C.
4. Electrophoresis marker IV: To prepare marker IV (200 ng/µL) in sample buffer, add the following reagents to a microcentrifuge tube:

   160 µL marker IV (Marker IV, 250 ng/µL, Boehringer Mannheim)
   80 µL 1X TE buffer (*see* **Subheading 2.1., item 4**)
   40 µL 5X DNA sample buffer (*see* **Subheading 2.2.1., item 4**)

   Mix and store in small aliquots of 50 µL at –20°C for up to 1 yr. For direct use, store one aliquot at 4°C.

2.6. Southern Blotting

2.6.1. Preparation of the Gel for Southern Blotting

1. 1 *M* HCl: Add 85.5 mL concentrated HCl to 914.5 mL water. Store at room temperature for up to 6 mo.
2. 0.25 *M* HCL: Prepare directly for use by diluting 1 *M* HCL in distilled water.
3. 4 *M* NaOH: Dissolve 160 g NaOH in 800 mL distilled water. Adjust the volume to 1000 mL (*see* **Note 10**). Store at room temperature for up to 3 mo.
4. 0.4 *M* NaOH: Prepare directly for use by diluting 4 *M* NaOH 1:10 in distilled water.

2.6.2. Southern Blotting—Two Methods

2.6.2.1. Transfer of DNA by Vacuum Blotting

1. Agarose.
2. Marking mix (*see* **Note 11**): Collect the leftovers of the DNA samples of **Subheading 3.5., item 4** in one microcentifuge tube. Mix 200 µL of these leftovers with 16 µL 4 *M* NaOH and 13 µL of DNA of the mycobacterial reference strain (1000 µg/mL). Vortex and incubate overnight at 4°C. Note that the leftovers and the mycobacterial DNA should be of the species of the RFLP typing method dealing with (*see* **Table 1**).
3. 10X SSPE: 0.1 *M* $Na_2HPO_4.2H_2O$ (17.8 g/L), 1.8 *M* NaCl (105.12 g/L), 10 m*M* EDTA (3.7 g/L). The pH should be 7.4. Autoclave. Store at room temperature for up to 1 yr.
4. Filter paper for blotting.

5. Hybond N+ membrane (Amersham International, Buckinghamshire, UK).
6. Blow-dryer.
7. Small brush.
8. Vacuum blot apparatus and vacuum pump (Miliblot-V system, Millipore, Bedford, MA).
9. Microwave or boiling water bath.
10. Water bath set at 70°C.

2.6.2.2. Transfer of DNA by Capillary Blotting

1. 1.25 *M* Tris-acetate: Dissolve 151.4 g Tris in 800 mL distilled water. Add acetic acid (100%) to adjust the pH to 8.0 (about 30 mL). Adjust the volume to 1 L. Autoclave. Store at room temperature for up to 1 yr.
2. 0.25 *M* Tris-acetate-0.1 *M* NaCl: Add 200 mL of 1.25 *M* Tris-acetate (*see* **Subheading 2.6.2.2., step 1**) and 20 mL of 5 *M* NaCl (*see* **Subheading 2.1., step 9**) to 780 mL distilled water. Autoclave. Store at room temperature for up to 1 yr.
3. 0.025 *M* Tris-acetate-0.01 *M* NaCl: Dilute 0.25 *M* Tris-acetate-0.1 *M* NaCl (*see* **Subheading 2.6.2.2., step 2**) 1:10 in distilled water. Prepare just before use.
4. 70% ethanol (*see* **Subheading 2.1., item 13**).
5. Materials for Southern blotting (*see* **Subheading 2.6.2.1., items 2, 4–7**).
6. Thin filter paper.

2.6.3. Treatment of the DNA Membrane After Southern Blotting

1. 20X SSC: 3 *M* NaCl (175.3 g/L), 0.3 *M* Na-citrate (88.2 g/L) in distilled water. Adjust the pH to 7.0 with 5 *M* NaOH. Autoclave. Store at room temperature for up to 1 yr.
2. 5X SSC: Add 1 vol of 20X SSC (*see* **Subheading 2.6.3., item 1**) to 3 vol of distilled water.
3. Filter paper.

2.7. Preparation of DNA Probes (see Note 6)

2.7.1. Preparation and Purification of PCR Products

1. 10X Super *Taq* PCR buffer (HT Biotechnology Ltd., Cambridge, UK).
2. Super *Taq* DNA polymerase (5 U/µL) (HT Biotechnology Ltd.).
3. DNAse-free water (Sigma, St. Louis, MO).
4. dNTP mix: add 10 µL of dNTP (dATP, dCTP, dGTP, dTTP) stock solution (100 m*M*) to 360 µL DNAse free water. Store in small aliquots at –20°C for up to 1 yr.
5. Primers. The primers to be used depend on the probe that is to be prepared. The primer sequences required for the different probes are listed in **Table 2**. Dilute the primers in DNAse free water to prepare a concentrated stock solution. Dilute this stock solution in DNAse free water to 50 ng/µL. Store at –20°C.
6. Target DNA: Depending on the probe that is to be prepared either plasmid pMA12 *(2)* or one of the following mycobacterial reference strains should be used (these strains can be obtained upon request from the authors) (*see* **Table 2**):

Table 2
Primer Sequences and PCR Conditions to Prepare the PCR-Amplified Probes (*see* Note 12)

	Primer sequence (5'-3')		PCR[a]		
Probe	Forward	Reverse	Target DNA[b]	Size product (bp)	Ref.
IS*6110*	CGT GAC GGC ATC GAG GTG GC	GCG TAG GCG TCG GTG ACA AA	P3	245	***1***
IS*1081*	TCG CGT GAT CCT TCG AAA GG	GCC GTT GCG CTG ATT GGA CC	P3	236	***33***
B9	GGC CTG GAC TCC GGT AGC CTA	TCT CGT GGC GAC TGT TAT GAC A	Mt 14323	150	***34***
mtp40	CAA CGC GCC GTC GGT GG	CCC CCC ACG GCA CCG C	Mt14323	396	***37***
IS*1245*	GCC GCC GAA ACG ATC TAC	AGG TGG CGT CGA GGA AGA C	pMAl2	427	***2***
IS*901*	GCA ACG GTT GTT GCT TGA AA	TGA TAC GGC AAT CGC GT	R13	1,108	***73***
IS*900*	ACG CCG CGG GTA GTT A	GGG GCG ITT GAG GTT IC	ATCC 19698	707	***62***

[a]All of the probes, except one, can be prepared by using the standard PCR program. The preparation of the *mtp40* probe requires a two-step PCR program. *See* **Subheading 2.7.1.2., steps 8** and **9**.

[b]*See* **Subheading 2.7.1.1., item 7**.

M. tuberculosis Mt14323
M. bovis BCG P3
M. avium R13
M. paratuberculosis ATCC 19698

7. Dilute the required target DNA (*see* **Table 2** and **Note 12**) in DNAse-free water to a final concentration of 5 ng/µL, just before use.
8. Mineral oil (Sigma).
9. Electrophoresis marker lambda-phi (*see* **Subheading 2.5., step 3**).
10. QIAquick PCR Purification kit (Qiagen, Hombrechtikon, Switzerland).
11. Thermocycler.

2.7.2. Preparation of PCR Product for Use as a DNA Probe

2.7.2.1. Preparation of PCR Product

1. Prepare the PCR mix, with the following volumes per PCR reaction (*see* **Notes 13** and **14**):
   5.0 µL 10X Super *Taq* PCR buffer
   4.0 µL dNTP mix (2.5 m*M* of each dNTP)
   5.0 µL forward primer (50 ng/µL) (*see* **Table 2**)
   5.0 µL reverse primer (50 ng/µL) (*see* **Table 2**)
   0.1 µL Super *Taq* DNA polymerase (5 U/µL)
   0.9 µL water
2. Vortex and keep the mix on ice.
3. Transfer the PCR mix to PCR tubes in aliquots of 20 µL.
4. Add 30 µL of target DNA to the PCR tubes. Include a negative control by adding 30 µL of water to one PCR tube, instead of target DNA.
5. Add approx 75 µL (2 drops) of mineral oil to each PCR tube (*see* **Note 15**).
6. Vortex and centrifuge for 5 s in a microcentrifuge at 11,000*g*.
7. Place the tubes in a PCR thermocycler and perform (*see* **Table 2**) either the standard- or the two-step PCR program, depending on the probe.
8. Standard PCR program: 3 min 96°C; 30 cycles of 1 min 96°C, 1 min 65°C, 2 min 72°C; and a final extension period of 6 min 72°C.
9. Two-step PCR program: 3 min 96°C; 30 cycles of 1 min 96°C, 2 min 74°C; and a final extension period of 6 min 74°C.
10. Prepare a 1% agarose gel as described in **Subheading 3.2.1., steps 1–8**.
11. Pool the PCR products from five PCR reactions together and vortex.
12. Add 2.5 µL 5X DNA sample buffer for each 10 µL of PCR product and load the samples onto the agarose gel.
13. Load 5 µL of electrophoresis marker lambda-phi to the first and the last wells of the gel.
14. Electrophorese at 100 V for 1 h and take a picture of the gel (**Subheading 3.2.1., steps 11–13**).
15. Evaluate the yield, purity, and size (*see* **Table 2**) of the PCR product on a UV transilluminator. The lane with the negative control should not show any trace of a PCR product.

2.7.2.2. Purification of the PCR Products Using the QIAquick PCR Purification Kit (*see* Note 16)

1. Add 500 µL PB buffer to 100 µL of PCR product (*see* **Note 17**).
2. Place a spin column in a collection tube.
3. Apply the sample to the column and centrifuge for 1 min at 11,000*g*.
4. Discard flow-through and place the column back into the collection tube (*see* **Note 18**).
5. Add 750 µL buffer PE to the column and centrifuge for 1 min at 11,000*g*.
6. Discard flow-through and place the column back into the collection tube.
7. Centrifuge for 1 min at 11,000*g*.
8. Place the column in a clean microcentrifuge tube.
9. Add 50 µL distilled water to the center of the column (*see* **Note 19**).
10. Centrifuge for 1 min at 11,000*g*.
11. Determine the DNA concentration of the purified probe by measuring a 1:50 dilution as described in **Subheading 3.2.**
12. Evaluate the specificity and the hybridization intensity of the probe by hybridizing a DNA membrane containing digested DNA of the external markers of the respective RFLP typing method the probe was prepared for (*see* **Table 1**). Preferably, use a membrane that has been shown to provide optimal RFLP patterns when hybridizing with a previously prepared probe. The RFLP patterns of the external markers should match those shown in **Fig. 6**.

2.7.3. Preparation of Plasmid Insert for Use as a Probe

2.7.3.1. Preparation of Plasmid Insert

1. Isolate the plasmid according to the protocol described by Maniatis et al. ***(71)***. Alternatively, a commercially available plasmid isolation kit can be used, e.g., the Qiagen Plasmid Purification System (Qiagen).
2. Prepare the following digestion mix in a microcentrifuge tube:
   10 µg plasmid pYZ55***(45)***
   5 µL 10X digestion buffer L
   3 µL restriction enzyme *Kpn*I
   distilled water to a final volume of 50 µL.
3. Incubate at 37°C for at least 1 h.
4. Prepare a 1% agarose gel as described in **Subheading 3.2.1., steps 1–8**.
5. Add 12.5 µL of 5X DNA sample buffer to the digested plasmid.
6. Load the digested plasmid sample and 5 µL of electrophoresis marker lambda-phi onto the gel.
7. Electrophorese at 80 V until the bands are clearly separated (at least 1 h) and take a picture of the gel (**Subheading 3.2.1., steps 11–13**).
8. Cut the insert (size DNA fragment: 4.5 Kb) from the gel on the UV transilluminator, using a clean scalpel knife, and add the gel slices from two lanes (approx 100 mg) in one microcentrifuge tube.

2.7.3.2. Isolation of the Insert from the Agarose Using the QIAquick Gel Extraction Kit (*see* **Note 16**)

1. Add 300 µL of buffer QG to each tube containing approx 100 mg of gel slices.
2. Incubate at 50°C for 10 min, while vortexing the tube every 2–3 min (*see* **Note 22**).
3. Add 100 µL isopropanol and vortex.
4. Carry on as in **Subheading 2.7.2.2., steps 2–12**.

*2.7.4. Using an Oligonucleotide as a Probe (*see ***Note 20***)*

1. The oligonucleotide sequences of the oligo probes that are described in this protocol are:

   DR: GTC GTC AGA CCC AAA ACC CCG AGA GGG GAC GGA AAC *(41)*;
   $(GTG)_5$: GTG GTG GTG GTG GTG *(12)*;
   MPTR: GCC GGT GTT G GCC GGT GTT G GCC GGT GTT G *(42)*;
   PGRS: CCG CCG TTG CCG CCG TTG CCG CCG CCG CCG TTG CCG CCG TTG CCG CCG *(30)*.
2. Dissolve the oligonucleotide in DNAse-free water (*see* **Subheading 2.7.1., item 3**) to prepare a concentrated stock solution.
3. Evaluate the newly generated probe by testing the specificity and hybridization signal on a DNA membrane containing digested DNA of the external markers of the RFLP typing method the probe was prepared for (*see* **Table 1**). Preferably, use a membrane that has been shown to provide optimal RFLP patterns when hybridizing with a previously prepared probe. The RFLP patterns of the external markers should match those shown in **Fig. 6**.

*2.7.5. Using a Plasmid as a Probe (*see ***Note 21***)*

1. Plasmid pYZ55 *(45)*.
2. Restriction enzyme *Kpn*I and digestion buffer (Boehringer, Mannheim).
3. Electrophoresis marker lambda-phi (*see* **Subheading 2.5., item 3**).
4. QIAquick Gel Extraction kit (Qiagen).
5. Water bath set at 37°C and 50°C.

2.8. Hybridization and Detection

2.8.1. Labeling of the Probe

1. Enhanced Chemiluminecense Direct Nucleic Acid Labeling and Detection System kit (ECL kit) (Amersham).
2. PCR machine, or water baths set at 37°C and 100°C.

2.8.2. Hybridization

1. Hybridization buffer (ECL kit, Amersham): Pour the buffer supplied by Amersham into a 1 L bottle and place it onto a magnetic stirrer. Add blocking agent (supplied with the kit) in small amounts to prevent clumping, to 5% (w/v), while stirring. Add 60 mL of 5 *M* NaCl (*see* **Subheading 2.1., item 9**) to obtain a

Table 3
Labeling of the Probe, Hybridization Temperature, and Posthybridization Washing Conditions for the Various Probes

	Labeling of the probe				Posthybridization wash	
Nature of the probe[a]	Amount of probe (ng)	Labeling conc. (ng/μL)	Denaturation required	Hybridization T (°C)	Primary washbuffer	T (°C)
PCR product	200	10	yes	42	UREA	42
Insert	200	10	yes	42	UREA	42
Internal size marker	100	10	yes	42	UREA	42
Oligol	400	20	no	40	SSC/SDS	35
Oligo2	600	30	no	40	SSC/SDS	35
Oligo3	600	30	no	35	SSC/SDS	30

[a]*See* **Table 1** for the nature of the various probes.

final concentration of 0.5 *M* NaCl. Warm the solution to 42°C to dissolve the blocking agent completely. This takes about 1 h. Store in aliquots of 10 mL for up to 3 mo at –20°C.
2. Roller bottle or plastic bag.
3. Hybridization incubator or shaking water bath.

2.8.3. Washing the DNA Membrane After Hybridization

1. Primary wash buffer: Depending on the RFLP typing method, use urea buffer or SSC/SDS buffer (*see* **Table 3** and **Note 6**).
2. Urea primary wash buffer: Add 360 g urea and 4 g SDS to 25 mL of 20X SSC (*see* **Subheading 2.6.3., item 1**) and adjust the volume to 1 L with distilled water. Do not autoclave. Either prepare just before use or sterilize by filtration through a 0.2 μm filter and store at room temperature for up to 1 yr.
3. SSC/SDS primary wash buffer: 3X SSC, 0.1% SDS. Add 150 mL of 20X SSC (*see* **Subheading 2.6.3., item 1**) and 10 mL of 10% SDS (*see* **Subheading 2.1., item 6**) to 840 mL distilled water.
4. Secondary wash buffer: 2X SSC. Dilute 20X SSC (*see* **Subheading 2.6.3., item 1**) ten times in distilled water. Prepare just before use.
5. Shaking platform.

2.8.4. Detection

1. Detection reagent 1 (ECL kit, Amersham).
2. Detection reagent 2 (ECL kit, Amersham).
3. Red light bulbs (darkroom light).
4. Clingfilm or Saran Wrap (Dow Chemical Company, Midland, MI).
5. DNA membrane support. Moisten a used film with tap water and wrap it in clingfilm.

6. Light protected cassette: hypercassette (Amersham).
7. Hyperfilm ECL (Amersham).
8. Film developer.
9. Seal apparatus.

2.8.5. Stripping of the DNA Membrane

1. Strip buffer: 0.1X SSC, 0.1% SDS. Add 5 mL of 20X SSC (*see* **Subheading 2.6.3., item 1**) and 10 mL of 10% SDS (*see* **Subheading 2.1., item 6**) to 985 mL distilled water.
2. Shaking water bath, 65°C.

3. Methods

3.1. Isolation of High-Molecular-Weight Genomic DNA from Mycobacteria

Caution: for mycobacteria pathogenic to humans, appropriate containment facilities should be used while handling before heat-inactivation.

1. Transfer at least two loopfuls of mycobacteria into a microcentrifuge tube containing 400 µL of 1X TE buffer (*see* **Notes 23** and **24**).
2. Kill the cells by heating for 20 min at 80°C, and cool at room temperature (*see* **Note 25**).
3. Put the CTAB/NaCl solution at 65°C, for use in **step 6**.
4. Add 50 µL of 10 mg/mL lysozyme to cells, vortex and incubate, while shaking, for at least 1 h at 37°C (*see* **Notes 3** and **26**).
5. Add 75 µL of 10% SDS/proteinase K solution, vortex, and incubate for 10 min at 65°C (*see* **Note 3**).
6. Add 100 µL of 5 *M* NaCl and 100 µL of prewarmed CTAB/NaCl solution, and vortex until the liquid content becomes white ("milky"). Incubate for 10 min at 65°C (*see* **Notes 3** and **27**).
7. Add 750 µL of chloroform/isoamyl alcohol and vortex for at least 10 s (*see* **Notes 2**, **3**, and **28**).
8. Centrifuge for 8 min at 11,000*g*.
9. Transfer the aqueous phase (top) to a fresh microcentrifuge tube, by pipeting a small volume, e.g., 180 µL, at a time (*see* **Note 29**).
10. Carefully add 0.6 vol (450 µL) of isopropanol (*see* **Note 30**).
11. Manually move the tube slowly upside down to precipitate the nucleic acids and estimate the amount of 1X TE in which the DNA should be redissolved in **step 21**. Write the estimated volume on the tube (*see* **Note 31**).
12. Place at –20°C for at least 30 min (*see* **Note 32**).
13. Centrifuge for 15 min at 11,000*g*.
14. Discard most of the supernatant; leave about 20 µL (3 mm height) above the pellet (*see* **Note 4**).
15. Add 1 mL of cold 70% ethanol (from the –20°C freezer) and turn the tube upside down a few times to wash the DNA pellet.

16. Centrifuge for 5 min at 11,000*g*.
17. Discard most of the supernatant; leave about 20 µL (3 mm height) above the pellet (*see* **Note 4**).
18. Centrifuge for 1 min at 11,000*g*.
19. Remove the remaining supernatant from above the pellet by pipeting very carefully with a 20 µL pipet (*see* **Note 33**).
20. Permit the pellet to dry for 15 min at room temperature. Check whether all ethanol is evaporated. If not, then extend the drying time.
21. Dissolve the pellet in the amount of 1X TE estimated in **step 11** (*see* **Note 34**).

3.2. Quantification of the Extracted DNA — Three Methods (see Note 35)

3.2.1. Estimation of the DNA Concentration in an Agarose Gel by Ethidium Bromide Straining and UV Irradiation

Caution: Beware of ethidium bromide, since it is mutagenic. Wear gloves when preparing solutions and handling gels. Discard ethidium bromide-containing waste in an appropriate way.

1. Prepare a bottle of 0.8% w/v agarose in 1X TBE buffer for a small gel (*see* **Notes 36** and **37**).
2. Transfer the bottle to a 70°C water bath until needed.
3. Seal the edges of a clean gel tray with tape and place on a horizontal platform.
4. Add ethidium bromide to the dissolved agarose to a final concentration of 0.5 µg/mL, swirl, and pour the agarose immediately on the tray.
5. Carefully place a comb in the tray, 2 mm from the bottom. Let the agarose solidify (*see* **Notes 38** and **39**).
6. When solidified, remove the tape from the gel tray and place the tray in an electrophoresis tank (*see* **Note 40**).
7. Fill the electrophoresis tank with 1X TBE containing 0.5 µg/mL ethidium bromide. The agarose gel must be covered to a depth of about 2 mm (*see* **Note 41**).
8. Remove the comb from the gel by lifting on both sides at the same time.
9. Vortex the extracted DNA (*see* **Subheading 3.1., step 21**) briefly and pipet 1 µL of the DNA to 9 µL of 1X DNA sample buffer (*see* **Notes 42** and **43**).
10. Apply these 10 µL samples to the slots of the gel.
11. Close the lid of the electrophoresis tank and connect the electrical leads to a power supply. Switch on the power supply and verify the orientation of the gel (*see* **Note 44**).
12. Electrophorese for about 15 min at 6.5 V/cm (100 V) (*see* **Note 45**).
13. Place the gel on a UV transilluminator and make a picture of the gel (*see* **Note 46**).
14. Estimate the concentration of the DNA samples, and choose the required volume (comparable to 4.5 µg DNA) for digestion (*see* **Fig. 1** and **Note 47**).

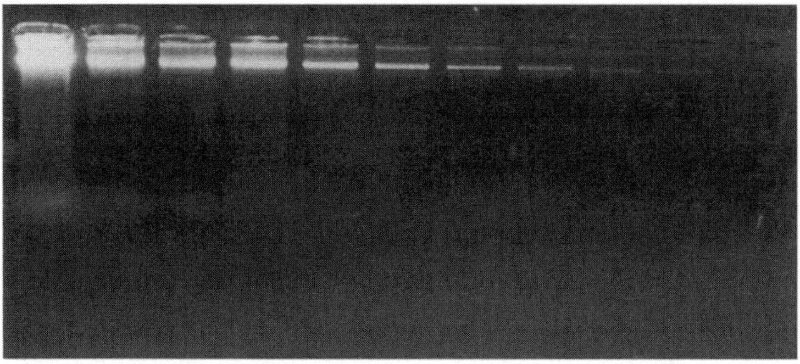

Fig. 1. Estimation of the concentration of the extracted DNA by electrophoresis. Dilutions of 1 µL mycobacterial genomic DNA in 10 µL of sample buffer were electrophoresed and visualized by ethidium bromide staining and UV transillumination. Lanes 1 to 8 contain about 2.25, 0.90, 0.55, 0.55, 0.45, 0.40, 0.30, and 0.25 µg of DNA, respectively. Therefore, for these samples 2, 5, 8, 8, 10, 12, 15, and 18 µL should be used for digestion (about 4.5 µg). The DNA concentration of the samples in **lane 9** to **11** is too low for use in RFLP typing.

3.2.2. Estimation of the DNA Concentration Using a GeneQuant Spectrophotometer

1. Vortex the DNA samples briefly and add 2 µL of each DNA sample to 200 µL of 1X TE (*see* **Notes 42** and **43**).
2. Switch the apparatus on. To check whether the apparatus is installed for double-stranded DNA, press the SET-UP-key followed by the ENTER-key until the setup factor "dsDNA50" appears on the display. If it does not, adjust the installation to "dsDNA 50" with the SELECT-key. Press the ENTER-key.
3. Pipet 100 µL 1X TE as the blank into a clean quartz cuvet.
4. Press the SET REF-key and insert the cuvet with the blank, after the apparatus displays "Insert reference."
5. Empty the cuvet (*see* **Note 4**).
6. Press the SAMPLE-key and insert the cuvet containing 100 µL of the first DNA sample, directly after the apparatus displays "Insert sample."
7. Remove the cuvet after the apparatus displays "Remove sample."
8. Press the CONC-key.
9. Write the DNA concentration depicted on the display on an appropriate form (*see* **Note 48**).
10. Remove the DNA sample from the cuvet (*see* **Notes 4** and **49**).
11. Repeat **steps 6–10** (excluding **step 8**) until all samples have been measured (*see* **Note 50**).
12. The amount of DNA needed for the digestion (4.5 µg) can be calculated from the formula: 4500/DNA concentration (µg/mL) = µL DNA for digestion (*see* **Note 51**).

3.2.3. Estimation of the DNA Concentration Using a General Spectrophotometer

1. Vortex the DNA samples briefly and add 2 µL of each DNA sample to 200 µL of 1X TE (*see* **Notes 42** and **43**).
2. Switch the apparatus on.
3. Adjust the wavelength to 260 nm.
4. Pipet 100 µL of 1X TE in the cuvet and measure the absorbance of the blank.
5. Empty the cuvet (*see* **Note 4**).
6. Measure the absorbance of all the samples, and empty the cuvet in between (*see* **Notes 4** and **49**).
7. Use the following formula to calculate the DNA concentration: (absorbance sample – absorbance blank) × 50 = DNA concentration in µg/mL (*see* **Notes 50** and **51**).
8. The amount of DNA needed for the digestion (4.5 µg) can be calculated from the formula: 4500/DNA concentration (µg/mL) = µL DNA for digestion (*see* **Note 51**).

3.3. Digestion of Chromosomal DNA by a Restriction Enzyme

1. Always include DNA for the appropriate external markers in the digestion experiment (*see* **Table 1** and **Note 6**). For digestion of the DNA samples pipet the following reagents into a microcentrifuge tube for each sample (*see* **Notes 51** and **52**):

   distilled water to 20 µL final volume
   2 µL digestion buffer
   1 µL restriction enzyme (10 U/µL) (*see* **Table 1**)
   4.5 µg DNA in volume
2. Vortex briefly and centrifuge for 5 s at 11,000*g*.
3. Incubate for 1 h at 37°C (*see* **Notes 6** and **53**).
4. If necessary, inactivate the enzyme by incubating for 15 min at 65°C (*see* **Table 1** and **Note 54**).

3.4. Estimation of the DNA Concentration in the Samples After Digestion

Caution: Beware of ethidium bromide, since it is mutagenic. Wear gloves when preparing solutions and handling gels. Discard ethidium bromide-containing waste in an appropriate way.

1. Prepare a small 0.8% (w/v) agarose gel as described in **Subheading 3.2.1., steps 1–8**.
2. Add 5 µL of 5X DNA sample buffer containing the appropriate internal size marker to the 20 µL of digested DNA sample (*see* **Table 1** and **Notes 6** and **8**).
3. Centrifuge for 5 s at 11,000*g*.
4. Apply 5 µL of the DNA samples to the slots of the gel (*see* **Note 55**).
5. Close the lid of the electrophoresis tank and connect the electrical leads to a power supply. Switch on the power supply and verify the orientation of the gel (*see* **Note 44**).

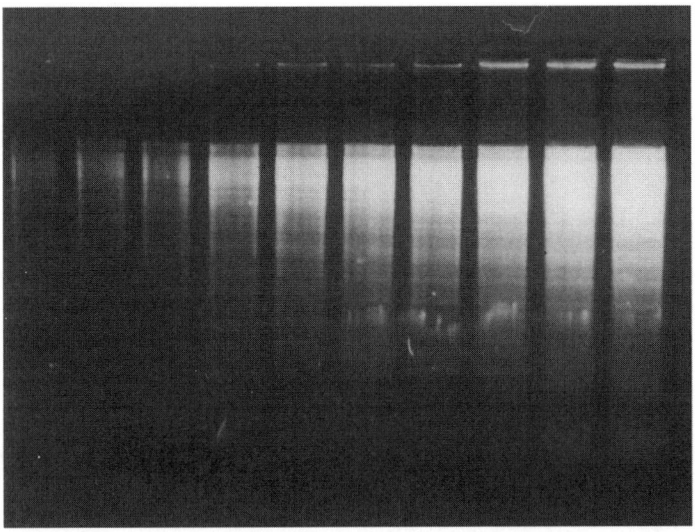

Fig. 2. Estimation of the concentration of the digested DNA by a short electrophoresis. Five microliters of 25 μL *Pvu*II-digested DNA sample in sample buffer was electrophoresed and visualized. **Lanes 1** to **10** contain about 0.5, 0.55, 0.65, 0.85, 1.0, 1.25, 1.45, 1.65, 2.0, and 2.5 μg of digested DNA. From the samples in **lane 1** to **10** it is recommended to apply respectively 20, 18, 15, 12, 10, 8, 7, 6, 5, and 4 μL to the slots of the gel for Southern blotting. This will result in approximately equal amounts of DNA in each lane (about 2 μg/lane).

6. Electrophorese for about 25 min at 6.5 V/cm (100 V) (*see* **Note 45**).
7. Place the gel on a UV transilluminator and take a picture of the gel.
8. Estimate the volume of the DNA samples that is required to get an equal DNA concentration of about 2 μg in each lane on the Southern blot gel, by comparing the intensity of the ethidium bromide stained DNA fragments of the samples on a UV transilluminator (*see* **Fig. 2** and **Note 47**).

3.5. Electrophoresis

1. Prepare an agarose gel of the size and % (wt/vol) according to the recommendations listed in **Table 1** as described in **Subheading 3.2.1., steps 1–8** (*see* **Notes 6** and **36**).
2. Load 5 μL of the electrophoresis marker in the first slot (*see* **Table 1** and **Note 6**).
3. Load the DNA samples in the second to the second-to-last slot (as estimated under **Subheading 3.4., step 8**).

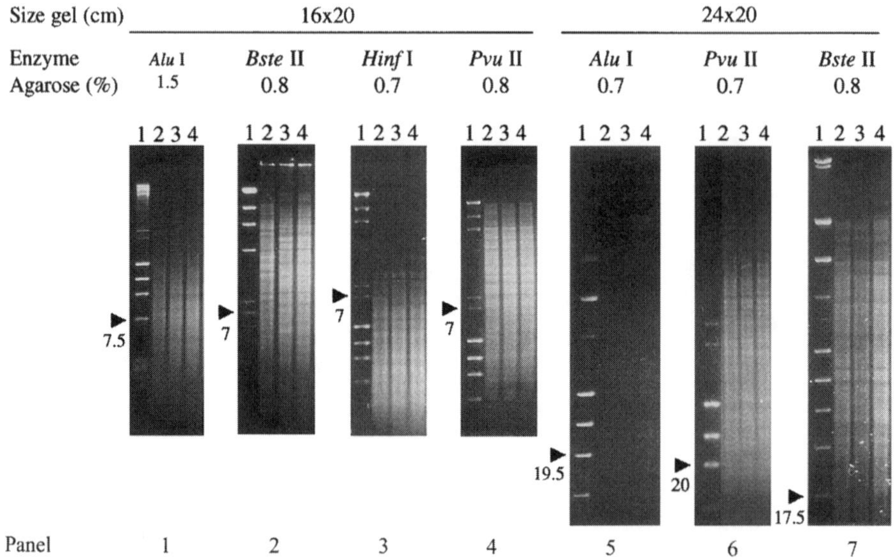

Fig. 3. Examples of agarose gels for Southern blotting containing electrophoresed restriction fragments of the various RFLP typing methods. The DNA was digested by the indicated restriction enzyme, and separated on an agarose gel of the appropriate %, and thereafter visualized by ethidium bromide staining and UV transillumination. **Lanes 1** in each gel contains the relevant electrophoresis markers. The indicator band marked by an arrow and the required electrophoresis distance of this marker from the slots in cm are also given. Panels 1–4 and 6 contain electrophoresis marker lambda-phi, panels 5 and 7 contain marker IV. **Lanes 2–4** of panels 1, and 3 to 5 contain DNA of *M. tuberculosis* complex strains. **Lanes 2–4** of panel 2 show DNA of *M. kansasii* strains, and panels 6 and 7 show DNA of *M. avium* and *M. paratuberculosis* strains, respectively.

4. Save the leftovers of the loaded DNA samples at 4°C to prepare marking mix (*see* **Subheading 2.6.2.1., step 2** and **Note 11**).
5. Electrophorese at 3.2 V/cm (100 V) until the DNA samples have run into the gel (for about 5–10 min), and thereafter decrease the voltage to the appropriate voltage (*see* **Table 1** and **Note 6**).
6. Electrophorese overnight for the appropriate time (*see* **Note 56**).
7. Check the migration of the DNA in the gel on an UV transilluminator and measure the migration distance of the indicator band of the external marker (*see* **Fig. 3**). Electrophorese further until this band has reached the required distance (*see* **Table 1** and **Note 6**).
8. Make a picture of the gel on the UV transilluminator and paste this photograph on the work form (*see* **Note 51**). Examples of overnight run gels are shown in **Fig. 4**.

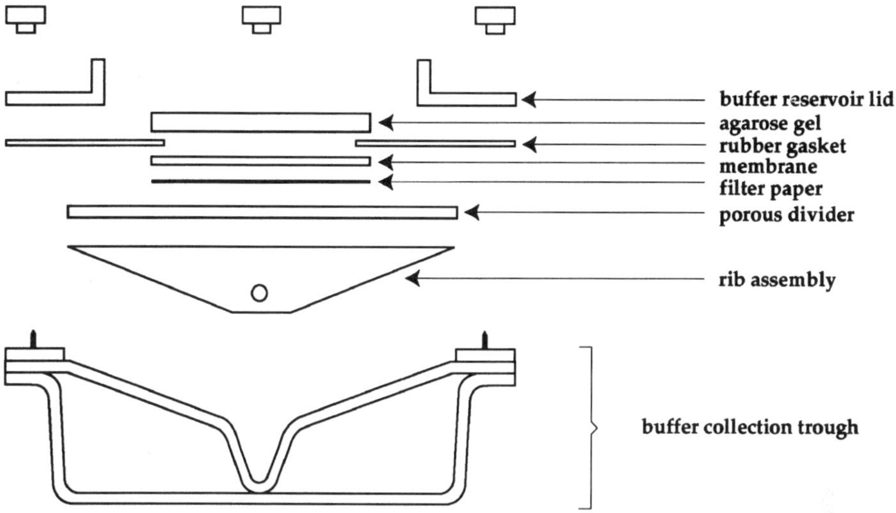

Fig. 4. Schematic representation of the use of a vacuum blotter for Southern blotting.

3.6. Southern Blotting (see Note 57)

3.6.1. Preparation of the Gel for Southern Blotting

1. Place the gel on a UV transilluminator until the fluorescence of the ethidium bromide has almost faded completely (for about 5 to 15 min).
2. Place the gel in 0.25 *M* HCl for 10 min (*see* **Note 58**).
3. Rinse with distilled water.
4. Place the gel in 0.4 *M* NaOH for 20 min (*see* **Note 58**).
5. Repeat **steps 3** and **4**.

3.6.2. Southern Blotting — Two Methods

3.6.2.1. Transfer of DNA from the Gel onto a Membrane by Vacuum Blotting

1. Build a blot construction as shown in **Fig. 4**.
2. Prepare 50 mL agarose 1% (wt/vol) and keep at 70°C in a water bath (*see* **Note 37**).
3. Put the porous divider in a sink filled with tap water until it is completely saturated and thereafter place it on the rib assembly.
4. Cut a filter paper to the appropriate size (*see* **Note 59**), saturate it with distilled water, and place on the center of the porous divider (*see* **Note 60**).
5. Cut a DNA membrane of the appropriate size (*see* **Note 59**) and mark it with a number and additional spots using a ball-point pen. Apply marking mix on the code with a small brush to enable visualization of the number and the spots during the detection. Dry the wetted spots using a blow-dryer (*see* **Notes 11**, **61**, and **62**).

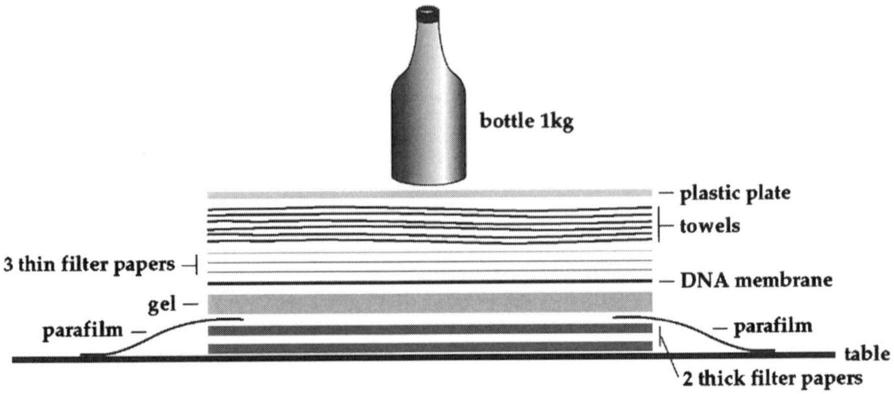

Fig. 5. Schematic representation of the use of a capillary method for Southern blotting.

6. Wet the membrane with distilled water and place it on the filter paper (*see* **Note 60**).
7. Place a rubber gasket on the edges of the membrane (0.5 cm overlap at all sides).
8. Place a ruler 1 cm from the edge of the rubber gasket and place the gel *in one move* (do not shove) onto the membrane with one side against the ruler (*see* **Note 63**).
9. Remove the excess buffer from the gel and the area surrounding the gel carefully using a tissue.
10. Put the cover on the vacuum blot apparatus and turn the screws hand-tight.
11. Apply 7 µL marking mix to the third gel slot from the left and third gel slot from the right (*see* **Notes 11, 61,** and **64**).
12. Cover the slots and the four sides of the gel with 1% agarose and let it solidify.
13. Pour 10X SSPE on the gel until the gel is covered with about 1 cm height of buffer.
14. Connect the tube with the vacuum pump and switch the pump on.
15. Adjust the vacuum to –3 kPa and check for leakage (*see* **Note 65**).
16. Increase the vacuum to –17 kPa after 5 min.
17. Blot until more than 100 mL 10X SSPE has been sucked through the gel (for about 20–30 min) (*see* **Notes 66** and **67**).

3.6.2.2. Transfer of DNA from the Gel onto a Membrane by Capillary Blotting

1. Incubate the gel in 0.25 *M* Tris-acetate-0.1 *M* NaCl for 15 min manually shaking occasionally (*see* **Note 58**).
2. Incubate the gel in 0.025 *M* Tris-acteate-0.01 *M* NaCl for 15 min manually shaking occasionally (*see* **Note 58**).
3. Clean the table with 70% ethanol and build a blot-construction as shown in **Fig. 5**.
4. Cut two pieces of thick filter paper, three pieces of thin filter paper, and a DNA membrane to the appropriate size (*see* **Notes 59** and **62**).

5. Mark the DNA membrane with a number and additional spots using a ball-point pen. Apply marking mix on the code with a small brush to enable visualization of the number and the spots during detection. Dry the wetted spots using a blow-dryer (*see* **Notes 11**, **61**, and **62**).
6. Saturate the two thick filter papers, the membrane, and one of the thin filter papers in 0.025 *M* Tris-acteate-0.01 *M* NaCl.
7. Place two thick filter papers on the table.
8. Cover all sides of the filter paper 1 cm with 5 cm broad slides of parafilm.
9. Subsequently, place the gel, the membrane (with marked side facing the gel), the three filter papers, paper towels, a plastic plate and a 1 kg weight on top (*see* **Notes 59**, **60**, and **62**).
10. Blot the gel for 60–90 min (*see* **Note 67**).

3.6.3. Treatment of the DNA Membrane After Southern Blotting

1. To fix the DNA, place the membrane with the DNA-side up for 2 min on a filter paper saturated with 0.4 *M* NaOH.
2. Rinse the membrane with 5X SSC.
3. The membrane can either be used directly for hybridization experiments, or be stored at 4°C in wet condition sealed in plastic (*see* **Note 68**).

3.7. Hybridization and Detection (see Note 69)

3.7.1. Labeling of the Probe

1. Dilute the probe with water from the ECL-kit to obtain the desired concentration (*see* **Table 3**).
2. If necessary, heat-denature the probe at 99.9°C for 5 min and chill on ice immediately for 1 min (*see* **Table 3** and **Note 70**).
3. Centrifuge for a few seconds at 11,000*g*.
4. Add an equal volume of DNA labeling reagent and mix by pipeting.
5. Add the same volume glutaraldehyde and vortex briefly.
6. Spin the solution for a few seconds in a microcentrifuge at 11,000*g*.
7. Incubate for 10 min at 37°C (*see* **Notes 70** and **71**).

3.7.2. Hybridization (see **Note 72**)

1. Prehybridize the membrane in 10 mL hybridization buffer in a roller bottle for at least 10 min at the appropriate temperature in a hybridization oven (*see* **Table 3** and **Note 6**).
2. Pour the hybridization buffer into a tube and add the labeled probe to the buffer (*see* **Table 1** and **Note 6**). Mix by turning the tube a few times upside down and pour the buffer-probe-mix back into the roller bottle.
3. Hybridize the membrane overnight at the appropriate temperature (*see* **Table 3**) in the hybridization oven, while rolling the bottle at 6 rpm (*see* **Note 73**).

3.7.3. Washing the DNA Membrane After Hybridization

1. Discard the hybridization solution.

2. Add about 50 mL primary wash buffer to the membrane in the roller bottle and place the bottle in the hybridization oven at the washing temperature for 20 min, while rolling the bottle at 6 rpm (*see* **Table 3** and **Note 72**).
3. Discard the primary wash buffer and repeat **step 2**.
4. Place the DNA membrane in a clean plastic box by using forceps and cover it with about 500 mL secondary wash buffer (2X SSC) (*see* **Note 74**).
5. Wash the filter for 5 min at room temperature on a shaking platform.
6. Repeat **step 5**.

3.7.4. Detection

1. Mix equal volumes of the ECL detection reagents 1 and 2 in a bottle. Use 10 mL of each ECL-detection reagent for each membrane. Pour the mix into a clean plastic box.
2. Turn off the light and switch on the red light (*see* **Note 75**).
3. Drain the membrane and transfer it from the secondary wash buffer to the box containing the ECL-detection reagent mix, using forceps, with the DNA-side facing up. Shake the box carefully until the membrane is completely soaked with the detection reagent mix.
4. Incubate the membrane, while moving the box manually, for exactly 1.5 min (*see* **Note 76**).
5. Drain the membrane and place on a membrane support. For example, for this purpose an old film wrapped with Saran Wrap can be used.
6. Wrap the membrane with the membrane support in cling film and place it, with the DNA-side facing up, in a light-protected cassette.
7. Take a film, fold one of its corners, and place it on the membrane with the folded corner on the right top of the filter (*see* **Note 77**).
8. Expose the membrane for 5–120 min depending on the expected intensity of the reaction (*see* **Note 78**).
9. Develop the film by incubating it for 0.5–2 min in developer, rinsing for 2 s in a sink with tap water, incubating for 1 min in fixer, and rinsing with tap water (*see* **Note 79**).
10. If necessary, expose another film for a longer or shorter period.
11. Store the membrane in moist condition, wrapped in cling film at 4°C (*see* **Notes 68** and **80**).

*3.7.5. Stripping of the DNA Membrane for Direct Reuse (*see ***Note 67***)*

1. Prewarm the strip buffer at 65°C.
2. Pour about 500 mL strip buffer in a clean plastic box and place the DNA membrane in it.
3. Strip the membrane for 30 min at 65°C, while shaking, in a water bath.
4. Drain the membrane and use directly for a new hybridization.

3.8. Quality Control

To check the whole RFLP typing procedure, including digestion, separation of the DNA fragments, Southern blotting, hybridization, and detection, check

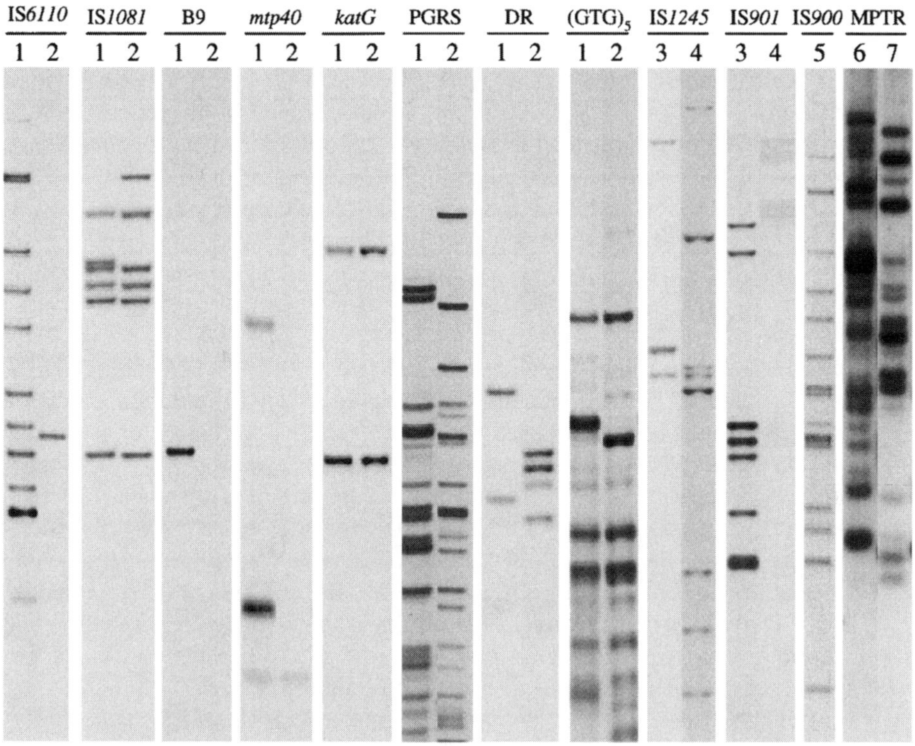

Fig. 6. RFLP patterns of the external markers (mycobacterial reference strains) of the RFLP typing methods described in this protocol (*see* **Table 1**). Text on top indicates the probe used for hybridization. **Lanes 1**, *M. tuberculosis* strain Mt14323; **lanes 2**, *M. bovis* BCG strain P3; **lanes 3** and **4**, *M. avium* strains R13 and IWGMT 49 respectively; **lane 5**, *M. paratuberculosis* strain ATCC 19698; **lane 6**, *M. kansasii* strain MkG59; **lane 7**, *M. gordonae* strain ATCC 19277.

the correctness of the RFLP patterns of the mycobacterial reference strains (external markers). **Figure 6** shows the correct RFLP patterns of the external markers of the RFLP typing methods described in this protocol.

4. Notes

1. Prevent inhalation of SDS when handling solid SDS. Use an exhaust hood and a mask.
2. Be careful with chloroform. Do not inhale. Always use an exhaust hood. Do not spill chloroform on plastic racks, as it can damage certain plastics.
3. For all incubations during the DNA isolation procedure a water bath can be used. If shaking is required, use 45 rpm. Alternatively, a thermomixer can be used. This is an apparatus that heats and shakes the tubes simultaneously (*see* **Subheading**

2.1., item 15). For shaking incubations use position 7, for vortexing use the highest shaking position. This apparatus can be used for the entire DNA isolation procedure, but it is important to check whether the vortexing went well after addition of CTAB/NaCl. We recommend avoiding this apparatus for heat-killing bacteria or the vortex step after the addition of chloroform/isoamylalcohol. These steps should be done manually.

4. It is more convenient to use an aspirator. Alternatively a pipet can be used.
5. Always wear gloves when handling ethidium bromide, as it is mutagenic.
6. Different RFLP typing methods require different restriction enzymes, external markers, internal size markers, electrophoresis markers and conditions, probes, and hybridization and posthybridization conditions. The conditions for the various RFLP typing methods described in this protocol are listed in **Table 1**. The hybridization and posthybridization conditions are listed in **Table 3**.
7. External markers are mycobacterial strains that serve as a control for the whole RFLP procedure including cleavage by a restriction enzyme, Southern blotting and hybridization. The DNA fingerprints of such strains also serve as external markers for computer-assisted analysis to control the normalization procedure with the internal size markers by matching the band positions of this pattern with those of previously scanned patterns of the external marker ***(14)***. They can also be used to test the comparability of DNA fingerprints originating from different autoradiograms and different institutes. If digested DNA of an external marker is applied on the gel at least three times, then the patterns can be used for the normalization of the fingerprints during the computer-assisted analysis.
8. Internal markers are added to each DNA sample for use as internal molecular weight markers. To visualize the marker DNA, the membrane is rehybridized with a probe derived from the internal marker DNA. The use of this size marker allows a precise estimation of the molecular size of the DNA fragments by superimposing the autoradiogram of internal marker and the RFLP patterns. These internal size marker patterns are critical when a reliable computer-assisted analysis of large numbers of strains is needed (*see* **Fig. 6**).
9. All DNA fragments of the supercoiled DNA ladder are supercoiled. By digesting this DNA with *Pvu*II, all fragments become linear, except for the smallest component of 2.07 kb, which contains no *Pvu*II restriction site. During digestion about 30% of this supercoiled circular DNA usually becomes open circular. Under the described electrophoresis conditions, this open circular component migrates with a mobility corresponding to that of linear DNA with a size of 2.0 kb. The 2.07 kb supercoiled DNA has, under the described conditions, a mobility corresponding to that of linear DNA of about 1.25 kb (*see* **Fig. 6**).
10. Dissolving NaOH is an exothermic reaction. Beware of heat production.
11. It is convenient to mark the DNA membrane with a code indicating the number of the blot and the year in which it was prepared with a ball-point pen. In addition, it is useful to mark it with symbols, for example, a small cross or short vertical or horizontal lines, in all four corners. When these marking points are covered with marking mix (a mixture of mycobacterial and internal marker DNA), these points

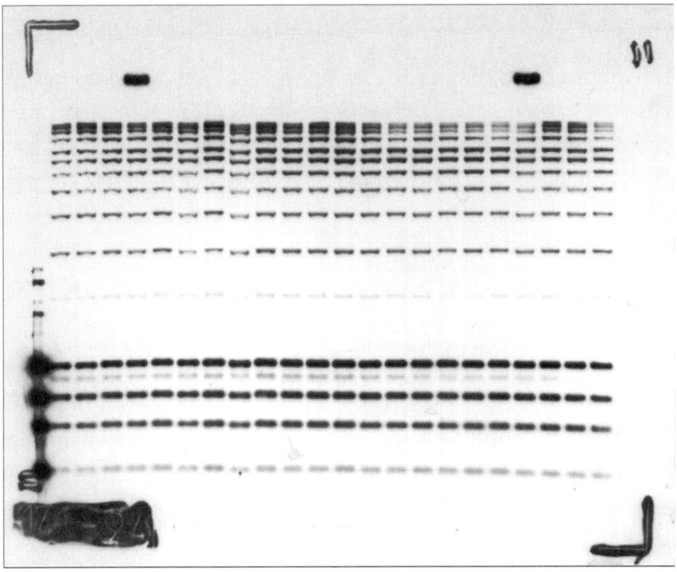

Fig. 7. Example of an autoradiogram with marking points. The membrane was marked with a ball-point pen before using marking mix. Besides two slots, the membrane was marked at all the corners, and in addition with a serial number. Marking of the slots was achieved by adding marking mix to the slots prior to the blotting. Marking of the corners and the blot number at the left bottom was achieved by drawing lines with a ball-point pen and putting marking mix on the membrane with a small brush. Thereafter the wetted spots were dried using a blow-dryer. All of these marking points on the membrane allow an accurate superimpositioning of the internal size marker autoradiogram and the autoradiogram containing the IS*6110* banding patterns. Accurate superimpositioning of these two autoradiograms is essential for reliable computer-assisted analysis.

will be visible after detection, because the DNA mix will not attach to the membrane at the ball-point marks but only to the surrounding area. After detection, these marking points appear as white marks within black spots (*see* **Fig. 7**). The code is useful for file systems (identification). The information on the blot can be listed elsewhere (*see* also **Note 27**) to make the blot and films are recognizable. Furthermore, the marking points are necessary to superimpose the autoradiogram of the internal marker patterns onto the autoradiogram of the RFLP patterns for computer-assisted analysis ***(14)***.

12. DNA from any other strain that contains the target DNA sequence for amplification can also be used.
13. We recommend preparing a large batch of probe using 30–50 PCR reactions. Therefore, prepare a PCR mix for that amount of PCR reactions.

14. Alternatively PCR beads (Ready to go PCR beads, Amersham) can be used for PCR amplification of the PCR products, according to the instructions of the manufacturer. These beads already contain the PCR buffer, the DNA polymerase, and the dNTPs. In our hands, *mtp40* PCR product prepared using the PCR beads are purer in comparison with products prepared using a home-made PCR mix. On the contrary, if the IS*6110* probe is prepared using the PCR beads, then many nonspecific products are obtained.
15. The PCR reaction mixture should be covered with mineral oil to prevent evaporation.
16. We describe the use of QIAquick DNA purification kits (Qiagen). These kits contain spin columns, collection tubes, and the following reagents: buffer PB, which allows the efficient binding of single- or double-stranded PCR products as small as 100 bp and the removal of primers up to 40 bp; buffer QG, which solubilizes the agarose gel slice and provides the appropriate conditions for binding of DNA to the column; buffer PE to wash and buffer EB to eluate the DNA from the column. Buffer EB may contain factors that influence the labeling of the probe; therefore, we advise the use of distilled water to elute the DNA. The pH of the water should be between 7.0 and 8.5 for efficient elution. We prefer the use of the Qiagen kit because in our hands it is provides the best results. Some other PCR purification kits severely inhibit the labeling of the probe.
17. It is not necessary to remove the oil before adding buffer PB; however, it is convenient to remove most of the oil using an aspirator. The 100 µL should not include oil.
18. The Qiaquick spin columns fit onto luer connectors, and vacuum protocols are available. The outlets nozzles of the columns fit into any commercial vacuum manifold with luer connectors. This reduces time and allows easy and convenient handling of up to 24 samples.
19. Alternatively, for increased DNA concentration, add 30 µL distilled water and leave the column for 1 min.
20. In this protocol we use the ECL DNA labeling kit to label the probes. In principle, the positively charged peroxidase that is used for labeling of the probe can, due to its size, only bind to the probe at every 40 bp. Consequently, only one or two peroxidase labels can bind to a short oligonucleotide sequence. Using an oligo as a probe in the ECL-labeling and detection system is therefore only successful when the oligo is at least 30 bp in length and when its sequence is directed to repetitive DNA.
21. The only probe that should be prepared from an insert described in this protocol is *katG*. The conditions and reagents necessary to prepare the *katG* probe are described in **Subheading 2.7.3.** *(45)*. If another insert is to be used as a probe, change or adjust the following variables where appropriate: the plasmid containing the insert, the restriction enzyme, the digestion buffer and the temperature, and the size of the insert fragment that should be isolated from the gel.
22. The color of the mixture should be of the same color of yellow as buffer QG. This indicates the correct pH for DNA binding. During this step all the agarose should dissolve.

23. If mycobacteria are isolated which grow well on solid media, such as, e.g., *M. tuberculosis*, then use at least two loops (0.5 cm diameter) of bacteria. Alternatively, in case of, e.g., *M. avium* complex strains, or other mycobacteria growing into the surface of the media, take a well-grown 50 mL liquid culture. Transfer the liquid culture to a suitable centrifuge tube and centrifuge for 15 min at 3000*g* using aerosol-containment buckets. Discard the supernatant and add 200 µL of 1X TE buffer to the tube. Resuspend the pellet by vortexing, transfer 200 µL to a microcentrifuge tube and add 200 µL of 1X TE.
24. Do not use a mycobacterial culture grown on 7H10 medium, because for unknown reasons DNA isolated from mycobacteria grown on this medium is not well digested by restriction enzymes.
25. Use microcentrifuge tubes with a safe-lock, or jam the microcentrifuge tubes in such a way that the lids cannot open spontaneously.
26. Incubation should preferably be overnight, especially when DNA is isolated from *M. bovis* or *M. microti* strains.
27. Prewarming the CTAB/NaCl solution in a water bath at 65°C will make the solution less viscous and therefore more appropriate to pipet. The aim of CTAB treatment is to remove cell wall debris, denatured protein, polysaccharides that complex to CTAB, although retaining the nucleic acids in solution. Adding salt is very important, since a CTAB-nucleic acid precipitate will form if the salt concentration drops below about 0.5 *M* at room temperature ***(72)***.
28. The chloroform/isoamyl alcohol extraction precipitates the CTAB-protein/polysaccharide complexes. A white interface should be visible after centrifugation.
29. Be careful not to transfer any of the interface, as this will result in impure DNA.
30. There is no need to add salt for precipitation of the DNA since the NaCl concentration is already sufficient.
31. While turning the tube upside-down precipitated DNA may or may not become visible, depending on the amount present. Stop shaking when a precipitate is formed and the solution becomes clear. If there is no precipitate of nucleic acids visible, then dissolve the pellet in 20 µL of 1X TE. If there is a small precipitate visible, then dissolve the pellet in 35 µL. Medium and large precipitates require 50 and 80 µL, respectively.
32. This step is not essential, but does ensure that all the DNA is precipitated. The incubation time can be extended as long as it is convenient, since DNA can be kept in these conditions for years.
33. Be sure that all traces of ethanol are removed, otherwise the pellet cannot dry and the precipitated DNA may redissolve.
34. Dissolving the DNA pellet at room temperature may take some time. To dissolve the DNA more quickly, incubate in a dry incubator at 37°C for 1 h. Alternatively, incubate overnight at 4°C. Dissolved DNA can be stored at 4°C. For longer periods of time (years) the DNA can be stored at –20°C.
35. Three methods to quantify the amount of extracted DNA are described. Using a GeneQuant (*see* **Subheading 2.2.2., step 2**) or a general spectrophotometer is more accurate than estimation of the DNA concentration by ethidium bromide staining.

The most convenient way is using the GeneQuant spectrophotometer or another dedicated apparatus, since these apparatus display the DNA concentration directly.

36. To prepare a small agarose gel (measuring 9 × 13 cm with 30 slots) use 50 mL of 1X TBE. For a large gel (24 slots), measuring 16 × 20 cm, use 150 mL. For a gel measuring 24 × 20 cm use 300 mL.
37. Dissolve the agarose by heating the buffer in a microwave. Always wear a face shield when working with a microwave. Alternatively, a boiling water bath can be used. Swirl and ensure that all agarose is completely dissolved. The agarose is well-dissolved if, while swirling, solid agarose is no longer visible.
38. The presence of ethidium bromide allows the gel to be examined by ultraviolet illumination at any stage during electrophoresis. The fluorescent dye intercalates between stacked base pairs reducing the electrophoretic mobility of linear DNA by about 15%. Do not add ethidium bromide until the temperature of the agarose solution has decreased to 70°C.
39. Make sure that no bubbles are trapped underneath the combs and that all bubbles on the surface of the agarose are removed before the gel sets. This can be achieved by tipping the bubbles briefly with a pipet tip.
40. The comb should be on the side of the cathode (negative electrode, black).
41. It is important to use the same batch of 1X TBE in both the electrophoresis tank and the gel. Small differences in ionic strength or pH create fronts in the gel that can effect the mobility of the DNA fragments.
42. Use a dedicated pipet, for small volumes.
43. If many samples are to be pipetted it is convenient to use a microtiter plate to prepare the dilutions in.
44. Always check the current. If the electrical leads have been attached correctly, bubbles should be generated at the anode and cathode (due to electrolysis), and, within a few minutes, the bromophenol blue should migrate from the wells into the agarose.
45. The electrical field strength (V/cm) can be calculated with the following formula:

$$E = \frac{\Delta V}{\Delta X}$$

E = electrical field strength
ΔV = potential difference (V)
ΔX = distance between the electrodes (cm)

46. Ultraviolet radiation is harmful for the skin, and in particular to the eyes. Wear a face shield.
47. For standardization purposes, we recommend preparing a similar picture using the equipment present in your own laboratory in order to have a reliable estimation of the DNA concentration.
48. The absorbance of the blank will be automatically subtracted and the corrected DNA concentration of the sample is automatically measured.
49. When an aspirator is used, it is not necessary to wash the cuvet in between two samples.
50. The DNA concentration should be between 0.2 and 2 mg/mL. If the DNA concentration of a sample is higher than 2 mg/mL, dilute the sample twofold in 1X

TE. If the DNA concentration of a sample is less than 0.2 mg/mL, the DNA is not suitable for RFLP typing and a new DNA preparation should be made.

51. If the DNA concentration is determined, it is convenient to calculate the amount of DNA and the amount of water needed for the digestion automatically by using the appropriate formulas in a spreadsheet (e.g., Excel, Microsoft Co., Redmond, WA). The different parameters can be printed directly onto a work form in separate columns. In addition, it may be useful to stick a photograph of the gel for Southern blotting on this form and to write the results of the hybridization on it. In this way, all the information related to one DNA membrane can be put on one form. It is also possible to prepare computer-printed stickers containing the sample number, DNA concentration, and isolation date from the same spreadsheet. These stickers can be pasted on the microcentrifuge tubes containing the respective DNA samples.
52. It is convenient to prepare one digestion mix for all samples containing 2 μL distilled water, 2 μL digestion buffer, and 1 μL restriction enzyme per sample (pipet for two samples more to compensate for loss during pipeting). Pipet in the indicated order, because restriction enzymes are very sensitive to buffer conditions. The amount of water needed for the digestion is 15-X μL. First pipet the distilled water to all the tubes, then add 5 μL digestion mix, and finally the required amount of DNA. In this case, the pipet tips only have to be changed in between the DNA samples.
53. The incubation time may be extended, but be aware that samples may partially evaporate. The optimum temperature for *Bste*II is 60°C, however, this causes very quick evaporation of the samples. Therefore, incubate *Bste*II digests at 37°C for an extended period of 4 h.
54. In some RFLP typing methods, the restriction enzyme will digest the internal marker. To avoid this, the restriction enzyme is inactivated by heating (*see* **Table 1**).
55. Mix each sample by pipeting before applying it to a slot.
56. To obtain an optimum separation of DNA fragments, it is preferable to electrophorese overnight, especially with chromosomal digests. Small gels can be electrophoresed at high voltage for shorter time periods, but the resolution decreases as the voltage gradient increases.
57. The DNA is exposed to UV light and treated with HCl and NaOH to break the DNA into smaller fragments, which are transferred to the membrane more efficiently. The acid treatment partially depurinates the DNA and these depurinated sites are cleaved during the alkali treatment, resulting in smaller DNA fragments. In the capillary transfer method, DNA fragments are carried from the gel in a flow of liquid and deposited on the surface of the solid support. The liquid is drawn through the gel and membrane by capillary action that is established and maintained by a stack of dry, absorbent paper towels. In a vacuum transfer device, the gel is placed in contact with the filter supported on a porous screen over a vacuum chamber. Buffer, drawn from an upper reservoir, elutes nucleic acids from the gel and deposits them on the membrane. Vacuum transfer is more efficient and more rapid than capillary transfer.

58. The gel should be completely covered.
59. The size of both the filter paper and the DNA membrane should be the same as the size of the gel that is blotted.
60. Avoid air bubbles between the gel and the filters.
61. Note that the marking mix to be used should contain both DNA of the internal marker and DNA of strains of the mycobacterial species being typed.
62. Always wear gloves when handling the DNA membrane because DNAses and other inhibitory factors may be present on bare hands.
63. The gel should be placed against the ruler either at the top or the bottom depending on where the DNA fragments of interest are positioned.
64. The marking mix is applied to the slots to identify the start point of electrophoresis and the first and last lane of the gel.
65. If the buffer collector is filled too quickly (within a few minutes), the blot construction is leaking.
66. When the blotting is finished the gel should be thin in the center in comparison with the edges. Check this, with a gloved finger, before turning off the vacuum. If not, continue the blotting.
67. Thinner gels can be transferred more rapidly than thicker ones. Similarly, smaller DNA fragments transfer more rapidly than larger ones.
68. Always keep the membrane moist. The membrane can be stored for short periods of time, wrapped in plastic, at 4°C. For longer periods of time (>1 wk) the membrane should be sealed in plastic. A membrane that is to be stored for years should be kept at –20°C. If a membrane is stored well, it can be hybridized repeatedly (up to 10–20 times).
69. The ECL system involves direct labeling of probe DNA with the enzyme horseradish peroxidase (HRP). This is achieved by completely denaturing the probe so that it is single-stranded and therefore negatively charged. HRP, which has been complexed with a positively charged polymer, is added and forms a loose attachment to the DNA by charge attraction. Addition of glutaraldehyde causes the formation of chemical crosslinks so that the enzyme is covalently bound to the probe. Once labeled, the probe is used in hybridization with target DNA immobilized on a membrane. HRP catalyzes the oxidation of the substrate luminol which, in the presence of a chemical enhancer, results in a large and sustained blue light emission, that is readily detected on film.
70. It is convenient to use a PCR machine for this incubation. Alternatively, a waterbath can be used.
71. The probe can be used directly for hybridization or can be stored at –20°C in a final concentration of 50% (v/v) glycerol.
72. Preferably, conduct the hybridization in a roller bottle in a hybridization oven. However, hybridization can be carried out in a plastic bag in a shaking waterbath. In this case use 30 mL of hybridization buffer and 400 mL of primary wash buffer.
73. The hybridization temperature should not exceed 42°C to prevent inactivation of the peroxidase.
74. The filter should not be incubated for more than 30 min in the secondary wash buffer.

75. If other light colors than red are used in the dark room, then this often results in background shading on the films.
76. It is important to work swiftly, because the reaction weakens fast (optimum after 1 min).
77. It is convenient to fold one corner of the film in order to know the orientation of the film on the blot after development.
78. If the intensity of the reaction is unknown, expose the first film for 10 min. The exposure time of the second film depends on the intensity of the RFLP patterns on the first.
79. Alternatively, a film developer machine can be used.
80. If a membrane is to be hybridized again within 24 h after detection, then it is necessary to "strip" the filter, in order to inactivate the peroxidase. Because peroxidase loses activity within 24 h, it is not necessary to strip the membrane when reused after more than 24 h after detection.

Acknowledgments

We gratefully acknowledge Piet Overduin for his tips on RFLP typing of *M. paratuberculosis*.

References

1. Van Embden, J. D. A., Crawford, J. T., Dale, J. W., Gicquel, B., Hermans, P. W. M., McAdam, R., Shinnick, T., and Small, P. M. (1993) Strain identification of *Mycobacterium tuberculosis* by DNA fingerprinting: recommendations for a standardized methodology. *J. Clin. Microbiol.* **31,** 406–409.
2. Van Soolingen, D., Bauer, J., Ritacco, V., Cardoso Leao, S., Pavlik, I., Vincent, V., Rastogi, N., Gori, A., Bodmer, T., Garzelli, C., and Garcia, M. J. (1998) IS*1245* restriction fragment length polymorphism typing of *Mycobacterium avium* isolates: proposal for standardization. *J. Clin. Microbiol.* **36,** 3051–3054.
3. Friedman, C. R., Stoeckle, M. Y., Johnson Jr., W. D., and Riley, L. W. (1995) Double repetitive element PCR method for subtyping *Mycobacterium tuberculosis* clinical isolates. *J. Clin. Microbiol.* **33,** 1064–1069.
4. Haas, W. H., Butler, W. R., Woodley, C. L., and Crawford, J. T. (1993) Mixed-linker polymerase chain reaction: a new method for rapid fingerprinting of isolates of the *Mycobacterium tuberculosis* complex. *J. Clin. Microbiol.* **31,** 1293–1298.
5. Kamerbeek, J., Schouls, L., Kolk, A., van Agterveld, M., van Soolingen, D., Kuijper, S., Bunschoten, A., Molhuizen, H., Shaw, R., Goyal, M., and van Embden, J. (1997) Rapid detection and simultaneous strain differentiation of *Mycobacterium tuberculosis* for diagnosis and tuberculosis control. *J. Clin. Microbiol.* **35,** 907–914.
6. Otal, I., Samper, S., Asensio, M. P., Victoria, M. A., Rubio, M. C., Gómez-Lus, R., and Martín, C. (1997) Use of a PCR method based on IS*6110* polymorphism for typing *Mycobacterium tuberculosis* strains from BACTEC cultures. *J. Clin. Microbiol.* **35,** 273–277.
7. Plikaytis, B. B., Crawford, J. T., Woodley, C. L., Butler, W. R., Eisenach, K. D., Cave, M. D., and Shinnick, T. M. (1993) Rapid, amplification-based fingerprinting of *Mycobacterium tuberculosis*. *J. Gen. Microbiol.* **139,** 1537–1542.

8. Van Soolingen, D., de Haas, P. E. W., Haagsma, J., Eger, T., Hermans, P. W. M., Ritacco, V., Alito, A., and Van Embden, J. D. A. (1994) Use of various genetic markers in differentiation of *Mycobacterium bovis* strains from animals and humans and for studying the epidemiology of bovine tuberculosis. *J. Clin. Microbiol.* **32,** 2425–2433.
9. Van Soolingen, D., de Haas, P. E. W., Hermans, P. W. M., Groenen, P., and van Embden, J. D. A. (1993) Comparison of various repetitive DNA elements as genetic markers for strain differentiation and epidemiology of *Mycobacterium tuberculosis*. *J. Clin. Microbiol.* **31,** 1987–1995.
10. Van Soolingen, D., de Haas, P. E. W., Hermans, P. W. M., and van Embden, J. D. A. (1994) DNA fingerprinting of *Mycobacterium tuberculosis*. *Methods Enzymol.* **235,** 196–205.
11. Van Soolingen, D., Hermans, P. W. M., de Haas, P. E. W., and van Embden, J. D. A. (1992) Insertion element IS*1081*-associated restriction fragment length polymorphism in *Mycobacterium tuberculosis* complex species: a reliable tool to recognize *Mycobacterium bovis* BCG. *J. Clin. Microbiol.* **30,** 1772–1777.
12. Wiid, I. J. F., Werely, C., Beyers, N., Donald, P., and van Helden, P. D. (1994) Oligonucleotide $(GTG)_5$ as a marker for *Mycobacterium tuberculosis* strain identification. *J. Clin. Microbiol.* **32,** 1318–1321.
13. Kremer, K., van Soolingen, D., Frothingham, R., Haas, W. H., Hermans, P. W. M., Martin, C., Palittapongarnpim, P., Plikaytis, B. B., W. Riley, L., Yakrus, M. A., Musser, J. M., and van Embden, J. D. A. (1999) Comparison of methods based on different molecular epidemiological markers for typing of *Mycobacterium tuberculosis* complex strains: interlaboratory study of discriminatory power and reproducibility. *J. Clin. Microbiol.* **37,** 2607–2618.
14. Heersma, H. F., Kremer, K., and van Embden, J. D. A. (1998) Computer analysis of IS*6110* RFLP patterns of *Mycobacterium tuberculosis*, in *Methods in Molecular Biology*, vol. 101: *Mycobacteria Protocols* (Parish, T. and Stoker, N. G., eds.) Humana, Totowa, NJ, pp. 395–422.
15. Beck-Sagué, C., Dooley, S. W., Hutton, M. D., Otten, J., Breeden, A., Crawford, J. T., Pitchenik, A. E., Woodley, C., Cauthen, G., and Jarvis, W. R. (1992) Hospital outbreak of multidrug-resistant *Mycobacterium tuberculosis* infections. Factors in transmission to staff and HIV-infected patients. *JAMA* **268,** 1280–1286.
16. Coronado, V. G., Beck-Sagué, C. M., Hutton, M. D., Davis, B. J., Nicholas, P., Villareal, C., Woodley, C. L., Kilburn, J. O., Crawford, J. T., Frieden, T. R., Sinkowitz, R. L., and Jarvis, W. R. (1993) Transmission of multidrug-resistant *Mycobacterium tuberculosis* among persons with human immunodeficiency virus infection in an urban hospital: epidemiologic and restriction fragment length polymorphism analysis. *J. Infect. Dis.* **168,** 1052–1055.
17. Edlin, B. R, Tokars, J. I., Grieco, M. H., Crawford, J. T., Williams, J., Sordillo, E. M., Ong, K. R., Kilburn, J. O., Dooley, S. W., Castro, K. G., Jarvis, W. R., and Holmberg, S. D. (1992) An outbreak of multidrug-resistant tuberculosis among hospitalized patients with the acquired immunodeficiency syndrome. *N. Engl. J. Med.* **326,** 1514–1521.

18. Greifinger, R., Grabau, J., Quinlan, A., Loeder, A., DiFerdinando, G., Jr., and Morse, D. L. (1992) Transmission of multidrug-resistant tuberculosis among immunocompromised persons in a correctional system in New York, 1991. *MMWR* **41,** 507–509.
19. Small, P. M., Hopewell, P. C., Singh, S. P., Paz, A., Parsonnet, J., Ruston, D. C., Schecter, G. F., Daley, M. P. H. C. L., and Schoolnik, G. K. (1994) The epidemiology of tuberculosis in San Francisco. *N. Engl. J. Med.* **330,** 1703–1709.
20. Alland, D., Kakut, G. E., Moss, A. R., McAdam, R. A., Hahn, J. A., Bosworth, W., Drucker, E., and Bloom, B. R. (1994) Transmission of tuberculosis in New York City. An analysis by DNA fingerprinting and conventional epidemiologic methods. *N. Engl. J. Med.* **330,** 1710–1716.
21. Yang, Z. H., de Haas, P. E. W., Wachman, C. H., van Soolingen, D., van Embden, J. D. A., and Andersen, Å. B. (1995) Molecular epidemiology of tuberculosis in Denmark in 1992. *J. Clin. Microbiol.* **33,** 2077–2081.
22. Van Deutekom, H., Gerritsen, J. J. J., Van Soolingen, D., Van Ameijden, E. J. C., Van Embden, J. D. A., and Coutinho, R. A. (1997) Molecular epidemiological approach to studying the transmission of tuberculosis in Amsterdam. *Clin. Infect. Dis.* **25,** 1071–1077.
23. Pfyffer, G. E., Strässle, A., Rose, N., Wirth, R., Brändli, O., and Shang, H. (1998) Tuberculosis in the Metropolitan Area of Zurich; A 3-year survey based on DNA fingerprinting. *Eur. Respir. J.* **11,** 804–808.
24. Van Soolingen, D., Borgdorff, M. W., de Haas, P. E. W., Sebek, M. M. G. G., Veen, J., Dessens, M., Kremer, K., and van Embden, J. D. A. (1999) Molecular epidemiology of tuberculosis in The Netherlands: a nationwide study from 1993 through 1997. *J. Infect. Dis.* **180,** 726–736.
25. Samper, S., Martin, C., Pinedo, A., Rivero, A., Blazquez, J., Baquero, F., van Soolingen, D., and van Embden, J. D. A. (1997) Transmission between HIV-infected patients of multidrug-resistant tuberculosis caused by *Mycobacterium bovis*. *AIDS* **11,** 1237–1242.
26. Hermans, P. W. M., Massadi, F., Guebrexabher, H., van Soolingen, D., de Haas, P. E. W., Heersma, H., de Neeling, H., Ayoub, A., Portaels, F., Frommel, D., Zribi, M., and van Embden, J. D. A. (1995) Analysis of the population structure of *Mycobacterium tuberculosis* in Ethiopia, Tunisia, and the Netherlands: usefulness of DNA typing for global tuberculosis epidemiology. *J. Infect. Dis.* **171,** 1504–1513.
27. Van Soolingen, D., Qian, L., de Haas, P. E. W., Douglas, J. T., Traore, H., Portaels, F., Qing, H. Z., Enkhasaikan, D., Nymadawa, P., and van Embden, J. D. A. (1995) Predominance of a single genotype of *Mycobacterium tuberculosis* in countries of East Asia. *J. Clin. Microbiol.* **33,** 3234–3238.
28. Fomukong, N. G., Dale, J. W., Osborn, T. W., and Grange, J. M. (1992) Use of gene probes based on the insertion sequences IS*986* to differentiate between BCG vaccine strains. *J. Appl. Bacteriol.* **72,** 126–133.
29. Van Soolingen, D., van der Zanden, A. G. M., de Haas, P. E. W., Noordhoek, G. T., Kiers, A., Foudraine, N. A., Portaels, F., Kolk, A. H. J., Kremer, K., and van Embden, J. D. A. (1998) Disclosure of *Myobacterium microti* infections among humans using novel genetic markers. *J. Clin. Microbiol.* **36,** 1840–1845.

30. Ross, B. C., Raios, K., Jackson, K., and Dwyer, B. (1992) Molecular cloning of a highly repeated DNA element from *Mycobacterium tuberculosis* and its use as an epidemiological tool. *J. Clin. Microbiol.* **30,** 942–946.
31. Sahadevan, R., Narayanan, S., Paramasivan, C. N., Prahakar, R., and Narayanan, P. R. (1995) Restriction fragment length polymorphism typing of clinical isolates of *Mycobacterium tuberculosis* from patients with pulmonary tuberculosis in Madras, India, by use of direct-repeat probe. *J. Clin. Microbiol.* **33,** 3037–3039.
32. Van Embden, J. D. A., Schouls, L. M., and van Soolingen, D. (1995) Molecular techniques: applications in epidemiologic studies, in *Mycobacterium bovis* Infection in Animals and Humans (Thoen, C. O. and Steele, J. H., eds.), Iowa State University Press, Ames, IA, pp. 15–27.
33. Collins, D. M. and Stephens, D. M. (1991) Identification of insertion sequence, IS*1081*, in *Mycobacterium bovis*. *FEMS Lett.* **83,** 11–16.
34. Musa, M., Zainuddin, Z. F., and Ramayah, S. (1994) A new DNA probe for identification and differentiation of *Mycobacterium tuberculosis* complex. *Asia Pac. J. Mol. Biol. Biotech.* **2,** 353–360.
35. Li, H., Ultrup, J. C., Jonassen, T. O., Melby, K., Nagai, S., and Harboe, M. (1993) Evidence for absence of the MPB64 gene in some substrains of *Mycobacterium bovis* BCG. *Infect. Immunol.* **61,** 1730–1734.
36. Van Soolingen, D., Hoogenboezem, T., de Haas, P. E. W., Hermans, P. W. M, Koedam, M. A., Teppema, K. S., Brennan, P. J., Besra, G. S., Portaels, F., Top, J., Schouls, L. M., and van Embden, J. D. A. (1997) A novel pathogenic taxon of the *Mycobacterium tuberculosis* complex, canetti: characterization of an exceptional isolate from Africa. *Int. J. Sys. Bacteriol.* **47,** 1236–1245.
37. Del Portillo, P., Murillo, L. A., and Patarroyo, M. E. (1991) Amplification of a species-specific DNA fragment of *Mycobacterium tuberculosis* and its possible use in diagnosis. *J. Clin. Microbiol.* **29,** 2163–2168.
38. Vera-Cabrera, L., Howard, S. T., Laszlo, A., and Johnson, W. M. (1997) Analysis of genetic polymorphism in the phospholipase region of *Mycobacterium tuberculosis*. *J. Clin. Microbiol.* **35,** 1190–1195.
39. Liébana, E., Aranaz, A., Francis, B., and Cousins, D. (1996) Assessment of genetic markers for differentiation within the *Mycobacterium tuberculosis* complex. *J. Clin. Microbiol.* **34,** 933–938.
40. Weil, A., Plikaytis, B. B., Butler, W. R., Woodley, C. L., and Shinnick, T. M. (1996) The *mtp40* gene is not present in all strains of *Mycobacterium tuberculosis*. *J. Clin. Microbiol.* **34,** 2309–2311.
41. Hermans, P. W. M., van Soolingen, D., Bik, E. M., de Haas, P. E. W., Dale, J. W., and van Embden, J. D. A. (1991) The insertion element IS*987* from *Mycobacterium bovis* BCG is located in a hot spot integration region for insertion elements in *Mycobacterium tuberculosis* complex strains. *Infect. Immunol.* **59,** 2695–2705.
42. Hermans, P. W. M., van Soolingen, D., and van Embden, J. D. A. (1992) Characterization of a major polymorphic tandem repeat in *Mycobacterium tuberculosis* and its potential use in the epidemiology of *Mycobacterium kansasii* and *Mycobacterium gordonae*. *J. Bacteriol.* **174,** 4157–4165.

43. Fang, Z., Morrison, N., Watt, B., Doig, C., and Forbes, K. J. (1998) IS*6110* transposition and evolutionary scenario of the direct repeat locus in a group of closely related *Mycobacterium tuberculosis* strains. *J. Bacteriol.* **180,** 2102–2109.
44. Mariani, F., Piccolella, E., Colizzi, V., Rappuoli, R., and Gross, R. (1993) Characterization of an IS-like element from *Mycobacterium tuberculosis. J. Gen. Microbiol.* **139,** 1767–1772.
45. Zhang, Y., Heym, B., Allen, B., Young, D., and Cole, S. (1992) The catalase-peroxidase gene and isoniazid resistance of *Mycobacterium tuberculosis. Nature* **358,** 591–593.
46. Cole, S. T., Brosch, R., Parkhill, J., Garnier, T., Churcher, C., Harris, D., Gordon, S. V., Eiglmeier, K., Gas, S., Barry III, C. E., Tekaia, F., Badcock, K., Basham, D., Brown, D., Chillingworth, T., Connor, R., Davies, R., Devlin, K., Feltwell, T., Gentles, S., Hamlin, N., Holroyd, S., Hornsby, T., Jagels, K., Krogh, A., McClean, J., Moule, S., Murphy, L., Oliver, K., Osborne, J., Quail, M. A., Rajandream, M. A., Rogers, J., Rutter, S., Seeger, K., Skelton, J., Squares, R., Squares, S., Sulston, J. E., Taylor, K., Whitehead, S., and Barrell, B. G. (1998) Deciphering the biology of *Mycobacterium tuberculosis* from the complete genome sequence. *Nature* **393,** 537–544.
47. Gordon, S. V., Heym, B., Parkhill, J., Barrell, B., and Cole, S. T. (1999) New insertion sequences and a novel repeated sequence in the genome of *Mycobacterium tuberculosis* H37Rv. *Microbiology* **145,** 881–892.
48. Von Reyn, C. F., Maslow, J. N., Barber, T. W., Falkinham III, J. O., and Arbeit, R. D. (1994) Persistent colonisation of potable water as a source of *Mycobacterium avium* infection in AIDS. *Lancet* **343,** 1137–1141.
49. Yajko, D. M., Chin, D. P., Gonzalez, P. C., Nassos, P. S., Hopewell, P. C., Reingold, A. L. Horsburgh, Jr., C. R., Yakrus, M. A., Ostroff, S. M., and Hadley, W. K. (1995) *Mycobacterium avium* complex in water, food, and soil samples collected from the environment of HIV-infected patients. *J. Acquir. Immune Defic. Syndr.* **9,** 176–182.
50. Horsburgh Jr., C. R., Chin, D. P., Yajko, D. M., Hopewell, P. C., Nassos, P. S., Elkin, E. P., Hadley, W. K., Stone, E. N., Simon, E. M., Gonzalez, P., Ostroff, S., and Reingold, A. L. (1994) Environmental risk factors for acquisition of *Mycobacterium avium* complex in persons with human immunodeficiency virus infection. *J. Infect. Dis.* **170,** 362–367.
51. Eaton, T. W., Falkinham III, J. O., and van Reyn, C. F. (1995) Recovery of *Mycobacterium avium* from cigarettes. *J. Clin. Microbiol.* **33,** 2757–2758.
52. Bono, M., Jemmi, T., Bernasconi, C., Burki, D., Telenti, A., and Bodmer, T. (1995) Genotypic characterization of *Mycobacterium avium* strains recovered from animals and their comparison to human strains. *Appl. Environ. Microbiol.* **61,** 371–373.
53. Ritacco, V., Kremer, K., Pijnenburg, J. E. M., van der Laan, T., de Haas, P. E. W., and van Soolingen, D. (1998) Usefulness of insertion sequence IS*1245* in restriction fragment length polymorphism typing of *Mycobacterium avium-intracellulare*: relatedness among serovar reference strains, human and animal isolates. *Int. J. Tuberc. Lung Dis.* **2,** 242–251.

54. Engel, H. W. B., Groothuis, D. G., Wouda, W., Koning, C. D. W., and Lenfders, L. H. H. M. (1978) "Pig compost" as a source of *Mycobacterium avium* infection in swine. *Zbl. Vet. Med. B.* **25,** 373–382.
55. Guero, C., Bernasconi, C., Burki, D., Bodmer, T., and Telenti, A. A. (1995) Novel insertion element from *Mycobacterium avium*, IS*1245*, is a specific target for analysis of strain relatedness. *J. Clin. Microbiol.* **33,** 304–307.
56. Komijn, R. E., de Haas, P. E W., Schneider, M. M. E., Eger, T., Nieuwenhuis, J. H. M., van den Hoek, R. J., Bakker, D., van Zijderveld, F. G., and van Soolingen, D. (1999) Prevalence of *Mycobacterium avium* in slaughter pigs in the Netherlands, and comparison of IS*1245* restriction fragment length polymorphism patterns of porcine and human isolates *J. Clin. Microbiol.* **37,** 1254–1259.
57. Schneider, M. M. E., de Haas, P., Konijnenburg, Y., Komijn, R., van den Hoek, R., Borleffs, J. C. C., Hoepelman, A. I. M., and van Soolingen, D. (1999) A 1-year nationwide study of the molecular epidemiology and clinical significance of *Mycobacterium avium* complex in humans. Thesis, University of Utrecht, The Netherlands.
58. Roiz, M. P., Palenque, E., Guerrero, C., and Garcia, M. J. (1995) Use of restriction fragment length polymorphism as a genetic marker for typing *Mycobacterium avium* strains. *J. Clin. Microbiol.* **33,** 1389–1391.
59. Moss, M. T., Malik, Z. P., Tizard, M. L. V., Green, E. P., Sanderson, J. D., and Hermon-Taylor, J. (1992) IS*902*, an insertion element of the chronic-enteritis-causing *Mycobacterium avium* subsp. silvaticum. *J. Gen. Microbiol.* **138,** 139–145.
60. Hernandez Perez, M., Fomukong, N. G., Hellyer, T., Brown, I. N., and Dale, J. W. (1994) Characterisation of IS*1110*, a highly mobile genetic element from *Mycobacterium avium. Mol. Microbiol.* **12,** 717–724.
61. Collins, D. M., Cavaignac, S., and de Lisle, G. W. (1997) Use of four DNA sequences to characterize strains of the *Mycobacterium avium* complex isolated from animals. *Mol. Cell. Probes* **11,** 373–380.
62. Green, E. P., Tizard, M. L. V., Moss, M. T., Thompson, J., Winterbourne, D. J., McFadden, J. J., and Hermon-Taylor, J. (1989) Sequence and characteristics of IS*900*, an insertion element identified in a human Crohn's disease isolate of *Mycobacterium paratuberculosis. Nucleic Acids Res.* **17,** 9063–9073.
63. Rita, M. A., Paolicchi, F., Morsella, C., Martin, Z., Angel, C., Bigi, F., Alito, A., Overduin, P., van Soolingen, D., and Romano, M. I. (1999) Distribution of IS*900* restriction fragment length polymorphism types among animal *Mycobacterium paratuberculosis* isolates from Argentina and Europe. *Vet. Microbiol.* **70,** 251–259.
64. Picardeau, M., Prod'hom, G., Raskine, L., Lepennec, M. P., and Vincent, V. (1997) Genotypic characterization of five subspecies of *Mycobacterium kansasii. J. Clin. Microbiol.* **35,** 25–32.
65. Yang, M., Ross, B. C., and Dwyer, B. (1993) Identification of an insertion sequence-like element in a subspecies of *Mycobacterium kansasii. J. Clin. Microbiol.* **31,** 2074–2079.
66. Picardeau, M., Bull, T. J., and Vincent, V. (1997) Identification and characterization of IS-like element in *Mycobacterium gordonae. FEMS Microbiol. Lett.* **154,** 95–102.

67. Collins, D. M. (1994) DNA fingerprinting of *Mycobacterium xenopi* strains. *Lett. In: Appl. Microbiol.* **18,** 234–234.
68. Picardeau, M., Varnerot, A., Rauzier, J., Gicquel, B., and Vincent, V. (1996) *Mycobacterium xenopi* IS*1395*. a novel insertion sequence expanding the IS*256* family. *Microbiology* **142,** 2453–2461.
69. Kikuchi, K., Bernard, E. M., Kiehn, T. E., Armstrong, D., and Riley, L. W. (1994) Restriction fragment length polymorphism analysis of clinical isolates of *Mycobacterium haemophilum. J. Clin. Microbiol.* **32,** 1763–1767.
70. Allen, B. W. (1998) Mycobacteria; general culture methodology and safety precautions, in *Methods in Molecular Biology*, vol. 101: *Mycobacteria Protocols* (Parish, T. and Stoker, N. G., eds.) Humana, Totowa, NJ, pp. 15–30.
71. Maniatis, T., Fritsch, E. F., and Sambrook, J. (1989) *Molecular Cloning: A Laboratory Manual.* Cold Spring Harbor Laboratory, Cold Spring Harbor, NY.
72. Murray, M. G., and Thompson, W. F. 1980. Rapid isolation of high molecular weight plant DNA. *Nucleic Acids Res.* **8,** 4321–4325.
73. Kunze, Z. M, Portaels, F., and McFadden, J. J. (1992) Biologically distinct subtypes of *Mycobacterium avium* differ in possession of insertion sequence IS*901*. *J. Clin. Microbiol.* **30,** 2366–2372.

13

Preparation of Culture Filtrate Proteins from *Mycobacterium tuberculosis*

Ida Rosenkrands and Peter Andersen

1. Introduction

1.1. Mycobacterium Tuberculosis *Culture Filtrate Proteins*

Culture filtrates obtained by in vitro cultivation of *Mycobacterium tuberculosis* have been studied for more than 20 years to identify and characterize proteins of immunological relevance. Culture filtrate preparations have been shown to induce a protective immune response in mice and guinea pigs by several groups *(1–4)*. Stimulated by these findings, the isolation and evaluation of culture filtrate antigens have been the subjects of intensified effort in several laboratories in recent years. This work has resulted in an increasing number of novel antigens such as MPT59 *(5–7)*, ESAT-6 *(8)*, MPT64 *(9)*, MTB12 *(10)*, MTB8.4 *(11)*, CFP29 *(12)*, TB10.4 *(13)*, among several others.

The nature of the extracellular proteins present in culture filtrate has been discussed extensively and proteins predicted to have a signal sequence are numerous in culture filtrate, e.g., MPT59, MPT44 and MPT45, MPT64, MPT51, MPT32, and MPT53. Recently, proteins which apparently are exported by other mechanisms were also found in culture filtrates as described for superoxide dismutase and glutamine synthetase *(14,15)*.

In addition to the "true" extracellular components, proteins such as the 38 kDa protein PstS and the 19 kDa lipoprotein are released slowly from the cell envelope to the culture medium *(16)* (**Fig. 1**). Several proteins expected to have an intracellular localization such as GroES and the ribosomal protein L7/L12 are also found in culture filtrates *(5,17)*. This could indicate that even though cultures of *M. tuberculosis* are less prone to autolysis than *M. bovis* BCG *(18)*, early culture filtrates will inevitably contain some cytoplasmic components.

From: *Methods in Molecular Medicine*, vol. 54: *Mycobacterium Tuberculosis Protocols*
Edited by: T. Parish and N. G. Stoker © Humana Press Inc., Totowa, NJ

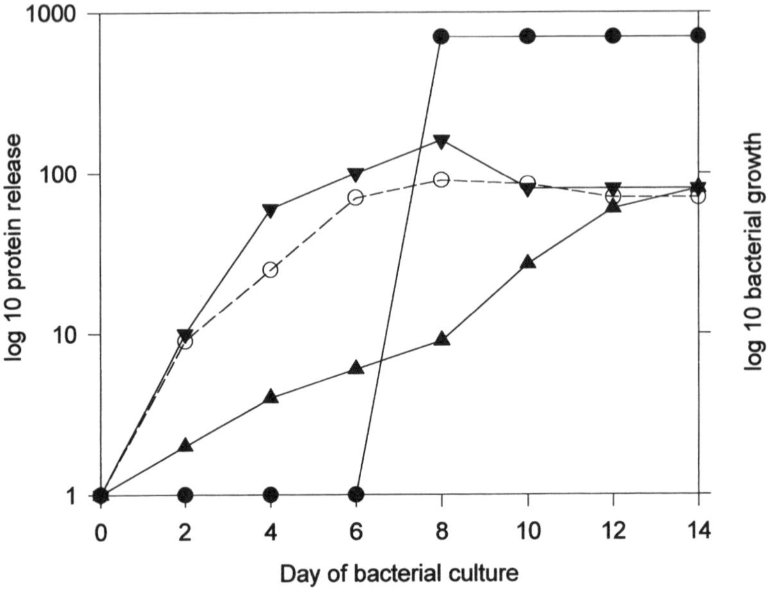

Fig. 1. Schematic representation of protein release during growth of *M. tuberculosis*. Based on the quantities of individual proteins in culture filtrates at different time points, the culture filtrate proteins have been divided into three major groups: The excreted proteins (▼), the cell wall proteins (▲), the cytoplasmic proteins (●). The bacterial growth is indicated (○).

For proteins such as GroES, however, the abundance at very early time points of culture ***(5,16)*** would suggest an alternative mechanism. To characterize proteins with respect to their localization, a "localization index" (LI) was suggested by Wiker and Harboe. In this system, concordance between a high LI value (>10) and the presence of a signal sequence was observed ***(19)***.

A definitive overview of culture filtrate proteins is not yet available, and is complicated by the variation in culture conditions (and thereby protein profiles) used in different studies. Mapping of known proteins by two-dimensional polyacrylamide gel electrophoresis (2D PAGE) enables comparison of different preparations of culture filtrate proteins and has been performed in several studies ***(5,20–22)***. The completion of the *M. tuberculosis* genome sequencing project ***(23)*** has facilitated proteome studies on *M. tuberculosis* to define the proteins expressed under various conditions and two recent proteome studies performed on culture filtrates have taken advantage of the information provided by the complete genome sequence ***(17,24)***.

This chapter gives a detailed protocol for production of culture filtrate suitable for protein identification, e.g., recognition by various monoclonal antibodies (Mabs) or proteome studies, protein characterization and protein purification (by chromatography or preparative electrophoresis) as well as cell cultures and animal experiments. The protocol has been optimized in our laboratory to handle large volumes of culture filtrate (4–5 L), but works well on a smaller scale.

1.2. Culturing M. tuberculosis *for Culture Filtrate Preparation*

Several parameters need to be considered before the preparation of culture filtrate proteins, e.g., the strain of *M. tuberculosis* (H37Rv, Erdman, or a clinical isolate), the inoculum used, the cultivation time (to avoid extensive autolysis the medium should be harvested in the mid to late logarithmic growth phase), the choice of medium, the temperature (usually 37°C), and shaking or no shaking. Although highly relevant, a systematic investigation of the influence of these parameters on protein composition has not yet been published. For protein purification and characterization, we strongly recommend the use of a synthetic medium to avoid the presence of foreign proteins derived from the addition of protein-based enrichment. Only when radioactive labeling is used for protein detection will the enrichment not contribute to the protein composition observed, but it may still affect the resolution obtained in SDS-PAGE and 2D PAGE. Several synthetic media have been used for culture filtrate protein preparation: modified Sauton's medium ***(5,16)***, the glycerol-alanine salts (GAS) medium ***(21)***, Youmans medium ***(25)***, and Proskauer-Beck medium ***(4)***.

1.3. Culture Filtrate Analyses

Depending on the intended use of the culture filtrate proteins, we recommend that each batch of culture filtrate protein is carefully analyzed. As a minimum, the protein concentration and SDS-PAGE profile should be evaluated to check for batch-to-batch variation. It is also recommended to use Mabs for detection of cytoplasmic proteins like GroEL to get an estimate of the level of autolysis in the cultures. Another useful analysis is the detection of cell wall components such as lipoarabinomannan (LAM), e.g., by Mabs, which may interfere with the intended use of the culture filtrate in cell culture or for immunization. For a more detailed investigation of the culture filtrate proteins we suggest 2D PAGE, which resolves approx 400 spots ***(17)***; a 2D PAGE gel of *M. tuberculosis* culture filtrate is shown in **Fig. 2**. 2D PAGE is the analytical method for proteome studies and the high resolution obtained is also extremely useful for detection of batch-to-batch variations.

2. Materials

2.1. M. tuberculosis *Cultures*

1. Culture flasks with screw cap, 1000 mL (Corning, Acton, MA).
2. Modified Sauton's medium (*see* **Notes 1** and **2**): dissolve 16.0 g L(+)-asparagine-1-hydrate in 1 L of water. Make sure all the asparagine is dissolved before adding

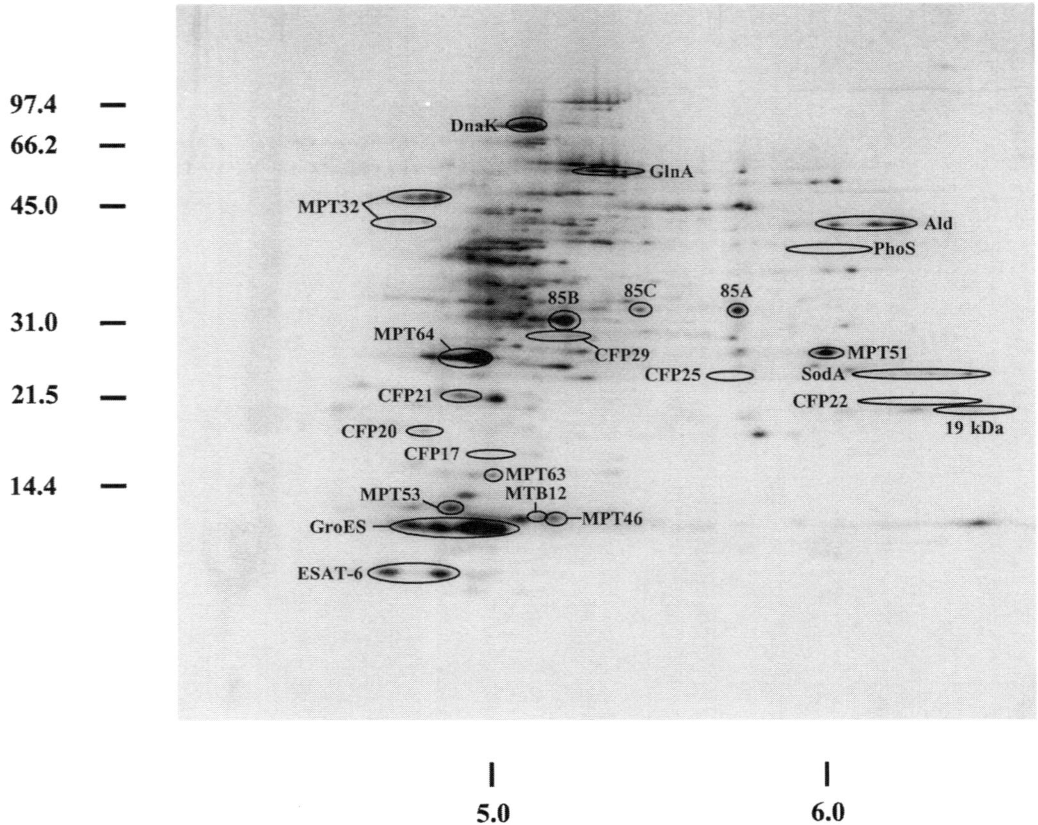

Fig. 2. 2D PAGE map of *M. tuberculosis* culture filtrate proteins visualized by silver staining. Spots representing some of the known culture filtrate proteins are indicated.

2 g of magnesium sulfate heptahydrate, 8 g of citric acid monohydrate, 2 g anhydrous di-potassium hydrogen phosphate, 0.2 g of ferric ammonium citrate, 19.3 g of D(+) glucose-monohydrate, and 19.3 g of pyruvic acid sodium salt. Finally, add 240 mL of 86–88% glycerol p.a. and 2.80 L of tap water (*see* **Note 3**). Adjust the pH to 6.8 with 32% ammonia solution. Autoclave for 20 min at 127°C, leave in the autoclave for at least 2 h to allow a slow cooling of the medium (*see* **Note 4**). Store at 4°C for up to 6 wk.
3. 4.5 mL sealed cuvets: 10 mm inner diameter (Greiner Labortechnik, Kremsmuenster, Austria).
4. 5% blood agar plates to control for contamination with other bacteria (Oxoid Limited, Basingstoke, Hampshire, England).

2.2. Harvest of Culture Filtrate

1. 150 mL or 1 L flasks for 0.2 μm filtration (Nalgene, Rochester, NY).
2. BACTEC 12B Mycobacterial Middlebrook 7H2 medium (Becton-Dickinson, Cockeysville, MD).

2.3. Ultrafiltration and Ammonium Sulfate Precipitation

1. Autoclaved Milli Q water.
2. Phosphate-buffered saline (PBS, pH 7.4): Dissolve 1.44 g di-sodium hydrogen phosphate dihydrate, 0.2 g potassium dihydrogen phosphate, 8 g sodium chloride, and 0.2 g potassium chloride, make up to 1 L with deionized water and autoclave.
3. Ammonium sulfate (Merck).
4. Dialysis membrane, cut-off 3.5 kDa (Spectrum, Houston, TX).
5. 10 or 150 mL stirred cells (Filtron Technology, Northborogh, MA) or the Prepscale 3 kD filter (Millipore, Bedford, MA) and the Prepscale module holder (Millipore) for ultrafiltration.
6. 150 mL flasks for 0.2 μm filtration (Nalgene).

2.4. Protein Quantification

Bicinchoninic acid (BCA) protein assay (Pierce, Rockford, IL).

3. Methods

3.1. Starter Culture of M. tuberculosis

1. *M. tuberculosis* is obtained either from a frozen stock or from agar plates (*see* **Notes 5** and **6**). Inoculate culture flasks containing 250 mL of preheated (37°C) modified Sauton's medium with approx 2×10^6 bacteria/mL. Place in an incubator at 37°C with gentle agitation.
2. Culture for 10–14 d or until an OD_{580} of 1.0–2.0 is reached. Take a 2 mL sample from each flask under sterile conditions. Inoculate two drops from the sample onto 5% blood agar plate to test for contamination by other bacteria, and incubate the plate for 24 h at 37°C.

3. The rest of the sample is used to measure the density of the culture. For each sample, measure the OD_{580} in a sealed cuvet using modified Sauton's medium as a reference. Make sure the sample is as homogeneous as possible before the analysis (*see* **Note 7**). Calculate the approximate concentration of bacteria assuming that an OD_{580} of 1 corresponds to approx 5×10^7 bacteria/mL.
4. The following day, inspect the blood agar plates, and if no colonies are observed, the corresponding flask can be used directly as starter culture or as the basis for frozen batches.

3.2. Culturing M. tuberculosis for Filtrate Production

For inoculation, the starter culture, prepared as described in **Subheading 3.1.**, is used.

1. Inoculate 250 mL of modified Sauton's medium (prewarmed to 37°C) with material from the starter culture corresponding to 2×10^6 bacteria/mL. Seal the flasks and incubate at 37°C with gentle agitation.
2. Grow to the mid- to late-log phase — with the described culture parameters this should be 6–7 d of culture, but ideally this should be investigated by the individual investigators (*see* **Notes 8** and **9**).

3.3. Harvest of Culture Filtrate

The culture medium is harvested after sterile filtration (*see* **Note 10**).

1. Allow the bacteria to settle and filter the culture medium using 150 mL or 1 L Nalgene flasks (0.2 µm filters).
2. To ensure that no live mycobacteria are present in the filtrate, withdraw a 0.9 mL sample from each filtration flask and analyze, e.g., by BACTEC. Meanwhile store the filtrate at –20°C (*see* **Note 11**).

3.4. Precipitation of Culture Filtrate Proteins

By combining ultrafiltration and ammonium sulfate precipitation, the filtrate is conveniently concentrated 100–200 times.

1. Thaw the mycobacterium-free filtrate and concentrate by ultrafiltration 15–20 times (*see* **Notes 12** and **13**).
2. Measure the volume of the concentrate and slowly add ammonium sulfate to 516 g/L (corresponding to 80% saturation at 4°C). Leave the solution overnight with slow magnetic stirring. Centrifuge at 13,000*g* for 1 h and dissolve the precipitate in PBS, pH 7.4, corresponding to approx 1/200 of the initial volume. To remove undissolved material, centrifuge at 13,000*g* for 30 min and collect the supernatant.
3. Dialyze the supernatant against PBS, pH 7.4, at 4°C with one or two exchanges of the buffer. Filter through a 0.2 µm filter and store at –80°C (*see* **Note 14**).

3.5. Analyses of Culture Filtrate Proteins

Depending on the application of the culture filtrate the following analyses are suggested:

1. Assay total protein concentration using the micro BCA-protein assay. Samples should normally be diluted approx 100 times to be in the range 20–100 µg/mL.
2. For comparison of culture filtrate batches, load 10–50 µg of total culture filtrate protein onto SDS-PAGE gels followed by silver staining (*see* **Note 15**). Batches with atypical band patterns are discarded or at least not pooled with the rest.
3. To detect specific mycobacterial antigens (e.g., LAM, GroEL, MPT64) perform Western blotting after SDS-PAGE of 10–50 µg total culture filtrate protein (*see* **Note 15**). For reduction of the LAM content, *see* **Note 16**.
4. To analyze the detailed protein pattern 2D PAGE of 25–250 µg of total culture filtrate is performed followed by silver staining (*see* Chapter 21 and **Note 17**).

4. Notes

1. Appropriate sterile techniques should be used when the medium is handled, aliquoting the medium in the hood, and so on.
2. Modified Sauton's medium is used here, but other media have also been used for culture filtrate production, as mentioned in **Subheading 1.2.** However, a synthetic medium without addition of bovine serum albumin or other proteins (so-called enrichment), is strongly recommended.
3. For preparation of the modified Sauton's medium we use tap water, which by direct comparison with distilled water results in an increased growth rate. The background for this empirical observation is unclear at present but is probably related to the presence of trace amounts of different metal ions in the tap water.
4. The slow cooling of the modified Sauton's medium after autoclaving should be emphasized (after which the medium acquires a brown color) as it has proved beneficial for the growth of *M. tuberculosis*.
5. As large-scale cultures of propagated *M. tuberculosis* are handled, this protocol should only be followed under biosafety level 3 facilities by a person trained in handling of this infectious agent and in emergency procedures.
6. For inoculation of starter cultures we recommend that a frozen stock of *M. tuberculosis* should be used for each batch to avoid serial passage from experiment to experiment. Starter cultures can also be inoculated directly from 7H11 plates or Lowenstein-Jensen tubes by transferring approx 60 mg of *M. tuberculosis* colonies from the plates to a sterile tube containing 3–4 autoclaved 4 mm glass beads and 3–4 drops of modified Sauton's medium, followed by vortexing of the sealed tube. A culture flask containing 250 mL modified Sauton's medium is inoculated with the homogenate. As a routine, we prepare three flasks of starter culture (each of 250 mL) for inoculation of 24 flasks (each of 250 mL) for culture filtrate preparation.

7. Extensive clumping is observed in stirred cultures without addition of detergent, which makes it difficult to quantitate the bacteria by optical methods; however, for measurement of growth of a culture we find the accuracy obtained sufficient.
8. Our routine production has been based on the strain ATCC 27294, and the culturing conditions may need to be optimized if other strains of H37Rv, Erdman, or clinical isolates are used or other parameters are changed. In any case, we recommend that a growth curve is established for the culture to ensure that it is harvested in the mid- to late-log phase where the amount of autolysis is expected to be low.
9. If large batches of culture filtrate based on many flasks are planned, it is worthwhile to check each flask for potential contamination by other bacteria one day before harvest as described in **Subheading 3.1.** In this way, the potential contamination of a large pooled batch of culture filtrate is avoided.
10. For large volumes of *M. tuberculosis* cultures (more than 1 L) we recommend a two-step filtration (0.5 μm followed by 0.2 μm) to avoid filter clotting. The 0.5 μm filtration system used in our laboratory consists of the Easy Load system (XX80EL0-05, Millipore), the motor (Millipore, XX8000230), Masterflex pump tubing (Millipore), Milligard Housing filter (Millipore), and the Milligard Housing (Millipore). After the 0.5 μm filtration step, the solution is filtered through a 0.2 μm Nalgene filter.
11. We recommend that the filter sterilized culture filtrate is checked for residual *M. tuberculosis* in the BACTEC system as described, or (undiluted) on Lowenstein-Jensen tubes or 7H11 plates, which are kept for 7 wk at 37°C. Although the culture filtrate is expected to be sterile, we have experienced leakage of the filters during use. As the following procedures with the culture filtrate are performed in an unclassified protein chemistry laboratory, we find it essential to include this control.
12. For smaller volumes of culture filtrate we recommend ultrafiltration in 10 or 150 mL stirred cells (Filtron Technology) under pressure from a nitrogen flask. The ultrafiltration system used in our laboratory is intended for large volumes of culture filtrate (usually 4–5 L) and consists of the Prepscale 3 kD filter, the Prepscale module holder (Millipore), and a motor.
13. For ultrafiltration the cut-off value should be considered: To recover all culture filtrate proteins, a cut-off of approx 3 kDa should be selected to ensure that low mass proteins like ESAT-6 are present in the concentrate. Lower cut-off values may give problems with filter clotting.
14. Other buffers could be used for dialysis depending on the expected use of the culture filtrate. A physiological buffer like PBS should be used when the culture filtrate is intended for animal experiments or cell cultures, but for fractionation purposes the relevant buffer for the first fractionation step (e.g., a Tris buffer) should be used.
15. Many different protocols exist for SDS-PAGE (including precast gels ready for use, e.g., NOVEX, San Diego, CA), silver staining, and Western blot analysis. From our experience, the detailed analysis of complex culture filtrate proteins of different masses demands large gradient gels (e.g., 16 × 16 cm), but for other purposes small gels of uniform acrylamide percentage may be sufficient.

16. Triton X-114 phase separation of proteins: The level of LAM in the early cultures described here is usually very low as compared to old cultures (as analyzed by Western blot). However, for some purposes it may be necessary to obtain a preparation essentially devoid of LAM. We have applied the method described by Hunter et al. ***(26)*** for this purpose: 900 µL of culture filtrate is added to 100 µL of 20% Triton X-114 to obtain a final concentration of 2%. The solution is mixed on ice for 30 min and then warmed to 37°C for 5 min to separate the phases followed by centrifugation (3000*g*, 5 min) at room temperature. The top-aqueous and the lower-detergent phases (containing the lipophilic LAM) are collected and the extraction is repeated on each phase (100 µL 20% Triton X-114 is added to the aqueous phase, and 900 µL PBS, pH 7.4 is added to the detergent phase). The pooled aqueous phases are collected. If the presence of small amounts of Triton X-114 interferes with the use of the culture filtrate preparation, Extractigels (Pierce) can be used for removal of detergent.
17. For 2D PAGE of culture filtrate proteins we use 13 cm IPG strips pH 4.0–7.0 (Amersham Pharmacia Biotech, Uppsala, Sweden) for the first dimension (isoelectric focusing) as described by the manufacturer. For the second dimension (SDS-PAGE) we use (160 × 160 × 1.00 mm) 10–20% gradient gels in the Protean IIxi system (Bio-Rad) according to the original protocol of Laemmli ***(27)***. The gels are silver stained as described by the method of Blum et al. ***(28)***, except that methanol is replaced with ethanol in all solutions.

Acknowledgments

We thank Dorthe Askgaard and Åse Bengård Andersen for their contribution to the initial development of these protocols, and Tove Slotved Simonsen and Annette Hansen for excellent technical assistance.

References

1. Andersen, P. (1994) Effective vaccination of mice against *Mycobacterium tuberculosis* infection with a soluble mixture of secreted mycobacterial proteins. *Infect. Immun.* **62,** 2536–2544.
2. Hubbard, R. D., Flory, C. M., and Collins, F. M. (1992) Immunization of mice with mycobacterial culture filtrate proteins. *Clin. Exp. Immunol.* **87,** 94–98.
3. Pal, P. G. and Horwitz, M. A. (1992) Immunization with extracellular proteins of *Mycobacterium tuberculosis* induces cell-mediated immune responses and substantial protective immunity in an guinea pig model of pulmonary tuberculosis. *Infect. Immun.* **60,** 4781–4792.
4. Roberts, A. D., Sonnenberg, M. G., Ordway, D. J., Furney, S. K., Brennan, P. J., Belisle, J. T., and Orme, I. M. (1995) Characteristics of protective immunity engendered by vaccination of mice with purified culture filtrate protein antigens of *Mycobacterium tuberculosis*. *Immunology* **85,** 502–508.
5. Nagai, S., Wiker, H. G., Harboe, M., and Kinomoto, M. (1991) Isolation and partial characterization of major protein antigens in the culture fluid of *Mycobacterium tuberculosis*. *Infect. Immun.* **59,** 372–382.

6. Andersen, P., Andersen, Å. B., Sørensen, A. L., and Nagai, S. (1995) Recall of long-lived immunity to *Mycobacterium tuberculosis* infection in mice. *J. Immunol.* **154,** 3359–3372.
7. Horwitz, M. A., Lee, B.-W. E., Dillon, B. J., and Harth, G. (1995) Protective immunity against tuberculosis induced by vaccination with major extracellular proteins of *Mycobacterium tuberculosis*. *Proc. Natl. Acad. Sci. USA* **92,** 1530–1534.
8. Sørensen, A. L., Nagai, S., Houen, G., Andersen, P., and Andersen, Å. B. (1995) Purification and characterization of a low-molecular-mass T-cell antigen secreted by *Mycobacterium tuberculosis*. *Infect. Immun.* **63,** 1710–1717.
9. Oettinger, T., Holm, A., Mtoni, I. M., Andersen, Å. B., and Hasløv, K. (1995) Mapping of the delayed-type hypersensitivity-inducing epitope of secreted MPT64 from *Mycobacterium tuberculosis*. *Infect. Immun.* **63,** 4613–4618.
10. Webb, J. R., Vedvick, T. S., Alderson, M. R., Guderian, J. A., Jen, S. S., Ovendale, P. J., Johnson, S. M., Reed, S. G., and Skeiky, Y. A. W. (1998) Molecular cloning, expression, and immunogenicity of MTB12, a novel low- molecular-weight antigen secreted by *Mycobacterium tuberculosis*. *Infect. Immun.* **66,** 4208–4214.
11. Coler, R. N., Skeiky, Y. A., Vedvick, T., Bement, T., Campos-Neto, A., Alderson, M. R., and Reed, S. G. (1998) Molecular cloning and immunologic reactivity of a novel low molecular mass antigen of *Mycobacterium tuberculosis*. *J. Immunol.* **161,** 2356–2364.
12. Rosenkrands, I., Rasmussen, P. B., Carnio, M., Jacobsen, S., Theisen, M., and Andersen, P. (1998) Identification and characterization of a 29-kilodalton protein from *Mycobacterium tuberculosis* culture filtrate recognized by mouse memory effector cells. *Infect. Immun.* **66,** 2728–2735.
13. Skjøt, R. L. V., Oettinger, T., Rosenkrands, I., Ravn, P., Brock, I., Jacobsen, S., and Andersen, P. (2000) Comparative evaluation of low mass T-cell antigens from *Mycobacterium tuberculosis* identify ESAT-6 family members as immunodominant. *Infect. Immun.* **68,** 214–220.
14. Harth, G., and Horwitz, M. A. (1999) Export of recombinant *Mycobacterium tuberculosis* superoxide dismutase is dependent upon both information in the protein and mycobacterial export machinery. A model for studying export of leaderless proteins by pathogenic mycobacteria. *J. Biol. Chem.* **274,** 4281–4292.
15. Harth, G., and Horwitz, M. A. (1997) Expression and efficient export of enzymatically active *Mycobacterium tuberculosis* glutamine synthetase in *Mycobacterium smegmatis* and evidence that the information for export is contained within the protein. *J. Biol. Chem.* **272,** 22,728–22,735.
16. Andersen, P., Askgaard, D., Ljungqvist, L., Bennedsen, J., and Heron, I. (1991) Proteins released from *Mycobacterium tuberculosis* during growth. *Infect. Immun.* **59,** 1905–1910.
17. Rosenkrands, I., Weldingh, K., Jacobsen, S., Hansen, C. V., Florio, W., Gianetri, I., and Andersen, P. (2000) Mapping and identification of *Mycobacterium tuberculosis* proteins by two-dimensional electrophoresis, microsequencing and immunodetection. *Electrophoresis* **21,** 935–948.

18. Wiker, H. G., Harboe, M., and Nagai, S. (1991) A localization index for distinction between extracellular and intracellular antigens of *Mycobacterium tuberculosis*. *J. Gen. Microbiol.* **137,** 875–884.
19. Wiker, H. G., Michell, S. L., Hewinson, R. G., Spierings, E., Nagai, S., and Harboe, M. (1999) Cloning, expression and significance of MPT53 for identification of secreted proteins of *Mycobacterium tuberculosis*. *Microb. Pathog.* **26,** 207–219.
20. Samanich, K. M., Belisle, J. T., Sonnenberg, M. G., Keen, M. A., Zolla-Pazner, S., and Laal, S. (1998) Delineation of human antibody responses to culture filtrate antigens of *Mycobacterium tuberculosis*. *J. Infect. Dis.* **178,** 1534–1538.
21. Sonnenberg, M. G. and Belisle, J. T. (1997) Definition of *Mycobacterium tuberculosis* culture filtrate proteins by two-dimensional polyacrylamide gel electrophoresis, N-terminal amino acid sequencing, and electrospray mass spectrometry. *Infect. Immun.* **65,** 4515–4524.
22. Weldingh, K., Rosenkrands, I., Jacobsen, S., Rasmussen, P. B., Elhay, M. J., and Andersen, P. (1998) Two-dimensional electrophoresis for analysis of *Mycobacterium tuberculosis* culture filtrate and purification and characterization of six novel proteins. *Infect. Immun.* **66,** 3492–3500.
23. Cole, S. T., Brosch, R., Parkhill, J., Garnier, T., Churcher, C., Harris, D., Gordon, S. V., Eiglmeier, K., Gas, S., Barry, C. E., 3rd, Tekaia, F., Badcock, K., Basham, D., Brown, D., Chillingworth, T., Connor, R., Davies, R., Devlin, K., Feltwell, T., Gentles, S., Hamlin, N., Holroyd, S., Hornsby, T., Jagels, K., and Barrell, B. G. (1998) Deciphering the biology of *Mycobacterium tuberculosis* from the complete genome sequence. *Nature* **393,** 537–544.
24. Jungblut, P. R., Schaible, U. E., Mollenkopf, H.-J., Zimny-Arndt, U., Raupach, B., Mattow, J., Halada, P., Lamer, S., Hagens, K., and Kaufmann, S. H. E. (1999) Comparative proteome analysis of *Mycobacterium tuberculosis* and *Mycobacterium bovis* BCG strains: towards functional genomics of microbial pathogens. *Mol. Microbiol.* **33,** 1103–1117.
25. Sinha, R. K., Verma, I., and Khuller, G. K. (1997) Immunobiological properties of a 30 kDa secretory protein of *Mycobacterium tuberculosis* H37Ra. *Vaccine* **15,** 689–699.
26. Hunter, S. W., Rivoire, B., Mehra, V., Bloom, B. R., and Brennan, P. J. (1990) The major native proteins of the leprosy bacillus. *J. Biol. Chem.* **265,** 14,065–14,068.
27. Laemmli, U. K. (1970) Cleavage of structural proteins during the assembly of the head of bacteriophage T4. *Nature* **227,** 680–685.
28. Blum, H., Beier, H., and Gross, H. J. (1987) Improved silver staining of plant proteins, RNA and DNA in polyacrylamide gels. *Electrophoresis* **8,** 93–99.

14

Analysis of the Capsule of *Mycobacterium tuberculosis*

Mamadou Daffé and Marie-Antoinette Lanéelle

1. Introduction

1.1. Evidence for a Mycobacterial Capsule

Mycobacterium tuberculosis and the other pathogenic mycobacteria examined so far by electron microscopy are seen to be surrounded within host cells by an electron-transparent zone (ETZ). For *Mycobacterium lepraemurium*, this space between the phagosomal membrane of the infected cellthe wall of the enclosed bacteria was called a "capsular space" *(1)*. Using light microscopic techniques *(2–4)*, Hanks demonstrated the presence of an unstainable "halo" around some pathogenic mycobacteria and pointed out *(5)* that what appeared to be a capsule could be seen in several published images of pathogenic mycobacteria within host cells as an ETZ.

More recently, the application of new microscopy techniques to mycobacteria has allowed the visualization of a thick capsule in specimen from axenic cultures of mycobacteria. Fréhel and colleagues *(6)* demonstrated that an extensive ETZ of bacterial origin resembling the intraphagosomal ETZ can be seen around in vitro-grown *M. tuberculosis* and *Mycobacterium avium* but not around nonpathogenic species (*Mycobacterium smegmatis* and *Mycobacterium aurum*), provided that the bacteria have either been coated with a specific antiserum or preembedded in gelatin prior to fixation for conventional electron microscopy studies to prevent the capsular material collapsing. Independent confirmation of the reality of this layer comes from sections of mycobacteria embedded by freeze-substitution *(7,8)*, a technique that avoids the shrinkage of hydrated structures which normally occurs during preparation for electron microscopy and minimizes extraction of soluble lipids during processing, by combining ultrarapid freezing with mild chemical fixation. The application of

From: *Methods in Molecular Medicine*, vol. 54: *Mycobacterium Tuberculosis Protocols*
Edited by: T. Parish and N. G. Stoker © Humana Press Inc., Totowa, NJ

such a method increases bonding and stabilizes the cell structureshas thus provided a much more accurate image of the morphological appearance of the mycobacterial capsule. Several mycobacteria processed in this way show an extensive translucent outer layer in which a weakly stained thin layer can also be seen *(7,8)*. When the same bacteria are instead processed by the conventional method commonly used to observe mycobacteria by electron microscopy, the translucent outer layer probably collapses by dehydration to give only a thin dark layer separated from the peptidoglycan layer by an electron-translucent layer *(7,8)*. This artefact may explain why the description of the mycobacterial cell envelope has been reduced, until recently *(9)*, to the plasma membrane and the cell wall. Finally, taking advantage of the possibility of extracting the outermost constituents of the mycobacterial cell envelope by gentle shaking of bacterial clumps with 4 mm diameter glass beads *(10)*, De Chastellier and Daffé's groups recently reinvestigated the occurrence of a capsule structure around in vitro-grown *M. avium*. Control and bead-treated bacteria were coated with antibodies to antigen 85 *(11)* prior to fixation for conventional electron microscopy. Untreated bacteria displayed a thin electron-dense layeran extended loosely-attached capsular layer while bead-treated bacteria showed only the thin dense layer *(12)*. It is therefore now well established that an extensive capsule surrounds some mycobacterial species grown in axenic media. At the present time it is not known whether or not this structure is restricted to pathogenic mycobacteria.

1.2. Chemical Nature of the Mycobacterial Capsule

For a long time, information about the nature of the ETZ was available for only two host-grown mycobacterial species, namely *Mycobacterium leprae* and *M. lepraemurium*. The capsule of the two species has been shown to contain large amounts of phenolic glycolipids (PGL) *(13)* and glycopeptidolipids (GPL) *(14)*, respectively. At the time the experiments were done there was no possibility of observing the situation with these species in culture media, since neither of them had been grown outside of animals or tissue culture. So it seemed that the ETZ represented an accumulation of distinctive lipids around the bacteria, although the simultaneous presence of other components could not be ruled out. Nevertheless, it was clear that accumulation of glycolipids was not a general explanation of the ETZ, first because in some PGL-positive species, such as *M. tuberculosis*, most strains do not synthesize significant amounts of PGL *(15)*; in other PGL-positive species, such as *Mycobacterium kansasii* and *Mycobacterium bovis (16)*, only small amounts of PGL are produced compared with *M. leprae* and *M. lepraemurium (9)*. Second, both GPL-positive and GPL-negative strains of *M. avium- Mycobacterium intracellulare* elaborate ETZ *(17,18)* with a transparency comparable to that of *M. leprae* and *M. lepraemurium*, whereas

M. smegmatis, a GPL-containing species ***(19)***, does not elaborate ETZ ***(20)***. Therefore, although the ETZ was assumed to be composed of lipids ***(21)***, the question of the chemical nature of the material remained open.

Because staining with ruthenium red revealed the presence of an outer layer whose thickness varied considerably among the mycobacterial species examined ***(22)***, it was suggested that the mycobacterial surface contains acidic polysaccharides. Immunocytochemistry ***(10,23–27)*** and cytometry ***(28–31)*** studies using specific antigenic capsular constituents have led to the identification of some capsular components. The outermost capsular components of in vitro-grown mycobacteria can be identified by chemical analysis of the isolated material obtained by the treatment of bacilli with glass beads ***(10)*** or the use of Tween-80 ***(32,33)***.

Data from the different methods have shown that the surface layers of *M. tuberculosis* and other mycobacteria are composed primarily of proteins and polysaccharides, with only tiny amounts of lipids ***(10,34)***. The ratio of protein to polysaccharide varies, however, depending on the species. Whereas the major surface capsular constituents of *M. tuberculosis*, *M. kansasii*, and *Mycobacterium gastri* are polysaccharides, those of *Mycobacterium phlei* and *M. smegmatis* are mainly proteins ***(10,34)***.

The major capsular polysaccharides consist mainly of a glucan, an arabinomannan (AM), and a mannan ***(10)***; small amounts of other, still uncharacterized, oligo-polysaccharides are also present. The glucan (which is quantitatively the major capsular polysaccharide of *M. tuberculosis*), is structurally related to the cytosolic glycogen of mycobacteria but has a much smaller molecular size and shorter branched chain length. It has an apparent molecular mass of 100 kDa, 1000-fold less than the latter ***(35)***, and is composed of repeating units of five or six -> 4-α-D-glucosyl residues substituted at position 6 with mono- or di-glucosyl residues ***(10,36)***.

The heteropolysaccharide, D-arabino-D-mannan (AM), has an apparent molecular mass of 13 kDa and a structure similar to that of lipoarabinomannan (LAM) of *M. tuberculosis* ***(37)***. LAM is absent or present in very small quantities in the capsule ***(38)***. Capsular AM possesses a mannan chain composed of a ->6-α-D-mannosyl-1-> core substituted at position 2 in some places with an α-D-mannosyl unit. The structure of the mannan segment of AM is apparently identical to that of the isolated capsular mannan, a free polysaccharide with an apparent molecular mass of 4 kDa.

The outermost capsular proteins of in vitro-grown *M. tuberculosis* are a complex mixture of polypeptides ***(10)***; some of them seem to be secreted proteins, being transported to the extracellular medium, but others may be either cell envelope-associated or cytoplasmic proteins ***(12)***. In fact, most of the 205 polypeptides recently visualized in the short-term culture filtrate of *M. tuber-*

culosis by 2D SDS-PAGE ***(39)*** are also present in substantial amounts in the material extracted by mild mechanical treatment of cells, suggesting that they have been shed from the surface of the cells into the medium ***(10)***. Indeed, in infected macrophages the secreted material would be confined around the bacilli in contact with the phagosomal membrane.

The outermost part of the capsule, i.e., glass-bead-extracted material, of *M. tuberculosis* and other mycobacteria examined so far contains rather little lipid (2–5% of the material), and progressive removal of the capsular material shows that most of the lipids are located in the inner rather than the outer part of the capsule ***(32)***. Although phospholipids (e.g., phosphatidylinositol mannosides), some of the species-specific lipids (e.g., phthiocerol dimycocerosate), and the type-specific glycolipids of mycobacteria (e.g., PGL, GPL ***[21]*** and lipooligosaccharides ***[40]***), are present on the cell surface, several other lipids (notably trehalose dimycolates) occur in the inner compartments of the capsule of the tubercle bacillus ***(32)***.

2. Materials

1. 0.2 µm cellulose acetate filter units (150 mL) (Nalgene Co., Rochester, NY).
2. HPLC grade solvents: chloroform, methanol, and ethanol.
3. Washed dialysis tubing: molecular weight cut off 6–8 kDa (kDa (The Spectrum Co, CA).
4. Rotatory shaker incubator.
5. Rotatory evaporator.
6. Sterile acid-washed glass beads: 4–5 mm diameter (Prolabo, Gradignan, France) for glass bead method.
7. Tween-80 (Sigma, Poole, Dorset, UK) for Tween method.
8. Distilled water.

3. Methods

3.1. Extraction of Surface-Exposed Capsular Constituents Using Glass Beads

1. Pour off as much of the growth medium as possible from pellicular-grown cells. Alternatively, harvest mycobacteria from culture by centrifugation at 2500*g* at 4°C for 15 min (*see* **Notes 1–3**).
2. Add 10 g of sterile glass beads per 2 g wet weight of cells.
3. Gently shake the mixture for 30–60 s to break up the cell clumps (*see* **Notes 4** and **5**).
4. Add 50 mL of distilled water to the cells (*see* **Notes 6** and **7**).
5. Filter the suspension through a 0.2 µm filter (*see* **Note 7**).

3.2. Extraction of Capsular Constituents Using Tween–80

1. Pour off as much of the growth medium as possible from pellicular-grown cells. Alternatively, harvest mycobacteria from culture by centrifugation at 2500*g* at 4°C for 15 min (*see* **Notes 1–3**).

2. Add fresh medium containing 1% (w/v) Tween-80 to the wet cells (*see* **Note 8**). Use a volume equivalent to the original culture volume.
3. Shake the mixture at 37°C for 1 h, 4 h, or 16 h on a rotary shaker at 125 rpm (*see* **Note 9**).
4. Transfer the bacterial suspension into appropriate sterile and safe centrifugation tubes.
5. Centrifuge at 8000*g* for 30 min.
6. Filter the suspension through a 0.2 μm filter (*see* **Note 10**).

3.3. Isolation of the Crude Capsular Macromolecules

1. Concentrate the sterile filtrate from glass-bead-treated bacilli (*see* **Subheading 3.1.**, and from Tween-80-treated cells (*see* **Subheading 3.2.**) to 1/10 of the original volume using a rotatory evaporator at 40°C (*see* **Note 11**).
2. Add 6 vol of cold ethanol and keep the suspension at 4°C for 1 h to overnight (*see* **Note 12**).
3. Centrifuge at 4°C at 14,000*g* for 1 h.
4. Dissolve the pellet in 1/10 the original volume of distilled water.
5. Repeat **steps 3** and **4**.
6. Dialyze against distilled water at 4°C for 1–3 d (*see* **Note 13**).
7. Concentrate the dialysate using a rotatory evaporator at 40°C (*see* **Note 11**).
8. Determine carbohydrateprotein concentrations (*see* **Notes 14** and **15**).

3.4. Analysis of Carbohydrates

1. Add chloroform and methanol to the concentrated dialysate (*see* **Subheading 3.3.**) to obtain an homogeneous phase of chloroform/methanol/water 1:2:0.8 (v/v/v).
2. Mix the solution and stand for 1 h (*see* **Note 16**).
3. Add 1 vol of chloroform and 1 vol of water to the homogeneous phase.
4. Mix and stand to obtain a partition phase (*see* **Note 17**).
5. Recover the aqueous phase, the organic phasethe interphase separately.
6. Concentrate the aqueous upper phase by rotatory evaporation at 40°C (*see* **Note 11**).
7. Extract the interphase three times with distilled water to obtain glucan-rich solutions. Pool the three extracts.
9. Add 6 vol of cold ethanol to the pooled extracts from the interphase (**step 7**) and to the concentrate of the aqueous phase (**step 6**).
10. Keep the suspensions at 4°C for 1 h to overnight (*see* **Note 12**).
11. Centrifuge at 4°C at 14,000*g* for 1 h.
12. Decant the supernatant and dissolve the pellet in 1/10 of the original volume of distilled water.
13. Repeat **steps 9–12**.
14. Dialyse against distilled water at 4°C for 1–3 d (*see* **Note 13**).
15. Concentrate the dialysate using a rotatory evaporator at 40°C.
16. Lyophilize and weigh (*see* **Notes 18** and **19**).

3.5. Analysis of Lipids

1. Add chloroform and methanol to the concentrated sterile filtrate (*see* **Subheading 3.3., step 1** and **Note 20**) to obtain an homogeneous phase of chloroform/methanol/water 1:2:0.8 (vol/vol/vol).
2. Mix the solution and stand for 1 h (*see* **Note 16**).
3. Add 1 vol chloroform and 1 vol water to the homogeneous phase.
4. Mix and stand to obtain a partition phase (*see* **Note 17**).
5. Recover the organic lower phase.
6. Dry under vacuum by rotatory evaporation at 40°C (*see* **Note 11**).
7. Weigh the crude lipid extract.
8. Analyze lipids (*see* Chapter 15 and **Note 21**)

4. Notes

1. Many different media can be used for the growth of mycobacteria. The synthetic medium defined by Sauton ***(41)*** is well-adapted to the study of capsular components since it contains only glycerol and asparagine as carbon and nitrogen sources, gives a good yield (roughly 2 g wet cells per 100 mL culture flask) and avoids the presence of large amounts of exogenous components such as bovine serum albumin and casitone which may interfere with the subsequent analyses. In addition, growth in any media supplemented with detergent-containing mixtures such as Tween-80 or oleic albumin dextrose catalase will result in the release of part of the outermost capsular constituents into the growth medium.
2. The property of *M. tuberculosis* to grow as surface pellicles allows an easy harvest of cells by permitting the medium to be poured off although the pellicles remain attached to the flasks. Most importantly, this method is safer than centrifugation when working with pathogenic mycobacteria such as *M. tuberculosis*. All the experiments should be done in a sterile and safe atmosphere (in a MSCIII) and the materials decontaminated by autoclaving.
3. To obtain substantial amounts of material for the different chemical analyses, cells from log-phase growth are generally used for the isolation of capsular constituents; however, it is necessary to check that only a minimal lysis occurred at this growth stage. Consequently, the sterilized growth medium should be analyzed for the presence of a lysis marker such as the cytosolic enzyme isocitrate dehydrogenase ***(33)***.
4. When untreated-control and glass-bead-treated cells were observed by scanning electron microscopy, treated cells were declumped and almost devoid of the amorphous material that covers the aggregated control cells in large clumps and obliterate individual bacilli ***(10)***. This material corresponds to the outermost capsular constituents.
5. The extent of cellular disruption can be checked by negative staining of a suspension of treated sample, followed by examination by electron microscopy. No paired fibrous structures usually typifying mycobacterial walls ***(42)*** should be visible, because in intact rod-shaped bacilli, these structures are masked by cap-

sular constituents. We have used chemical analysis of the filtrate derived from the bead-treatment to show the absence of cytosolic cell walls markers ***(10)***.

6. It is important to add the glass beads to wet cells first, shake the mixture and then add water. This gives a better yield of capsular material than by adding glass beads and water before shaking.
7. The answer to the question of the nature and the amount of the different families of constituents extracted with glass beads is essential for the validity of the method. Solvents of different polarities (water and light petroleum/diethyl ether) and various types of filters (Nalgene or Durieux filter paper) were used to ascertain this point ***(10)***. Both polar (e.g., phospholipids) and apolar lipids (e.g., phthiocerol dimycocerosate) were found among the extracted products ***(32)***. Some lipids, e.g., trehalose dimycolates, were not found among the surface-exposed constituents of *M. tuberculosis* but were identified among those of other mycobacterial species, e.g., *M. aurum*, using the same glass bead extraction method ***(32)***. In all of the experiments, carbohydrate and protein were the major constituents of the glass bead-extracted material and lipids were minor constituents.
8. Low concentrations of Tween-80 are generally used in culture media to achieve the declumping of cell aggregates; such treatment may affect both the morphology of colonies and the virulence of the bacilli ***(43)***. For instance, whereas a concentration from 0.02 to 1% Tween resulted in a small prolongation of the survival time of mice and affected the morphology of the colonies, the next two-fold increase (from 1 to 2%) had a very pronounced effect on the virulence of tubercle bacilli ***(44)***. Thus we use a concentration of 1% Tween-80 in our experiments, but different concentrations may be used to extract the capsular constituents of *M. tuberculosis*. The ease of removal of the outermost constituents from the different strains of tubercle bacilli is strain-dependent. It was shown that a higher concentration of Tween-80 was needed to convert the colonies of the virulent H37Rv strain from rough to smooth morphology than that required to achieve the conversion of the colony morphology of the attenuated strain *M. bovis* BCG; the conversion of the colony morphology of the avirulent strain H37Ra needed less Tween than either H37Rv or BCG ***(43)***.
9. The amount of capsular material extracted with Tween-80 depends on the length of the extraction time. More material is extracted with a 16 h-incubation time than with a 4 h-period of treatment with Tween-80 ***(32)***. Thus, depending on the components needed, i.e., surface-exposed or crude capsular material, one may use a 1–16 h period of treatment.
10. When the question to be solved is to know whether or not the constituents are surface-located, treatment with glass beads, and further analysis of the resulting material, may be sufficient. For localization purposes, however, one may need to obtain capsular components from different cell envelope compartments. This may be achieved by combining glass-bead-treatment with Tween-80-treatment ***(32,33)***, provided that large amounts of bacteria are available. To determine the precise cell envelope location of nonsurface-exposed compounds, one needs to

combine glass-bead-treatment with Tween-80 treatment for a given time (e.g., 1 h), followed by retreatment of the bacterial pellet with glass beads, then Tween-80 treatment for 4 h, and so on.

11. Because of the detergent property of Tween-80, it is necessary to evaporate the filtrate from Tween-80-treated samples very slowly to avoid a massive loss of material.
12. The precipitation step is crucial for Tween-80-treated samples and greatly help in the removal of most of the detergent. For this reason, additional precipitation steps are encouraged. The period needed to observe a precipitate greatly depends on the concentration of the filtrate in macromolecules. Thus, the sample will be kept at 4°C at least overnight for diluted samples but less for concentrated samples. If no precipitate is observed after an overnight incubation, the ethanolic solution should be dried and resuspended in a smaller volume of distilled water and reprecipitated with ethanol.
13. To achieve the complete removal of glycerol (the carbon source in Sauton's medium), it is necessary to extensively dialyse the precipitate. The length of dialysis required depends on the concentration of macromolecules. As a first step, it is also possible to use a filtration membrane with a low cut off (e.g., 2–4 kDa) prior to dialysis.
14. The carbohydrate and protein concentrations may be determined by various methods; the Dische method ***(45)*** is convenient for carbohydrate and the standard Lowry assay for protein; however, the bicinchroninic acid (BCA) protein assay has a greater tolerance to the presence of detergents than the Lowry assay and should be used when Tween-80-treated samples are analyzed.
15. The crude capsular macromolecule preparation contains mainly proteins and carbohydrates; this material is suitable for protein analysis by conventional SDS-PAGE and Western blot analyses ***(10)*** and for the determination of enzyme activities ***(33)***.
16. The extraction is conveniently performed in a separating funnel when large volumes of solvents are used.
17. The phase separation usually occurs in a few hours at room temperature; if not, an overnight incubation at 4°C may be necessary to achieve a complete phase separation.
18. The aqueous phase contains water-soluble polysaccharides and small amounts of proteins. Purification of the different classes of polysaccharides may be achieved by ion-exchange chromatography and gel filtration ***(10,34,36)***.
19. The interphase is rich in glucanproteins. Purification of the neutral polysaccharide glucan may be achieved by ion-exchange chromatography, followed by gel filtration ***(10,34,36,38)***.
20. It is important to use the untreated sterile filtrate rather than the ethanol-precipitated dialysate for lipid analysis because the filtrate contains all the classes of lipids present on the bacterial surface, whereas ethanol precipitation and subsequent dialysis may lead to the loss of some types of lipids, i.e., ethanol-soluble and short-chain fatty acid-containing lipids.

21. When the organic phase from Tween-80-extracted material is analyzed, the presence of large amounts of the detergent is expected; this will generally interfere with lipid analysis. A convenient way to identify the various classes of lipids is to fractionate the crude lipid extract on a Florisil or silicic acid column ***(15,40)***, followed by conventional lipid analysis (*see* Chapter 15).

References

1. Chapman, G. B., Hanks, J. H., and Wallace, J. H. (1959) An electron microscope study of the disposition and fine structure of *Mycobacterium leprae* and murium in mouse spleen. *J. Bacteriol.* **77,** 205–211.
2. Hanks, J. H. (1961) The problem of preserving internal structures in pathogenic mycobacteria by conventional methods of fixation. *Int. J. Leprosy* **29,** 175–178.
3. Hanks, J. H. (1961) Demonstration of capsules on *M. leprae* during carbol-fuchsin staining mechanism of the Ziehl-Neelsen stain. *Int. J. Leprosy* **26,** 179–182.
4. Hanks, J. H, Moore, J. T., and Michaels, J. E. (1961) Significance of capsular components of *Mycobacterium leprae* and other mycobacteria. *Int. J. Leprosy* **26,** 74–83.
5. Hanks, J. H. (1961) Capsules in electron micrographs of *Mycobacterium leprae. Int. J. Leprosy* 29, 84–87.
6. Fréhel, C., Rastogi, N., Bénichou, J.-C., and Ryter, A. (1988) Do test tube-grown pathogenic mycobacteria possess a protective capsule? FEMS *Microbiol. Lett.* **56,** 225–230.
7. Paul, T. R. and Beveridge, T. J. (1992) Reevaluation of envelope profiles and cytoplasmic ultrastructure of mycobacteria processed by conventional embedding and freeze-substitution protocols. *J. Bacteriol.* **174,** 6508–6517.
8. Paul, T. R. and Beveridge, T. J. (1994) Preservation of surface lipids and determination of ultrastructure of *Mycobacterium kansasii* by freeze-substitution. *Infect. Immunol.* **62,** 1542–1550.
9. Daffé, M. and Draper, P. (1998) The envelope layers of mycobacteria with reference to their pathogenicity. *Adv. Microbial Phys.* **39,** 131–203.
10. Ortalo-Magné, A., Dupont, M.-A., Lemassu, A., Andersen, A. B., Gounon, P., and Daffé, M. (1995) Molecular composition of the outermost capsular material of the tubercle bacillus. *Microbiology* **141,** 1609–1620.
11. Wiker, H. G. and Harboe, M. (1992) The antigen 85 complex: a major secretion product of *Mycobacterium tuberculosis. Microbiol. Rev.* **56,** 648–661.
12. Daffé, M. and Etienne, G. (1999) The capsule of *Mycobacterium tuberculosis*its implications for pathogenicity. *Tuberc. Lung Dis.* **79,** 153–169.
13. Hunter, S. W., Fujiwara, T., and Brennan, P. J. (1982) Structure and antigenicity of the major specific glycolipid antigen of *Mycobacterium leprae*. *J. Biol. Chem.* **257,** 15,072–15,078.
14. Draper, P. and Rees, R. J. W. (1973) The nature of the electron-transparent zone that surrounds *Mycobacterium leprae*murium. *J. Gen. Microbiol.* **77,** 79–87.
15. Daffé, M., Lacave, C., Lanéelle, M.-A., and Lanéelle, G. (1987). Structure of the major triglycosyl phenol-phthiocerol of *Mycobacterium tuberculosis* (strain Canetti). *Eur. J. Biochem.* **167,** 155–160.

16. Daffé, M. and Lanéelle, M-A. (1988) Distribution of phthiocerol diesters phenolic mycosides and related compounds in mycobacteria. *J. Gen. Microbiol.* **134,** 2049–2055.
17. Rastogi, N. and David, H. L. (1988) Mechanisms of pathogenicity in mycobacteria. *Biochimie* **70,** 1101–1120.
18. Rastogi, N., Lévy-Frebault, V., Blom-Potar, M.-C., and David, H. L. (1989) Ability of smooth and rough variants of *Mycobacterium aviumM. intracellulare* to multiply and survive intracellularly: role of C-mycosides. *Zbl. Bakt. Hyg.* **270,** 345–360.
19. Daffé, M., Lanéelle, M.-A., and Puzo, G. (1983) Structural elucidation by field desorption and electron-impact mass spectrometry of the C-mycosides isolated from *Mycobacterium smegmatis. Biochim. Biophys. Acta* **751,** 439–443.
20. Fréhel, C., Ryter, A., Rastogi, N., and David, H. L. (1986) The electron-transparent zone in phagocytized *Mycobacterium avium*other mycobacteria: formation, persistence and role in bacterial survival. *Ann. Inst. Pasteur/Microbiol.* **137B,** 239–257.
21. Draper, P. and Rees, R. J. W. (1970) Electron transparent zone of mycobacteria may be a defense mechanism. *Nature* **228,** 860–861.
22. Rastogi, N., Fréhel, C., and David, H. L. (1986) Triple-layered structure of mycobacterial cell wall: evidence for the existence of a polysaccharide-rich outer layer in 18 mycobacterial species. *Curr. Microbiol.* **13,** 237–242.
23. Espitia, C., Elinos, M., Hernandez-Pando, R., and Mancilla, R. (1992) Phosphate starvation enhances expression of the immunodominant 38-kilodalton protein antigen of *Mycobacterium tuberculosis*: demonstration by immunogold electron microscopy. *Infect. Immunol.* **60,** 2998–3001.
24. Rambukkana, A., Das, P. K. A., Chand, A., Baas, J. G., Groothuis, D. G., and Kolk, A. H. J. (1991) Subcellular distribution of monoclonal antibody defined epitopes on immunodominant *Mycobacterium tuberculosis* proteins in the 30-kDa region: identification and localization of 29/33-kDa doublet proteins on mycobacterial cell wall. *Scand. J. Immunol.* **33,** 763–775.
25. Harth, G., Lee, B.-Y., Wang, J., Clemens, D. L., and Horwitz, M. A. (1996) Novel insights into the genetics, biochemistry and immunocytochemistry of the 30-kilodalton major extracellular protein of *Mycobacterium tuberculosis. Infect. Immunol.* **64,** 3038–3047.
26. Menozzi, F. D., Rouse, J. H., Alavi, M., Laude-Sharp, M., Muller, J., Bischoff, R., Brennan, M. J., and Locht, C. (1996) Identification of a heparin-binding hemagglutinin present in mycobacteria. *J. Exp. Med.* **184,** 993–1001.
27. Cunningham, A. F. and Spreadbury, C. L. (1998) Mycobacterial stationary phase induced by low oxygen tension: cell wall thickening and localization of the 16-kilodalton α-crystallin homolog. *J. Bacteriol.* **180,** 801–808.
28. Ozanne, V., Ortalo-Magné, A., Vercellone, A., Fournié, J.-J., and Daffé, M. (1996) Cytometric detection of mycobacterial surface antigens: exposure of mannosyl epitopes and of arabinan segment of arabinomannans. *J. Bacteriol.* **178,** 7254–7259.
29. Harboe, M., Wiker, H. G., Ulvund, G., Lund-Pedersen, B., Bengard, A., Hewinson, R. G., and Nagai, S. (1998) MPB70MPB83 as indicators of protein localization in mycobacterial cells. *Infect. Immunol.* **66,** 289–296.

30. Lefèvre, P., Braibant, M., de Wit, L., Kalai, M., Röeper, D., Grötzinger, J., Delville, J.- P., Peirs, P., Ooms, J., Huygen, K., and Content, J. (1997) Three different putative phosphate transport receptors are encoded by the *Mycobacterium tuberculosis* genome and are present at the surface of *Mycobacterium bovis* BCG. *J. Bacteriol.* **179,** 2900–2906.
31. Cywes, C., Hoppe, H. C., Daffé, M., and Ehlers, M. R. W. (1997) Nonopsonic binding of *Mycobacterium tuberculosis* to complement receptor type 3 is mediated by capsular polysaccharides and is strain dependent. *Infect. Immunol.* **65,** 4258–4266.
32. Ortalo-Magné, A., Lemassu, A., Lanéelle, M.-A., Bardou, F., Silve, G., Gounon, P., Marchal, G., and Daffé, M. (1996) Identification of the surface-exposed lipids on the cell envelopes of *Mycobacterium tuberculosis* and other mycobacterial species. *J. Bacteriol.* **178,** 456–461.
33. Raynaud, C., Etienne, G., Peyron, P., Lanéelle, M.-A., and Daffé, M. (1998) Extracellular enzyme activities potentially involved in the pathogenicity of *Mycobacterium tuberculosis. Microbiology* **144,** 577–587.
34. Lemassu, A., Ortalo-Magné, A., Bardou, F., Silve, G., Lanéelle, M.-A., and Daffé, M. (1996) Extracellular and surface-exposed polysaccharides of nontuberculous mycobacteria. *Microbiology* **142,** 1513–1520.
35. Antoine, A. D. and Tepper, B. S. (1969) Characterization of glycogen from mycobacteria. *Arch. Biochem. Biophys.* **134,** 207–213
36. Lemassu, A. and Daffé, M. (1994) Structural features of the exocellular polysaccharides of *Mycobacterium tuberculosis. Biochem. J.* **297,** 351–357.
37. Chatterjee, D., Lowell, K., Rivoire, B., McNeil, M. R., and Brennan, P. J. (1992) Lipoarabinomannan of *Mycobacterium tuberculosis*. Capping with mannosyl residues in some strains. *J. Biol. Chem.* **267,** 6234–6239.
38. Ortalo-Magné, A., Andersen, A. B., and Daffé, M. (1996) The outermost capsular arabinomannans and other mannoconjugates of virulent and avirulent tubercle bacilli. *Microbiology* **142,** 927–935.
39. Sonnenberg, M. G. and Belisle, J. T. (1997) Definition of *Mycobacterium tuberculosis* culture filtrate proteins by two-dimentional polyacrylamide gel electrophoresis, N-terminal amino-acid sequencing and electrospray mass spectrometry. *Infect. Immunol.* **65,** 4515–4524.
40. Daffé, M., McNeil, M., and Brennan, P. J. (1991) Novel type-specific lipooligosaccharides from *Mycobacterium tuberculosis. Biochemistry* **30,** 378–388.
41. Sauton, B. (1912) Sur la nutrition minérale du bacille tuberculeux. *C R Acad Sci Ser III Sci Vie* **155,** 860–863.
42. Draper, P. (1982) The anatomy of mycobacteria, in *The Biology of The Mycobacteria* (Ratledge, C. and Stanford, J. L., eds.), Academic Press, London New York, pp. 9–49.
43. Middlebrook, G., Dubos, R. J., and Pierce, C. (1947) Virulence and morphological characteristics of mammalian tubercle bacilli. *J. Exp. Med.* **86,** 175–184.
44. Bloch, H. and Noll, H. (1953) Studies on the virulence of tubercle bacilli. Variations in virulence effected by Tween-80 and thiosemicarbazone. *J. Exp. Med.* **97,** 1–16.
45. Dische, Z. (1962) Color reaction of hexoses. *Methods Carbohydr. Chem.* **1,** 488–494.

15

Analysis of the Lipids of *Mycobacterium tuberculosis*

Richard A. Slayden and Clifton E. Barry, 3rd

1. Introduction

1.1. Characteristics of the Lipids and Cell Wall of M. tuberculosis

Mycobacterial cell wall ultrastructure has been studied through the use of negative staining, electron microscopy *(1,2)*, freeze fracture *(3)*, X-ray diffraction *(4)*, differential scanning calorimetry *(5,6)*, and electron spin resonance spectroscopy. Through the use of these techniques, the cellular envelope has been shown to be highly ordered and organized in a tripartite structure *(2,3,7,8)*. Classical freeze-fracture and freeze-etch electron microscopy studies have established that fragmentation takes place along extended lipid-rich nonaqueous domains. Applied to mycobacteria, these techniques have revealed two fracture sites, an inner cleavage plane within the plasmalamellar membrane and an outer cleavage plane between the mycolic acids and the tenuous outer leaflet *(1)*. These two cleavage sites represent the two domains containing the majority of the lipid material of the bacillus.

The organizational arrangement underlying these features was first proposed by Minnikin and depends critically upon the predominantly lipid components of the matrix, especially mycolic acids *(9)*. He suggested that mycolic acids are aligned perpendicular to the inner surface of the cell, allowing the hydrocarbon chains to form a tightly associated permeability barrier. The mycolic acids of mycolyl-arabinogalactan-peptidoglycan (mAGP) are the inner-leaflet of the pseudo-outer bacterial membrane. They interact with lipids and accessory molecules, which constitute the outer-leaflet of this asymmetric anchored membrane bilayer. Associated with the mAGP complex are a number of lipo-heteropolysaccharides, proteins, and free lipids *(10)*. The interior or "core"

From: *Methods in Molecular Medicine*, vol. 54: *Mycobacterium Tuberculosis Protocols*
Edited by: T. Parish and N. G. Stoker © Humana Press Inc., Totowa, NJ

hydrophobic domain is subtended by a covalently linked complex of peptidoglycan and arabinogalactan (AG), which serves as the foundation for the mycolic acids ***(11,12)***.

1.2. Mycolic Acids

Mycolic acids are found predominantly anchored as carboxylate esters to the 5-position of each arabinose residue present in a hexaarabinosyl motif of AG ***(13)***. In addition to these clusters, mycolic acids are also present within the fluid outer-lipid matrix in the form of trehalose dimycolate (TDM; "cord factor") and trehalose monomycolate (TM). TDM has long been implicated in the pathogenesis of tuberculosis, whereas TM is regarded as the precursor of the arabinan-linked mycolates ***(14–19)***. Mycolic acids also occur naturally attached to other sugars such as glucose and as components of polyprenol-linked carriers such as mycolylmannosylphosphorylheptaprenol (Myc-PL) ***(20)***.

In addition to Myc-PL there are an array of prenol-based glycolipid intermediates involved in sugar transfer reactions. The role of these polyprenol-phospho-sugars is the transport of activated glycosyl residues to the site of the growing cell wall. Thus far in mycobacteria a variety of prenol-based glycolipids have been identified that, unlike Myc-PL, are involved in polysaccharide biosynthesis rather than mycolic acid. These glycolipids have been found as monosaccharides and multiglycosylated forms ***(21,22)***.

There is considerable variety in mycolic acid structure; however, all variations share a common α-alkyl, β-hydroxy defining structure. The various types are generally considered as either α-mycolates or oxygenated mycolates, based upon whether they contain an oxygen moiety in addition to the β-hydroxy acid ***(23)***. Their structural variety is a result of functional groups introduced into the merochain, giving rise to two functional centers, proximal and distal to the ester linkage ***(24)***. The chemical moieties found in mycolic acids include olefins, cyclopropanes, ketones, methyl ethers, epoxides, and wax esters. Organisms of the *M. tuberculosis* complex contain only significant quantities of α-mycolates (di-cis cyclopropanated), methoxymycolates (a methyl ether and variable quantities of *cis* and *trans* cyclopropane), and ketomycolates (an α-methyl branched ketone and variable quantities of *cis* and *trans* cyclopropane) ***(23)***. These can be present in the proximal or the distal position, or both. The reason for structural variation among mycolic acids in a single organism is unknown; however, it may determine to some degree the extent of their cellular characteristics, such as permeability, structural integrity, and pathogenesis ***(25,26)***.

1.3. Loosely Associated Lipids and Glycolipids

The most prominent substance intercalating the cell wall core and associated with the mycolic acids are glycolipids based on phosphatidylinositol

(27,28). They are found in all mycobacteria and are a crucial component of the cell wall, although they do not have a covalent association ***(29)***. These glycolipids are separated into three biosynthetically related groups: (1) phosphatidylinositol mannosides (PIMs), (2) lipomannans (LMs) and (3) lipoarabinomannans (LAMs) ***(30–32)***. Recently, a novel inositol-P-capping motif has been identified on a minor portion of the uncapped arabinan termini of LAMs ***(33)***. The acylation consists of palmitic and tuberculosteric acids ***(34,35)***.

In addition to the phosphatidyl inositol anchored glycolipids are a number of complex, surface-exposed lipids. The wide range of complex lipids that form the outer leaflet of the cell wall include acylglycerols (mono-, di-, tri-acylglycerol), phthiocerol dimycocerosates (PDIMs), TM, TDM, and other acylated trehaloses ***(36–39)***. Also present in some species are the type-species specific lipids: glycopeptidolipids (GPLs), phenolic glycolipids (PGLs), and lipooligosaccharides (LOSs).

The abundant apolar acylglycerols are found in organisms grown in glycerol-rich medium ***(40)***. Interestingly, they are virtually absent or replaced by a glycosyl form when the organism is grown in glucose rich medium. A metabolic role has not been attributed to these fats due to the variation with growth medium. PDIMs are considered the "true" waxes of mycobacteria, and occur in three forms that differ in functionality in the diol, containing either phthiocerol A, phthiocerol B, or phthiodiolone ***(40,41)***.

In addition to the previously described TM and TDM, trehalose may also be found substituted with a combination of saturated straight chain (C_{16}–C_{18}), and mycocerosates, mycolipanolates, or mycolipenates, all multimethyl branched fatty acids ***(37)***. Included among these acyl-trehaloses are the sulfolipids. These polyanionic lipids are based on trehalose-2-sulfate and their variety is due to differences in acylation patterns ***(42,43)***. The sulfolipids have been associated with virulence ***(44)***, based on the observation that attenuation of virulent strains of *M. tuberculosis* is accompanied by the loss of sulfolipid production. Originally their role as virulence factors was based on the speculation that the charged glycolipids may promote intracellular survival by preventing endosomal-lysosomal fusion ***(43,45)***. However, there is also evidence that suggests that intracellular survival is promoted due to sulfatide-induced phagosomal inactivation ***(46)***. In addition to acyl groups, trehalose may also be substituted with other sugars. Although absent in the majority of tuberculosis strains a lipooligosaccharide (LOS) has been isolated from the Canetti strain ***(47)***. LOSs consist of distinct homologs of closely related acylated-trehalose, differing in acylation and glycosylation patterns. The acyl chains are present in various combinations at the 3-, 4-, 6-position of the terminal glycosyl residue of the trehalose core and the substitutions are composed of a mixture of tetradecanoic, hexadecanoic, and 2,4-dimethyleicos-2-enoic acids. In addition to the presence of LOS the unusual Canetti strain also produces PGLs *(48)*. PGLs consist of an oligosaccharide anchored to phenolphthiocerol dimycocerosate and have not been reported from other tuberculosis strains investigated to date *(49)*.

2. Materials

2.1. Total Lipid Extraction and Analysis

1. A suitable *Mycobacterium tuberculosis* culture can be grown in a variety of media including Middlebrook 7H9 with albumin-dextrose additions, Sauton's media, or glycerol-alanine-salts media (GAS) *(52)*. Cultures grown in the absence of detergent will be significantly clumpy so Tween-80 is typically included at 0.05% (*see* **Note 1**).
2. Methanol, petroleum ether, and chloroform (Aldrich, St. Louis, MO) (*see* **Note 2**).
3. 0.3% (w/v) aqueous sodium chloride.

2.2. Polar Lipids: PIMs, LM, and LAM

1. Mycobacterial culture (*see* **Subheading 2.1., item 1**).
2. Chloroform, methanol, and phenol (*see* **Note 2**).
3. 0.01 *M* HCl.
4. Dialysis membrane, 2500 molecular weight cutoff.

2.3. Extraction of Mycolic Acid-Containing Glycolipids

1. Mycobacterial culture (*see* **Subheading 2.1., item 1**).
2. Ethanol, chloroform, and methanol (*see* **Note 2**).
3. 0.1 *M* NaOH in ethanol.

2.4. Extraction of Polyprenol-Glycolipids

1. Mycobacterial culture (*see* **Subheading 2.1., item 1**).
2. Chloroform, methanol, and acetone (*see* **Note 2**).

2.5. Characterization of Fatty Acid Methyl Esters (FAME) and Mycolic Acid Methyl Esters (MAME)

1. Prepare 20% stock of tetrabutylammonium hydroxide (TBAH) from 40% stock solution by dilution with water (1:1, v/v).
2. Dichloromethane, diethyl ether, toluene, and acetonitrile (*see* **Note 2**).
3. Iodomethane (Aldrich).

2.6. Pyrolytic Cleavage and Oxidation of Mycolic Acids

1. 5 mL Reacti-Vial (Kontes Glass, Vineland, NJ) fitted with a ground glass condensation tube and a vacuum adapter tube attached directly to an oil diffusion vacuum pump.
2. 5% w/v silver (II) nitrate solution in 10% w/v NaOH, 2.5% v/v tetrahydrofuran, 2.5% v/v toluene, 50% v/v ethanol.

3. 0.1 *M* HCl.
4. Diethyl ether.

2.7. TLC Detection

2.7.1. TLC Plates

1. Thin layer chromatography plates: normal phase Silica gel 60F254 (EM Science, Gibbstown, NJ) (*see* **Note 3**).
2. Reversed-phase silica gel plates KC-18, 60A (Whatman, Clifton, NJ) (*see* **Note 3**).

2.7.2. TLC Detection Reagents (see **Note 4**)

1. 1,6-Diphenylhexatriene (DPHT) (Sigma, St. Louis, MO): 0.01% w/v in acetone: petroleum ether (1:1).
2. Rhodamine 6G (Sigma): 0.01% w/v in methylene chloride.
3. Rhodamine B (Sigma): 0.05% w/v in 95% ethanol.
4. Dittmer detection dip. Dissolve 4 g molybdenum (VI) oxide (molybdenum trioxide) in 100 mL of 12.5 *M* H_2SO_4. Dissolve 0.18 g molybdenum metal with heat in 50 mL of the molybdenum trioxide acid solution and then add the remaining 50 mL. Add 200 mL of distilled water and 300 mL of ethanol to the metal solution.
5. Phosphomolybdic acid (Sigma): 5% in ethanol.
6. 10% concentrated sulfuric acid in absolute ethanol.
7. Iodine crystals.
8. 2',7'-Dichloroflurescein (Sigma): 0.2% in ethanol.

2.7.3. Glycolipid Detection and Assay Reagents

1. α-Naphthol spray reagent for sugar detection. Dissolve 5 g of α-naphthol (Sigma) in 25 mL of concentrated sulfuric acid. Add 475 mL of 95% ethanol.
2. Concentrated sulfuric acid.
3. 5% w/v phenol in water.
4. 10 mg/mL dextran.

3. Methods

3.1. Total Lipid Extraction and Analysis (after [50])

1. Harvest cells from 0.5–1.0 L of culture by centrifugation at 750*g* for 15 min (for smaller cultures use proportionally less volumes) (*see* **Notes 5** and **6**).
2. Transfer cells to a glass bottle containing a stir bar using 20 mL of methanol: 0.3% aqueous sodium chloride (10:1).
3. Add 10 mL of petroleum ether and stir for 15 min, sufficiently vigorously to completely emulsify the two layers.
4. Allow mixture to separate and transfer the upper layer to a 50 mL bottle using a clean Pasteur pipet.
5. Add another 10 mL of petroleum ether to the lower aqueous phase and stir for another 15 min.

6. Allow the mixture to separate and add the upper layer to the previously removed upper layer. These combined layers contain the apolar lipids (*see* **Note 7**).
7. To the remaining lower layer add 17.3 mL of chloroform: methanol: 0.3% aqueous sodium chloride (9:10:3).
8. Stir vigorously for 1 h, pellet the cellular debris by centrifugation at 750*g* for 15 min and transfer the supernatant to a 50 mL tube.
9. Resuspend the pelleted material in 5.6 mL of chloroform: methanol: 0.3% aqueous sodium chloride (5:10:4).
10. Stir for 30 min, centrifuge at 750*g*, and combine with the previous supernatant.
11. To the combined supernatants add 9.75 mL of chloroform and 9.75 mL of 0.3% aqueous sodium chloride.
12. Mix for 5 min, centrifuge at 750*g* for 10 min and recover the lower phase. This phase contains the polar lipids (*see* **Note 8**). The remaining pellet contains the covalently associated cell wall skeleton, including peptidoglycan-arabinogalactan esterified to mycolic acids and other macromolecules.
13. Dry both the apolar and polar extracts by rotary vacuum evaporation or under a stream of air and store at –20°C for further analysis or purification.

3.2. Polar Lipids: PIMs, LM, and LAM

1. Harvest cells from 0.5–1.0 L culture and extract with 10 mL of chloroform: methanol: water (10:10:3) for 15 min stirring at 55°C (*see* **Note 9**).
2. Pellet the cellular material by centrifugation at 750*g* for 30 min and remove the organic layer.
3. Dry the organic layer by evaporation under a stream of air.
4. Hydrolyze the resulting organic residues in 3 mL of 0.01 *M* HCl for 5 min at 100°C.
5. After hydrolysis the intact PIMs can be separated from the saccharide constituents of the polyprenols by adding 12 mL of chloroform: methanol (2:1) to result in a final chloroform: methanol: water ratio of 8:4:3 (*see* **Note 10**).
6. Retrieve the lower organic phase and dry by evaporation. This is the crude PIM fraction (*see* **Note 11**).
7. Extract the remaining cellular pellet (from **Subheading 3.2., step 2**) two times with 5 mL phenol and 5 mL water for 30 min at 70°C with constant stirring (*see* **Note 12**).
8. Cool the phenol: water extract and centrifuge for 30 min at 750*g*. The mixture should become biphasic upon cooling and centrifugation.
9. Remove the phenol and aqueous fractions into separate tubes. The phenol layer contains additional PIM and the aqueous layer is a mixture of LM/LAM.
10. Dialyze the aqueous PIM and LM/LAM fractions against water with a membrane having a 2500 molecular weight cutoff until all the phenol is exchanged. Dry the aqueous phase containing PIM, resuspend in chloroform: methanol (2:1) and analyze by TLC (*see* **Note 11**). Analyze PIMLM/LAM by SDS-PAGE and periodate oxidation (*see* **Note 13**). Sugar analysis of the glycolipids can be done by GC/MS of the alditol acetate derivatized sugars (*see* **Note 14**).

3.3. Extraction of Polyprenol-Glycolipids

1. Harvest cells from 0.5–1.0 L of culture and extract with 10 mL of ethanol at 70°C for 30 min.
2. Pellet the cellular debris by centrifugation at 750*g* for 15 min.
3. Remove the organic extract and air-dry. Resuspend the residue by addition of 12 mL of chloroform: methanol (2:1) and partition by the addition of 3 mL water. Final ratio is chloroform: methanol: water 8:4:3. Remove the organic phase that contains the glycolipids (*see* **Note 15**).
4. Evaporate to dryness and subject residue to 1 mL of 0.1 *M* NaOH in ethanol for 45 min at 37°C.
5. Partition again as described in **step 3**. The organic extract contains the polyprenol-based glycolipids and can be visualized by thin-layer chromatography (TLC) (*see* **Note 11**). Sugar constituents can be determined by alditol acetate derivatization and GC/MS analysis (*see* **Note 14**).

3.4. Extraction of Mycolic Acid Containing Glycolipids

The mycolate containing glycolipids TDM, TM, and Myc-PL are extracted from cellular material with chloroform: methanol (2:1).

1. Harvest cells from 0.5–1.0 L of culture and add 10 mL of chloroform: methanol (2:1), stir vigorously for 2–16 h (overnight).
2. Remove the organic extract and add slowly to 500 mL of acetone at –20°C. In general acetone should be in 50–100 times excess. Place at –20°C for 12 h to allow for complete flocculation of material. Recover the precipitated mycolate containing material by centrifugation at 20,000*g* at 4°C for 15 min (*see* **Note 16**).
3. Resuspend the recovered material in 1–2 mL of chloroform: methanol (2:1).
4. Small scale separation of the mycolate glycolipids is achieved by preparative thin layer chromatography as follows. (Large scale separation can be performed with flash column chromatography) (*see* **Note 17**). Separate TDM, TM, and Myc-PL by preparative TLC on silica gel plates using the solvent system chloroform: methanol: ammonium hydroxide (80:20:2).
5. Visualize using DPHT *vide infra* (*see* **Note 18**). Individual species can be removed from the plate by scraping and extracting from the silica gel with chloroform: methanol (2:1). Anion exchange resin can be used to ensure the purity of Myc-PL from contaminating diacyl trehalose (*see* **Note 19**). Comigrating free fatty and mycolic acids can be removed from TDM by TLC (*see* **Note 20**).

3.5. Characterization of Fatty Acid Methyl Esters (FAME) and Mycolic Acid Methyl Esters (MAME)

1. Hydrolyze whole cells using 5 mL of 20% (w/v) TBAH per 1 L culture of cellular material (about 2–3 g wet weight) for 1–16 h at 100°C (*see* **Notes 21** and **22**).
2. After hydrolysis, cool the sample and add 2 mL of dichloromethane and 200 μL of iodomethane. Allow this to mix extensively for 30–60 min (*see* **Note 23**).

Table 1
Solvent Systems for TLC Analysis of Mycobacterial Lipids

Solvent System	Components	Lipids resolved[a]
I	1[b]: petroleum ether: ethyl acetate (98:2) × 3[c] 2: petroleum ether: acetone (98:2) × 1	PDIM, TAG, MQ
II	1: petroleum ether: acetone (92:8) × 3 2: toluene: acetone (95:5) × 1	AT, FA
III	1: chloroform: methanol (96:4) 2: toluene: acetone (80:20)	FA, GLY
IV	1: chloroform: methanol: water (100:14:0.8) 2: chloroform: acetone: methanol: water (50:60:2.5:3)	CF, SL, DAT
V	1: chloroform: methanol: water (60:30:6) 2: chloroform: acetic acid: methanol: water (40:25:3:6)	DPG, PE, PI, PIM
VI	acetonitrile: dioxane (1:1)	FAME, MAME
VII	petroleum ether: diethyl ether (85:15) × 3–5	MAME
VIII	1: hexane: ethyl acetate (95:5) × 2 2: petroleum ether: diethyl ether (85:15) × 3	MAME[d]

[a]PDIM, phthiocerol dimycoserosates; TAG, triacyl glycerides; MQ, menaquinones; AT, acylated trehalose; FA, fatty acids; GLY, glycosides; CF, cord factor; SL, sulfolipids; DAT, diacyltrehalose; DPG, diphosphatidyglycerol; PE, phosphatidylethanolamine; PI, phosphatidylinositol; PIM, phosphatidylinositol mannosides; FAME, fatty acid methyl esters; MAME, mycolic acid methyl esters.

[b]1 refers to the solvent used in the first dimension of silica gel TLC plates, 2 to the second dimension. For examples, *see* **ref. *50***.

[c]x = number of independent developments with the indicated solvent system.

[d]This solvent system requires specially prepared TLC plates that are square with 3/4 immersion of the plate in silver nitrate and activation as described in **Subheading 2.1.6.** The first dimension is without argentation. (For example, *see* **ref. *51*** and **Note 3**.)

3. Allow the biphasic mixture to separate and discard the aqueous phase (*see* **Note 24**).
4. Completely dry the remaining organic layer, which contains the methyl esters. The dry material will be a whitish-yellow crystalline and amorphous oily material. Add 2 mL of diethyl ether and break up the crystalline material into a fine powder and then allow it to settle and remove the diethyl ether to a new tube.
5. To separate the MAMEs from the FAMEs, dry the diethyl ether extract and dissolve the residue in 200 µL of toluene and 100 µL acetonitrile. Heat gently if necessary, transfer to a microcentrifuge tube and add an additional 200 µL of acetonitrile. Chill this sample to –20°C for at least 2 h and collect the precipitated MAME by centrifugation at 20,000*g* for 20 min in a refrigerated microfuge. Remove the toluene: acetonitrile mixture that contains the FAMEs from the pelleted MAMEs.

6. FAME can be analyzed by reversed phase TLC (*see* **Note 25**) or by GC/MS (*see* **Note 26**). The MAMEs can be visualized with either one-dimensional TLC using solvent system VII or by two-dimensional TLC using solvent system VIII (**Table 1**).
7. For high-resolution of MAME species HPLC may be employed with *p*-bromophenacyl ester preparation instead of methyl esterification starting from the TBAH lysate in **step 1** (*see* **Note 27**).

3.6. Pyrolytic Cleavage and Oxidation of Mycolic Acids

1. Place purified MAMEs (from **Subheading 3.5.**) into a small glass reaction vessel, dry, and heat to 300°C under vacuum of at least 26 in. Hg for 30 min (*see* **Note 28**).
2. Collect the resulting meroaldehyde at the bottom of the flask and condense on the side of the vessel (*see* **Note 29**).
3. Oxidize the aldehyde by the addition of 1–2 mL of the silver (II) nitrate solution at 25°C for 1 h.
4. Acidify the resulting solution with dilute HCl to pH 6.0 and extract three times with diethyl ether.
5. Dry the diethyl ether extract under a stream of air.
6. Derivatize the meromycolic acid to the MAME as described in **Subheadings 3.4.2–3.4.4.** The MAMEs can be purified further by HPLC (*see* **Note 27**).

3.7. TLC Detection Methods

3.7.1. TLC Lipid Detection Reagents

1. Use DPHT spray to detect lipid material and visualize under *UV* light. Separated material appears as bright spots. DPHT can be subsequently removed by redevelopment of the plate in toluene for visualizing and marking preparative TLC plates of suitably polar materials.
2. Use rhodamine 6G spray to detect most neutral lipids and phospholipids. Visualization can be enhanced by *UV* light. Lipids show red-purple on a pink-orange background.
3. Use rhodamine B as a spray to detect most neutral lipids and phospholipids. Visualization can be enhanced with *UV* light. Lipids show red-purple on a pink-orange background.
4. Use Dittmer detection reagent as a dip and heat briefly for enhanced visualization.
5. Use phosphomolybdic acid as a spray and heat to 120°C until charring is complete. Organic material appears as blue spots on a greenish background.
6. Dip TLC plates in 10% concentrated sulfuric acid in absolute ethanol and allow to air dry briefly before charring at 110°C for 1–2 min. Organic compounds form dark brown to black spots on a white background.
7. Most unsaturated lipids can be detected with iodine vapor. Place crystals of iodine in a tank and place the chromatogram in the tank with the vapor for 5–10 min. The lipids appear as yellow spots on a white background.

8. Use 2',7'-dichlorofluorescein as a spray to detect apolar lipids which are visible when irradiated with short-wave *UV* light after the chromatogram is sprayed.

3.7.2. Glycolipid Detection Reagents

1. Use α-naphthol spray reagent for sugar detection. Sprayheat to 120°C. Glycolipids appear as purple spots.
2. Phenol sulfuric acid assay for determination of total carbohydrate. Combine 200 µL of sample with 1 mL of sulfuric acid and 200 µL of 5% phenol in water. Allow 10 min for color development and read at 490 nm. Use dextran (10 mg/mL) to generate a linear calibration curve from 10 µg to 50 µg.

4. Notes

1. Detergents and associated molecules can significantly alter the apparent distribution of lipoidal materials in a strain being examined. Tween-80, for example, is included in the media at concentrations above the critical micelle concentration (0.05% is normal), thus the detergent will exist as mixed micelles which may preferentially associate with otherwise surface-associated lipids. Likewise, cultures produced with the addition of bovine serum albumin (BSA) may have significantly altered lipid distribution because of the lipid binding properties of BSA.
2. All organic solvents should be reagent grade or better. Organic solvents should be handled with caution in a chemical hood using protective clothing including gloves, safety glasses, and a laboratory coat. Many of the reagents used are highly flammable and/or reactive and the user should be familiar with their safety data which indicates the health effects, flammability, and reactivity hazards for each solvent.
3. Silica and reversed phase thin layer chromatography plates come as glass, plastic or aluminum mounted. In general, glass backed plates give fewer edge effects and are more stable to the heating that must often be done to visualize lipids. Cutting glass-backed plates to usable size requires some skill and practice. In general glass-backed plates are the most versatile for all applications. Silver TLC plates are prepared by immersing glass-backed silica gel plates in 5% aqueous silver nitrate very briefly ***(53)***. Following air drying for 1 h the plates are heated at 80°C for 1 h and then 110°C for 1 h and used immediately or stored desiccated for short periods of time.
4. Chemical-based detection reagents typically form colored compounds at the expense of oxidizing the material resolved on the plate. Since materials differ greatly in how easily they are oxidized and how well they form colored complexes it often pays to try several different development schemes for different compounds. Such detection methods can be very deceptive as far as quantitation is concerned and assessments of purity or composition should be made with caution, if at all. Somewhat more quantitative information can be obtained by radiolabeling using lipid precursors. The radiolabeled products can then be accurately quantitated by phosphorimager rather than chemical detection. Real estimates of purity can only be obtained by NMR or compositional elemental analysis.

5. In general total lipid analyses are quite complex and the number of components involved limits the usefulness of this technique. Selective radiolabeling of many individual constituent families can simplify the analysis considerably. Total lipids can be labeled with ^{14}C-acetic acid, methyl branched lipids can be labeled with ^{14}C-propanoic acid, ^{14}C-methyl methionine allows the specific labeling of methylated or cyclopropanated lipids.
6. Petroleum ether extraction should not be assumed to render *M. tuberculosis* non-viable. In general, cells from biohazardous organisms should be worked up through chloroform-methanol extraction before they are removed from containment. Performing these procedures on a large scale from virulent organisms requires the use of a total exhaust Biosafety Cabinet (Class II, Type B2) or a chemical hood within a containment facility. Many of the solvents used are volatile and flammable and should not be used in a recirculating type cabinet.
7. "Apolar lipids" as prepared using this protocol contain a relatively small number of individual components. The major components of this fraction seem to be phthiocerol dimycocerosates (PDIM), triacylglycerols, and menaquinones *(54)*. This fraction can be analyzed by TLC using solvent system I (**Table 1**) and detection can be accomplished as described in **Subheadings 2.2.** and **3.7.** PDIMs can be selectively labeled in this population by adding ^{14}C-propionic acid to the culture media for 12–24 h before extraction.
8. "Polar lipids" include a wide variety of components, including phospholipids such as phosphatidylethanolamine, phosphatidylglycerol, and various phosphatidylinositols, including mannosylated species, it also includes many trehalose-containing components such as sulfatides, cord factor (trehalose dimycolate), and various acylated trehaloses. This complex fraction also includes some level of free fatty acids and a wide variety of less abundant materials. Polar lipids can be analyzed by TLC using solvent systems, II, III, IV, or V and can be detected using the chemical methods outlined in **Subheadings 2.2.** and **3.7.** Carbohydrate containing polar lipids can also be detected by the methods outlined in **Subheadings 2.3.** and **3.7.** This fraction can be further purified by many methods including those outlined for the identification of specific materials below but also by high-pressure liquid chromatography (HPLC) or normal phase silica gel preparative chromatography.
9. If wet cells are used a biphasic mixture results, titrate in chloroform: methanol (1:1) to result in a final ratio of 10:10:3. With the correct ratio of chloroform: methanol to water this should form a monophasic solution.
10. This mild acid hydrolysis cleaves phosphodiester bonds of the polyprenol contaminating lipids.
11. TLC analysis of PIM and polyprenol glycolipids is performed with solvent systems of chloroform: methanol: water (65:25:4) or (60:30:6).
12. All phenol used in the extraction of phosphatidylinositol extractions should be presaturated with water or PBS.
13. 12–14% SDS-PAGE of PIMs, LM, and LAM can be carried out using the same procedures as for proteins. Following electrophoresis fix the gel with 40% metha-

nol and 10% acetic acid in water for 45 min. Remove fixative and add 200 mL of the same solution containing 0.7% sodium periodate for 10 min. Remove the periodate and add 200 mL of 5% methanol, 7% acetic acid for 10 min. Remove wash and add 200 mL of 2.5% glutaraldehyde (Aqueous) for 5 min. Wash the gel in water four times and then add 0.0025% dithiothreitol (DTT) solution for 5 min. Remove DTT solution and add 0.1% aqueous silver nitrate solution for 5 min. Pour off the silver nitrate solution and briefly rinse with water to remove excess silver nitrate. Add developing solution, and when the solution becomes slightly brown-orange colored pour off the developing solution. Add more developing solution and agitate until the desired intensity is obtained. (Developing solution: 6% sodium bicarbonate in 300 mL deionized water + 50 µL formaldehyde). Stop the development by adding 200 mL of 50% citric acid solution.

14. Hydrolyze the purified lipopolysaccharide with 2 *M* trifluoroacetic acid at 120°C for 2–3 h. Include a neutral sugar standard such as persitol so sugar integration can be performed. Dry samples under a stream of air in a 37°C heat block within a fume hood. Treat the hydrolyzed sugars with 10 mg/mL of freshly prepared $NaBD_4$ for 1 h. Add 30 µL of acetic acid, followed by 200 µL of 10% acetic acid in methanol and dry under a stream of nitrogen at 37°C. Further treat the samples with 200 µL of 10% acetic acid in methanol, evaporate and then add an additional 200 µL methanol and dry again. Add 50–100 µL of acetic anhydride to the residue and heat for 3–4 h at 120°C. Add 100 µL of toluene and dry as before. Repeat this step three times to remove excess acetic anhydride from the alditol acetates. Partition with chloroform: water (1:1) and discard the aqueous layer. Add 100 µL of toluene and dry as before. Add 25–50 µL toluene and analyze by GC/MS. GC/MS analysis is performed on polar columns (i.e., Supelco 2380, 30 meters, I.D. 0.25, 0.2 µ film, Bellefonte, PA). The injection temperature of 100°C with a ramp of 30°C/min to 200°C and 5°C/min to 260°C hold for 10 min ***(55)***.
15. The polyprenol glycolipids can be purified by ion exchange chromatography if desired. Load the organic material onto a DEAE-cellulose activated with sodium formate. Wash with four column volumes of chloroform: methanol (2:1) and elute the polyprenol-containing glycolipids with a step gradient of 0.05 *M*, 0.10 *M*, and 0.15 *M* formic acid in methanol. Analyze the resulting fractions by TLC.
16. Trituration with cold acetone only works well if the acetone is in excess and cold (–20°C). When the organic extract is added slowly, it is often obvious that the precipitation is taking place. Allow the material to precipitate for 10–12 h for best results. When recovering the precipitated material by centrifugation, a cold centrifuge and rotor is preferred so that the material is not warmed in the process.
17. Large scale separation (greater than 20 mg) is done with silica gel flash chromatography. The organic extract is applied directly to a silica gel flash column and eluted in a step gradient fashion with chloroform and chloroform containing 5%, 10%, 15%, 20%, and 30% methanol. The various fractions containing TDM, TM, and Myc-PL can be determined by TLC analysis in chloroform: methanol: ammonium hydroxide (80:20:2).

18. Visualization is done with DPHT under *UV* light as described in **Subheading 3.7.** The DPHT is removed by developing the plate in toluene. TDM R_f 0.75, TM R_f 0.2,and Myc-PL R_f 0.53.
19. To separate Myc-PL from diacyltrehalose (DAT), the extracted material is subjected to anion exchange chromatography using DEAE-cellulose activated with sodium formate. DAT is eluted off the column with four column volumes chloroform and four column volumes of chloroform: methanol (2:1). The Myc-PL is eluted with 0.1 *M* formic acid in methanol.
20. The band corresponding to TDM can be rechromatographed with chloroform: methanol: water (90:10:1). TDM run with an R_f 0.67 and fatty acids and free mycolates run with R_f of 0.9.
21. Tetrabutylammonium hydroxide (TBAH) is very caustic. Take care by using the appropriate laboratory clothing such as gloves, eye glasses, and a laboratory coat. 40% TBAH often crystallizes at room temperature, if this happens gently heat the solution in the bottle until freely dissolved. Dilution to the working (20%) concentration eliminates this concern. Hydrolysis with 20% TBAH is largely complete (>95%) within 1 h at > 100°C.
22. Polytetrafluroethylene (PTFE)-capped tubes should be used for manipulations with organic solvents at elevated temperatures. Be cautious not to use the caps repeatedly, as through continual use the tops become worn and tend to leak.
23. The reaction of free fatty acids with the phase transfer catalyst iodomethane to form methyl esters is a rapid reaction and is essentially complete in a few min. Be sure to mix the aqueous and organic phases well, as transfer of the acid and the iodomethane between phases is necessary to achieve esterification. Inverting the tubes rapidly is generally preferred.
24. If desired, treat the organic phase with 2 mL of 0.1 *M* hydrochloric acid to remove excess TBAH, resulting in the elimination of the crystalline material upon drying. Be sure that the solvent is as dry as possible and then add a small volume of diethyl ether. Dry the ether extract under mild heat with a stream of air.
25. Reversed phase TLC of FAMEs are performed on KC18 reversed phase glass plates (**Subheading 2.7.**) developed with dioxane: acetonitrile (1:1).
26. For GC/MS analysis of FAMEs a polar column is used (i.e., SGE-BPX5, 30 meter, I.D. 0.25 mm, 0.25 μ film). Typical parameters are 150–325°C with a temperature rate of 4°C/min. For more information on the application of GC analysis on mycobacterial lipids *see* **refs. *56*** and ***57***).
27. Reversed phase HPLC analysis of FAMEs and MAMEs is analyzed on a C18 reversed phase column (Regis C18 reversed phase, 25 cm × 4.6 mm I.D., Morton Grove, IL) with a continuous linear gradient of acetonitrile to dioxane. Apply sample to column equilibrated in 100% acetonitrile and wash with acetonitrile for 2 min. Follow this with a linear gradient to 100% dioxane over 50 min and then hold 100% dioxane for 10 min. Detection can be radioassay if the lipids are labeled with ^{14}C-acetate, or can be at 254 nm if the lipids are derivatized as para-bromophenacyl (PBPA) esters ***(58)***.

28. A glass reaction vessel with a ground glass fitting to a condensation tube can be used. Apply vacuum using a high-vacuum pump and heat with a conventional heat block. The reaction vessel should have a 2 cm diameter and 6 cm height and the glass condensation tube should be 13 cm long with a 7.5 cm glass elbow that connects to the vacuum pump.
29. The mero-aldehyde and α-alkyl fatty acids will be found throughout the reaction vessel and the condensation tube.

References

1. Barksdale, L. and Kim, K.-S. (1977) Mycobacterium. *Bacteriol. Rev.* **41,** 217–372.
2. Imaeda, T., Kanetsuna, F., and Galindo, B. (1968) Ultrastructure of cell walls of genus *Mycobacterium. J. Ultrastruct. Res.* **25,** 46–63.
3. Paul, T. R. and Beveridge, T. J. (1992) Reevaluation of envelope profiles and cytoplasmic ultrastructure of mycobacteria processed by conventional embedding and freeze-substitution protocols. *J. Bacteriol.* **174,** 6508–6517.
4. Nikaido, H., Kim, S.-H., and Rosenberg, E. Y. (1993) Physical organization of lipids in the cell wall of *Mycobacterium chelonae. Mol. Microbiol.* **8,** 1025–1030.
5. Liu, J., Barry, C. E., 3rd, Besra, G. S., and Nikaido, H. (1996) Mycolic acid structure determines the fluidity of the mycobacterial cell wall. *J. Biol. Chem.* **271,** 29,545–29,551.
6. Liu, J., Rosenberg, E. Y., and Nikaido, H. (1995) Fluidity of the lipid domain of cell wall from *Mycobacterium chelonae. Proc. Natl. Acad. Sci. USA* **92,** 11,254–11,258.
7. Paul, T. R. and Beveridge, T. J. (1993) Ultrastructure of mycobacterial surfaces by freeze-substitution. *Zbl Bakt* **279,** 450–457.
8. Paul, T. R. and Beveridge, T. J. (1994) Preservation of surface lipids and determination of ultrastructure of *Mycobacterium kansasii* by freeze-substitution. *Infect. Immun.* **62,** 1542–1550.
9. Minnikin, D. E. (1982) Lipids: complex lipids, their chemistry, biosynthesis and roles, in *The Biology of the Mycobacteria*, vol. 1 (Ratledge, C. and Standford, J., eds.), Academic Press, London, pp. 95–184.
10. Lane, S. J., Marshall, P. S., Upton, R. J., and Ratledge, C. (1998) Isolation and characterization of carboxymycobactins as the second extracellular siderophores in *Mycobacterium smegmatis. BioMetals* **11,** 13–20.
11. Daffe, M., Brennan, P. J., and McNeil, M. (1990) Predominant structural features of the cell wall arabinogalactan of *Mycobacterium tuberculosis* as revealed through characterization of oligoglycosyl alditol fragment by gas chromatography/mass spectrometry and by ^{1}H and ^{13}C NMR analyses. *J. Biol. Chem.* **265,** 6734–6743.
12. Daffe, M., McNeil, M., and Brennan, P. J. (1993) Major structural features of the cell wall arabinogalactans of *Mycobacterium*, *Rhodococcus*, and *Nocardia* spp. *Carb. Res.* **249,** 383–398.
13. McNeil, M., Daffe, M., and Brennan, P. J. (1991) Location of the mycolyl ester substituents in the cell walls of mycobacteria. *J. Biol. Chem.* **266,** 13,217–13,223.
14. Belisle, J. T., Vissa, V. D., Sievert, T., Takayama, K., Brennan, P. J., and Besra, G. S. (1997) Role of the major antigen of *Mycobacterium tuberculosis* in cell wall biogensis. *Science* **276,** 1420–1422.

15. Spargo, B. J., Crowe, L. M., Ioneda, T., Beaman, B. L., and Crowe, J. H. (1991) Cord factor (alpha, alpha-trehalose 6,6'-dimycolate) inhibits fusion between phospholipid vesicles. *Proc. Natl. Acad. Sci. USA* **88,** 737–740.
16. Crowe, L. M., Spargo, B. J., Ioneda, T., Beaman, B. L., and Crowe, J. H. (1994) Interaction of cord factor (alpha, alpha'-trehalose-6,6'-dimycolate) with phospholipids. *Biochim. Biophys. Acta.* **1194,** 53–60.
17. Kato, M. (1969) Studies of a biochemical lesion in experimental tuberculosis in mice. XI. Mitochondrial swelling induced by cord factor in vitro. *Am. Rev. Respir. Dis.* **100,** 47–53.
18. Behling, C. A., Perez, R. L., Kidd, M. R., Gerald, W., Staton, J., and Hunter, R. L. (1993) Induction of pulmonary granulomas, macrophage procoagulant activity, and tumor necrosis factor-alpha by trehalose glycolipids. *Ann. Clin. Lab. Sci.* **23,** 256–266.
19. Baba, T., Natsuhara, Y., Kaneda, K., and Yano, I. (1997) Granuloma formation activity and mycolic acid composition of mycobacterial cord factor. *Cell Mol. Life Sci.* **53,** 227–232.
20. Besra, G. S., Sievert, T., Lee, R. E., Slayden, R. A., Brennan, P. J., and Takayama, K. (1994) Identification of the apparent carrier in mycolic acid synthesis. *Proc. Natl. Acad. Sci. USA* **91,** 12,735–12,739.
21. Wolucka, B. A. and de Hoffmann, E. (1998) Isolation and charaterization of the major form of polyprenyl-phospho-mannose from *Mycobacterium smegmatis. Glycobiology* **8,** 955–962.
22. Wolucka, B. A. and de Hoffmann, E. (1995) The presence of beta-D-ribosyl-1-mannophosphodecaprenol in mycobacteria. *J. Biol. Chem.* **270,** 20,151–20,155.
23. Barry, C. E., 3rd, Lee, R. E., Mdluli, K., Sampson, A. E., Schroeder, B. G., Slayden, R. A., and Yuan, Y. (1998) Mycolic acids: structure, biosynthesis and physiological functions. *Prog. Lipid Res.* **37,** 143–179.
24. Yuan, Y., Mead, D., Schroeder, B. G., Zhu, Y., and Barry, C. E., 3rd (1998) The biosynthesis of mycolic acids in *Mycobacterium tuberculosis*. Enzymatic methyl(ene) transfer to acyl carrier protein bound meromycolic acid in vitro. *J. Biol. Chem.* **273,** 21,282–21,290.
25. Yuan, Y., Lee, R. E., Besra, G. S., Belisle, J. T., and Barry, C. E., 3rd (1995) Identification of a gene involved in the biosynthesis of cyclopropanated mycolic acids in *Mycobacterium tuberculosis. Proc. Natl. Acad. Sci. USA* **92,** 6630–6634.
26. Yuan, Y., Zhu, Y., Crane, D. D., and Barry, C. E., 3rd (1998) The effect of oxygenated mycolic acid composition on cell wall function and macrophage growth in *Mycobacterium tuberculosis. Mol. Microbiol.* **29,** 1449–1458.
27. Hunter, S. W. and Brennan, P. J. (1990) Evidence for the presence of a phosphotidylinositol anchor on the lipoarabinnomannan and lipomannan of *Mycobacterium tuberculosis. J. Biol. Chem.* **265,** 9272–9279.
28. Ballou, C. E., Vilkas, E., Lederer, E. (1963) Structural studies on the myoinositol phospholipids of *Mycobacterium tuberculosis. J. Biol. Chem.* **238,** 69–76.
29. Prinzis, S., Chatterjee, D., and Brennan, P. J. (1993) Structure and antigenicity of lipoarabinomannan from *Mycobacterium bovis* BCG. *J. Gen. Microbiol.* **139,** 2649–2658.

30. Chatterjee, D., Hunter, S. W., McNeal, M., Jardine, I., and Brennan, P. J. (1989) Structure and function of mycobacterial glycolipids and glycopeptidolipids. *Acta Leprologica* **7,** 81–84.
31. Chatterjee, D., Bozic, C. M., McNeil, M., and Brennan, P. J. (1991) Structural features of the arabinan component of the lipoarabinomannan of *Mycobacterium tuberculosis. J. Biol. Chem.* **266,** 9652–9660.
32. Chatterjee, D., Lowell, K., Rivoire, B., McNeil, M. R., and Brennan, P. J. (1992) Lipoarabinomannan of *Mycobacterium tuberculosis* (capping with mannosyl residues in some strains). *J. Biol. Chem.* **267,** 6234–6239.
33. Khoo, K.-H., Dell, A., Morris, H. R., Brennan, P. J., and Chatterjee, D. (1995) Inositol phosphate capping of the nonreducing termini of lipoarabinomannan from rapidly growing strains of mycobacterium. *J. Biol. Chem.* **270,** 12,380–12,389.
34. Tsumita, T., Matsumoto, R., Mizuno, D. (1960) Chemical and biological properties of the hemagglutination antigen, a lipopolysaccharide of *Mycobacterium tuberculosis. Jpn. J. Med. Sci.* **13,** 131–138.
35. Ohashi, M. and Tsumita, J. (1964) The fatty acid composition of the lipopolysaccharide of *Mycobacterium tuberculosis*, the hemagglutination antigen. *Jpn. J. Exp. Med.* **34,** 323–328.
36. Minnikin, D. E., Dobson, G., Goodfellow, M., Magnusson, M., and Ridell, M. (1985) Distribution of some mycobacterium waxes based on the phthiocerol family. *J. Gen. Microbiol.* **131,** 1375–1381.
37. Minnikin, D. E., Dobson, G., Sesardic, D., and Riedll, M. (1985) Mycolipenates and mycolipanolates of trehalose from *Mycobacterium tuberculosis. J. Gen. Microbiol.* **131,** 1369–1374.
38. Besra, G. S., Bolton, R. C., McNeil, M. R., Ridell, M., Simpson, K. E., Glushka, J., Halbeek, H. V., Brennan, P. J., and Minnikin, D. E. (1992) Structural elucidation of a novel family of acyltrehaloses from *Mycobacterium tuberculosis. Biochemistry* **31,** 9832–9837.
39. Daffe, M., Lacave, C., Laneelle, M.-A., Gillois, M., and Laneelle, G. (1988) Polyphthienoyl trehalose, glycolipids specific for virulent strains of the tubercle bacillus. *Eur. J. Biochem.* **172,** 579–584.
40. Brennan, P. J. (1988) Mycobacterium and other actinomycetes, in *Microbial Lipids*, vol. 1 (Rateledge, C. and Wilkinson, S. G., eds.), Academic Press, London, pp. 203–298.
41. Goren, M. B., Brokl, O., and Schaefer, W. B. (1974) Lipids of putative relevance to virulence in *Mycobacterium tuberculosis*: phthiocerol dimycocerosate and the attenuation indicator lipid. *Infect. Immunol.* **9,** 150–158.
42. Middlebrook, G., Coleman, C. M., and Schaefer, W. B. (1959) Sulfolipid from virulent tubercle bacilli. *Proc. Natl. Acad. Sci. USA* **45,** 1801–1804.
43. Goren, M. B., Hart, P. D. A., Young, M. R., and Armstrong, J. A. (1976) Prevention of phagosome-lysosome fusion in cultured macrophages by sulfatides of *Mycobacterium tuberculosis. Proc. Natl. Acad. Sci. USA* **73,** 2510–2514.
44. Goren, M. B., Brokl, O., and Schaefer, W. B. (1974) Lipids of putative relevance to virulence in *Mycobacterium tuberculosis*: correlation of virulence with elaboration of sulfatides and strongly acidic lipids. *Infect. Immun.* **9,** 142–149.

45. Goren, M. B., Vatter, A. E., and Fiscus, J. (1987) Polyanionic agents as inhibitors of phagosome-lysosome fusion in cultured macrophages: evolution of an alternative interpretation. *J. Leuk. Biol.* **41,** 111–121.
46. Goren, M. B., Vatter, A. E., and Fiscus, J. (1987) Polyanionic agents do not inhibit phagosome-lysosome fusion in cultured macrophages. *J. Leuk. Biol.* **41,** 122–129.
47. Daffe, M., McNeil, M., and Brennan, P. J. (1991) Novel type-specific lipooligosaccharides from *Mycobacterium tuberculosis*. *Biochemistry* **30,** 378–388.
48. Daffe, M., Lacave, C., Laneelle, M.-A., and Laneelle, G. (1987) Structure of the major triglycosyl phenol-phthiocerol of *Mycobacterium tuberculosis* (strain Canetti). *Eur. J. Biochem.* **167,** 155–160.
49. Daffe, M. (1991) Further sterochemical studies of phthiocerol and phenol phthiocerol in mycobacteria. *Res. Microbiol.* **142,** 405–410.
50. Dobson, G., Minnikin, D. E., Minnikin, S. M., Parlett, J. H., Goodfellow, M., Ridell, M., and Magnusson, M. (1985) Systematic analysis of complex mycobacterial lipids, in *Chemical Methods in Bacterial Systematics*, vol. 1 (Goodfellow, M. and Minnikin, D. E., eds.), Academic Press, London, pp. 237–265.
51. George, K. M., Yuan, Y., Sherman, D. R., and Barry, C. E., 3rd (1995) The biosynthesis of cyclopropanated mycolic acids in *Mycobacterium tuberculosis*: Identification and functional analysis of CMAS-2. *J. Biol. Chem.* **270,** 27,292–27,298.
52. Allen, B. W. (1998) Mycobacteria: general culture methodology and safety considerations, in *Methods in Molecular Biology*, vol. 101, *Mycobacteria Protocols* (Parish, T. and Stoker, N. G., eds.) Humana, Totowa, NJ, pp. 15–30.
53. Kennerly, D. A. (1986) Improved analysis of species of phospholipids using argentation thin-layer chromatography. *J. Chromatogr.* **363,** 462–467.
54. Minnikin, D. E., Dobson, G., and Hutchinson, I. G. (1983) Characterization of phthiocerol dimycocerosates from *Mycobacterium tuberculosis*. *Biochem. Biophys. Acta* **753,** 445–449.
55. York, W. S., Darvill, A. G., McNeil, M., Stevenson, T. T., and Albersheim, P. (1986) Isolation and characterization of plant cell wall components, in *Methods in Enzymology*, vol. 118 (Weissback, A. and Weissbach, H., eds.), Academic Press, Orlando, pp. 3–40.
56. Teng, L. J., Liaw, S. J., Hsueh, P. R., Fan, J. H., Luh, K. T., and Ha, S. W. (1997) Constituitive fatty acid and enzyme profiles of *Mycobacterium* species. *J. Formos. Med. Assoc.* **96,** 336–45.
57. Couderc, F. (1995) Gas chromatography/tandem mass spectrometry as an analytical tool for identification of fatty acids. *Lipids* **30,** 691–699.
58. Wong, M. Y. H., Steck, P. A., and Gray, G. R. (1979) The major mycolic acids of *Mycobacterium smegmatis*. *J. Biol. Chem.* **254,** 5734–5740.

16

In Vitro Model of Hypoxically Induced Nonreplicating Persistence of *Mycobacterium tuberculosis*

Lawrence G. Wayne

1. Introduction

1.1. In Vivo Evidence for Dormancy and Latency

Great progress has been made in the latter half of the twentieth century in the understanding of the immunology of tuberculosis and of strategies for chemotherapeutic management of this disease. Indeed, given the evidence that the dominant, and perhaps sole, ecologic niche of *Mycobacterium tuberculosis* is the infected human host, it seemed reasonable to hope that the disease could not only be controlled, but eradicated by the end of this century *(1)*. These hopes are dashed by the periodic resurgence of tuberculosis in various populations. Undoubtedly socioeconomic factors have played a major role in the failure to eradicate this disease, but another, neglected, factor is the apparent ability of the tubercle bacillus to remain in a relatively quiescent state in the host, neither replicating and causing progression of disease, nor dying off and disappearing from the host's tissues, in spite of apparently adequate immune responses and aggressive chemotherapy.

Evidence for the presence of tubercle bacilli in a nonreplicating persistent (NRP) state in mammalian hosts may be inferred from a number of observations in humans and experimental animals *(2)*. It has long been recognized that many years may intervene between the first evidence of infection of a person, as demonstrated by a positive tuberculin reaction, and actual development of tuberculous disease *(3,4)*; during this variable period of latency some bacilli must remain viable, even though they are not multiplying. Similarly, individuals with clear evidence of tuberculous disease may exhibit prolonged periods when the lesions appear to be stable and blocked so that there is no communi-

From: *Methods in Molecular Medicine*, vol. 54: *Mycobacterium Tuberculosis Protocols*
Edited by: T. Parish and N. G. Stoker © Humana Press Inc., Totowa, NJ

cation with a patent bronchus and access to air, yet which yield viable tubercle bacilli when the lesions are removed by surgery and subjected to bacteriologic examination *(5,6)*.

More direct evidence for the NRP state may be found with experimental animals, especially the mouse. In the latter animal, tubercle bacilli replicate logarithmically for a number of weeks after infection, until the cell-mediated immune mechanisms become activated, after which the count reaches a plateau, i.e., neither increasing nor decreasing, for many months *(7,8)*. As the mice age and immunity ebbs due to senescence, bacterial replication may resume. Similarly, chemotherapeutic treatment may cause a marked decline in numbers of tubercle bacilli in infected mice, even to the extent that they may not be detectable by culture for many months, but abrogation of the immune mechanisms may reactivate the infection *(9–12)*.

1.2. In Vitro Hypoxic Model of Nonreplicating Persistence

A number of factors, including pH changes, accumulation of inhibitory substances, depletion of specific nutrients, and depletion of oxygen might contribute to the NRP state of *M. tuberculosis* in the mammalian host. The effects of oxygen depletion have been the subject of considerable recent study, and the hypoxic model is the subject of this chapter. There is evidence that some very specific adaptations to oxygen depletion occur that make it possible for the hypoxic NRP state to exist. When *M. tuberculosis* is growing under well-aerated conditions, a very abrupt depletion of oxygen has a catastrophic effect on the bacilli, rapidly leading to their death and autolysis *(13)*. On the other hand, when the oxygen content of a culture is allowed to diminish gradually, the tubercle bacilli undergo specific inductions that enable them to survive without replicating under hypoxic conditions *(14–16)*. In our original hypoxic adaptation model, the hypoxic condition occurred along a self-generated gradient as the bacilli used up dissolved O_2 while settling through unstirred liquid culture medium *(14)*.

A problem inherent in the original, spatial gradient model of hypoxic shiftdown that depended on settling of the bacilli was that it did not permit isolation of events during that shiftdown, i.e., the bacilli in the middle layers, where the gradient was being established, represented a mixed population in different stages of shiftdown. An alternative model was then developed, that was based on a temporal gradient wherein the bacilli were maintained in a dispersed state, but under conditions such that the O_2 was depleted gradually but uniformly throughout the culture *(16)*. This was achieved by growing the organisms in sealed containers with a controlled ratio of air to culture medium, which we refer to as the head space ratio (HSR),with slow magnetic stirring that keeps the bacilli suspended in the medium without agitating the surface and affecting the slow equilibration between head space gas and liquid medium. This is the technique to be described in this chapter.

1.3. Markers of Hypoxic Shiftdown to NRP

1.3.1. Microaerophilic NRP Stage 1

Among the earliest changes that occur in actively growing tubercle bacilli as they adapt to hypoxia is the termination of replication of DNA synthesis, even as the optical density of the culture continues to rise slowly due to some nonreplicative cell enlargement ***(16,17)***. This occurs abruptly as the dissolved oxygen content drops below about 1% of that of a solution saturated with air, and the bacilli enter the microaerophilic NRP stage 1. It is while the bacilli are in NRP stage 1 that most of the presently recognized inductions occur, including that of an antigen ***(18)*** that appears to correspond to the α crystallin chaperone protein ***(19,20)***, of an enzyme that reductively aminates glyoxylate ***(15)***, and of a respiratory type of nitrate reductase activity ***(21)***.

1.3.1.1. Termination of Replication and DNA Synthesis

Young, slowly stirred cultures of *M. tuberculosis* in sealed 20 cm diameter tubes with a HSR of 0.5 initially replicate exponentially with a doubling time ranging from 16 to 18 h, just as well-aerated cultures do. When the dissolved oxygen concentration drops to about 1% relative saturation (using air saturated medium as reference) at an optical absorption level at 580 nm (OD_{580}) of 0.08 (corresponding to a viable cell count of 5×10^7 CFU per mL), the replication stops abruptly; however, the OD_{580} continues to rise, albeit at a sharply reduced rate, as long as the culture remains in the microaerophilic NRP stage 1. The viable count remains at plateau through the balance of the microaerophilic period. Concurrent with the termination of replication, DNA synthesis ceases abruptly as well, and the rate of RNA synthesis drops precipitously ***(16)***. The post replication rise in OD_{580} is a reflection of an increase in cell size ***(16)*** that has been demonstrated by electron microscopy to be due to outer cell wall thickening, and is unique to the hypoxic model; it does not occur in old aerated stationary phase cultures ***(17)***. This hypoxic cell wall thickening has also been seen in *Mycobacterium bovis* BCG but not in the rapid grower *Mycobacterium smegmatis* ***(17)***.

1.3.1.2. α Crystallin Protein

A dominant protein antigen designated URB-1 was found in hypoxically adapted cultures of *M. tuberculosis* but not in aerobic cultures ***(18)***. Subsequent studies identified a 16 kDa protein that is induced in *M. tuberculosis* under hypoxic conditions as the α crystallin chaperone protein, and it is believed that this corresponds to the URB-1 antigen ***(19)***. This protein is induced very soon after tubercle bacilli encounter hypoxic conditions, but is not induced under other stress conditions *(20)*. Furthermore, a direct correlation has been seen between the rate of depletion of the URB-1 antigen and the loss of tolerance to anaerobiosis when tubercle bacilli are induced to shift up from the NRP state to active growth by reinitiation of aeration *(15)*.

1.3.1.3. Glyoxylate Reductive Aminase

Tubercle bacilli in the NRP state have moderately elevated levels of isocitrate lyase, a key enzyme in the glyoxylate bypass of the tricarboxylic acid cycle, but no elevation of malate synthase, a downstream enzyme in that pathway. On the other hand, highly elevated levels were seen of an enzyme that catalyzes the reductive amination of glyoxylate to glycine, with concomitant oxidation of reduced nicotine adenine dinucleotide (NADH) to nicotine adenine dinucleotide (NAD) *(15)*. This enzyme was called glycine dehydrogenase when first recognized in *M. tuberculosis* *(22)*, but we have only been able to demonstrate the reaction in the direction of glyoxylate to glycine, and not the reverse. Representing, as it apparently does, an alternative exit pathway from the recognized glyoxylate cycle, this enzyme's main contribution to hypoxic survival of tubercle bacilli may be the regeneration of NAD from NADH, providing an energy source for synthesis of adenosine triphosphate (ATP) that may be needed to complete a round of replication before shiftdown can be completed successfully or to support essential inductions during the NRP state. Kinetic studies with the various components of the reaction mixture demonstrated that the rate of the reaction is essentially governed by the proportions of NAD and NADH in that mixture *(15)*.

1.3.1.4. Nitrate Reductase

When *M. tuberculosis* is grown aerobically in the presence of nitrate, it reduces the nitrate to nitrite at a slow to moderate rate that is proportional to the substrate concentration. On the other hand, when the bacilli are grown in a limited HSR configuration, immediately on entry into the microaerophilic NRP stage 1 they exhibit rapid induction of an apparent respiratory nitrate reductase (NAR) activity, which produces nitrite much more rapidly than the aerobic enzyme and that rate is not a function of substrate concentration *(21)*. This latter induction may be analogous to what is seen in *Escherichia coli*, which under anaerobic conditions, produces a respiratory NAR that reduces nitrate to provide energy for anaerobic growth, but differs in that *M. tuberculosis* adapts to anaerobic survival, but not growth.

1.3.2. Anaerobic NRP Stage 2

1.3.2.1. Susceptibility to Antimicrobial Agents

As the headspace oxygen depletion continues and the dissolved oxygen drops below about 0.06% saturation, the turbidity of the culture abruptly stops increasing and the bacilli enter anaerobic NRP stage 2. Only when they enter this stage do they exhibit susceptibility to the bactericidal action of nitroimidazole drugs *(16,23)*; they show little if any susceptibility to other antimicrobial agents *(16,23)* while in this stage. In NRP stage 2 the bacilli are killed at a concentration of 12 μg/mL of metronidazole, whereas under aerobic conditions they can grow unimpeded in concentrations of the drug as high as 200 μg/mL. There is also evidence of an additive bactericidal effect when rifampin is added to metronidazole-treated cells in NRP stage 2, suggesting that some necessary mRNA inductions are occurring even under these inhospitable conditions. Neither isoniazid nor ciprofloxacin, which are bactericidal to actively growing tubercle bacilli, exhibit toxic effects on bacilli in anaerobic NRP stage 2.

1.4. Aerobic Shiftup

1.4.1. Synchrony

The uniform physiologic condition of the bacillary population after induction of the NRP state is demonstrated by the observation that these bacilli exhibit synchronized replication upon resumption of aeration of the cells *(16,24)*. The sequence of events when the nonreplicating bacilli are exposed to air is an immediate initiation of RNA synthesis, which is followed by a round of synchronous cell doubling, and then the initiation of DNA synthesis *(24)*. The synchrony has been maintained through at least three cycles of cell division.

1.4.2. Dilution of Protein and Loss of Anaerobic Tolerance

As noted above (**Subheading 1.3.1.2.**) the URB-1 antigen that is produced on hypoxic shiftdown of tubercle bacilli is believed to correspond to the α crystallin chaperone protein. In this regard, the decline in concentration of this protein upon aerobic shiftup of hypoxic NRP cultures of the bacilli, which appeared to reflect dilution of the protein by other, freshly synthesized protein during shiftup rather than its destruction, closely parallels the decline in tolerance of the bacilli to the lethal effects of anaerobiosis *(18)*.

1.5. Relevance of the In Vitro Model to In Vivo Realities

For all of the effort being expended on the study of *M. tuberculosis* in the in vitro hypoxic NRP model, the question arises as to the relevance of this model to the condition of the bacilli in the lesions of the mammalian host. In view of the demonstrated rapid loss of viability of aerobically grown tubercle bacilli upon abrupt exposure to anaerobiosis without having had time to adapt *(13,15)*, and the fact that viable bacilli have been recovered from the contents of old blocked human lung lesions recovered at surgery *(5,6)*, it is evident that some adaptation to hypoxic conditions must occur in human tuberculosis. Segal has reviewed evidence that tubercle bacilli recovered directly (i.e., without subculture) from mouse lung lesions contain enzymes of anaerobic metabolism, further supporting the hypothesis that specific adaptations occur in vivo to hypoxic conditions ***(25)***. Among the strongest evidence that the model described here does reflect events in the in vivo adaptation are the observations that the α crystallin chaperone protein is induced by mild hypoxia but not by a variety of other stress conditions ***(19,20)***, and that antibody to this protein is found in the serum of most tuberculosis patients ***(20,26,27)***.

A question that remains to be resolved is that of the relative roles of NRP stage 1 and NRP stage 2 in latency of disease. To what extent are tuberculosis lesions completely anaerobic, and to what extent microaerophilic? The in vitro data suggest that survival is most favored under microaerophilic conditions, in which inductions of survival factors occur ***(16)***. The fact that tuberculosis may persist in a latent state for years without appearance of gross detectable lesions or symptoms would seem more compatible with a microaerophilic than an anaerobic milieu, i.e., it seems unlikely that a microscopic granuloma would be completely isolated from oxygen. On the other hand, there may well be some fluctuation between microaerophilic and anaerobic conditions within individual old blocked necrotic lesions, and these fluctuations may help determine the fate of the bacilli at any given site.

2. Materials

2.1. Media and Cell Washing and Processing Solutions

1. Liquid medium: Dubos Tween Albumin broth (DTA). Dissolve 2 g asparagine, 0.5 g casitone, 2.5 g Na_2HPO_4, 1 g KH_2PO_4, 50 mg ferric ammonium citrate, 10 mg $MgSO_4$, 0.5 mg $CaCl_2$, 0.1 mg $ZnSO_4$, 0.1 mg $CuSO_4$, 0.2 g Tween-80 in 800 mL of distilled water and autoclave. Dissolve 5 g bovine serum albumin fraction V and 7.5 g glucose in 200 mL of 0.85% sodium chloride and sterilize by filtration through a 0.22 μm membrane filter. Add this solution to the cooled basal medium. The final pH should be 6.6 ± 0.2 (*see* **Notes 1** and **2**).
2. Solid medium: Dubos Oleic Albumin (DOA) agar (*see* **Note 3**). Dissolve 1 g asparagine, 0.5 g casitone, 2.5 g Na_2HPO_4, 1 g KH_2PO_4, 50 mg ferric ammonium citrate, 10 mg $MgSO_4$, 0.5 mg $CaCl_2$, 0.1 mg $ZnSO_4$, and 0.1 mg $CuSO_4$ in 800 mL of distilled H_2O and autoclave. Dissolve 5 g of bovine serum albumin fraction V and 50 mg of sodium oleate in 200 mL of 0.8% sodium chloride and sterilize by filtration. Add this albumin-oleate complex to the autoclaved basal medium after it has cooled to 50°C and immediately dispense to appropriate sterile plates. Because of the presence of albumin, the complete medium cannot be remelted once it has set.
3. Screw-capped culture tubes: 20 mm diameter by 125 mm tall.
4. Conical screw-capped Nephelo flasks with 20 mm sidearms and flat (nonfluted) bases, of nominal 500 mL capacity (Wheaton Scientific Products, Millville, NJ). These have an actual total volume, including sidearms and neck, of 600 mL.

5. 8 mm and 50 mm long Teflon-coated magnetic stirring bars.
6. Paraplast (Oxford Labware, St. Louis, MO).
7. Tissue culture type of magnetic stirrer: Biostir 4 Heavy Duty Magnetic Stirrer (Wheaton Science Products).
8. Sterile 12-well tissue culture plate (Falcon, Becton Dickinson, Lincoln Park, NJ).
9. Phosphate buffered saline (PBS): add 100 mL of 0.1 *M* phosphate buffer, pH 7.5 to 900 mL of 0.85% NaCl, dispense in convenient aliquots, and autoclave (*see* **Note 4**).
10. 10% w/v Tween-80: undiluted Tween-80 is too viscous to measure volumetrically, so prepare a 10% w/v solution in water. Autoclave this concentrate, as the unsterilized solution will support the growth of molds, even when refrigerated.
11. Phosphate buffered Tween (PBS-T): 0.05% Tween-80 in PBS. Aseptically add 5 mL of 10% Tween-80 to 1000 mL PBS.
12. DTT/Mg buffer: 1 m*M* dithiothreitol, 5 m*M* $MgCl_2$ in PBS ***(15)***. This buffer is used for the preparation of sonic extracts of bacilli for assay of reductive amination of glyoxylate.
13. W-380 Cup Horn Sonicator (Heat Systems-Ultrasonics, Inc., Farmingdale, NY).
14. 22 µm pore-sized, low protein-binding membrane filter, e.g., Costar Spin-X (Corning Inc., Corning, NY).

2.2. Reagents for Assays

2.2.1. Estimation of Nucleic Acid Synthesis

1. Tritiated uracil. A sterile stock solution of either [6-^{3}H]uracil or [5,6-^{3}H]uracil at a specific concentration of 20 to 40 mCi/mmol should be used for labeling both the RNA and DNA that are synthesized by the bacilli ***(16,24)*** (*see* **Note 5**).
2. Unlabeled uracil stock solution, 10 µg/mL.
3. 25 mm, 0.45 µm pore size B-6 Bac-T-Flex membrane (Schleicher and Schuell, Keene, NH).
4. 2-Ethoxyethanol.
5. Scintillation fluid: Aquasol-2 (New England Nuclear, Boston, MA) or equivalent.
6. Potassium hydroxide, 3% stock solution.

2.2.2. Detection of α Crystallin Protein

1. 12% polyacrylamide gels.
2. Peptide molecular weight markers.
3. Western blot materials (widely commercially available).
4. Antibody to *M. tuberculosis* α crystallin (16 kDa) protein ***(19)***. Monoclonal antibody F24-2–3 (IT-4), obtained from the UNDP/World Bank/World Health Organization Special Program for Research and Training in Tropical Diseases.

2.2.3. Estimation of Reductive Amination of Glyoxylate

1. 0.5 *M* Glyoxylate substrate: this substrate solution may be prepared from either free glyoxylic acid or from its sodium salt. In either case, it must be made fresh

on the day of use, using precautions to protect the substrate from degradation (*see* **Note 6**). Dissolve 57 mg of the sodium glyoxylate, sodium salt monohydrate in 1.0 mL distilled H_2O ***or*** dissolve 46 mg of glyoxylic acid monohydrate in 1.0 mL 0.5 *N* NaOH.
2. 0.1 *M* phosphate buffer, pH 6.4.
3. 2 *M* ammonium sulfate: dissolve 6.6 g $(NH_4)_2SO_4$ in 15 mL of H_2O, adjust the pH to 6.4 with 0.1 *M* NaOH, transfer to a 25 mL volumetric flask, and bring to volume with more H_2O. This reagent is stable.
4. 0.8 m*M* nicotine adenine dinucleotide reduced form (NADH): add 3.5 mL of 0.01 *M* phosphate buffer, pH 6.4, to a preweighed 2 mg vial of NADH. To ensure that it is satisfactory for this assay, dilute 100 µL of the NADH solution with 470 µL H_2O and read the absorbance at 340 nm (A_{340}) in a UV-transparent 1 mL microcuvet. If the A_{340} is between 750 and 850, it is satisfactory to use. This solution must be prepared immediately before use.

2.2.4. Assay of Nitrate Reductase (NAR)

1. 250 µ*M* sodium nitrite standard. Prepare a 0.01 *M* stock solution of $NaNO_2$. Transfer 1.25 mL of this stock to a 50 mL volumetric flask and bring to volume with distilled H_2O to yield a 250 µ*M* solution.
2. 0.1 *M* HCl.
3. 0.2% sulfanilamide stock.
4. *N*-(1 naphthyl)-ethylene diamine·dihydrochloride (NEDD): 0.1% w/v aqueous solution.
5. 13 × 100 mm test tubes.

2.2.5. Assay of Adenosine Triphosphate (ATP)

1. *N*-(2-hydroxyethyl)piperazine-*N*'(2-ethanesulfonic acid) (HEPES) buffer: 0.025 *M*, pH 7.75.
2. HEPES buffered Tween-80 (HBT): 0.02% Tween-in HEPES. Prepare by diluting 0.2 mL of 10% Tween-80 in 100 mL of HEPES buffer.
3. Chloroform.
4. ATP standard, 80 ng/mL in HEPES buffer. Prepare fresh from a 10 µg/mL stock concentrate.
5. 13 × 100 mm disposable glass culture tubes.
6. Aluminum heating block with holes 13 mm diameter by 45 mm deep.
7. Luminometer and tubes (Turner model TD-20e, Turner Designs, Sunnyvale, CA or equivalent).
8. Luciferin/luciferase reagent (Turner Designs).

3. Methods

3.1. Culture of Bacilli

For a more complete review of dynamics of cultivation of tubercle bacilli, *see* **ref. *28***.

3.1.1. Strains and Inocula

If at all possible, we recommend that the H37Rv strain of *M. tuberculosis* be used as a reference culture for studies employing this model. Other species have been examined by this technique, but caution should be observed interpreting results with any species other than *M. tuberculosis* (*see* **Note 7**). Avoid serial passages of inocula of the strain to be tested.

1. Grow a large single seed lot aerobically in DTA medium until it attains an optical absorbance at 580 nm (OD_{580}) of 0.4. This corresponds to a cell density of about 2.5×10^8 CFU/mL.
2. Dispense the seed stock in small aliquots and maintain at –70°C.
3. When a working culture is needed, thaw a frozen seed and inoculate 100 µL into 10 mL of DTA. Incubate with agitation until it reaches an OD_{580} of 0.4 (2.5×10^8 CFU/mL) and use that culture as the inoculum for the actual experimental culture.
4. Discard excess thawed seed, and thaw a new one for subsequent experiments.

3.1.2. Aerobic Fully Replicating Control Cultures

Both working inocula and control reference cultures must be prepared under well-aerated conditions. We use two types of culture containers, depending on the volume needed.

3.1.2.1. Aerated Tubed Cultures

1. Dispense 10 mL of DTA into screw-capped 20 mm tubes and inoculate with 100 µL of seed stock.
2. Incubate at 37°C with shaking at 250 rpm. This shaking rate should produce a small vortex at the top surface of the medium, maximizing aeration.
3. Loosen the screw caps slightly (about 1/8 to 1/4 turn) and hold in place with a small strip of tape. Monitor the growth rate by daily reading of OD_{580}; a linear correction of readings for particle coincidence should be made for all readings of OD_{580} in excess of 0.20 ***(14)*** (*see* **Note 8**).

3.1.2.2. Aerated Flask Cultures

When large volumes of actively growing cultures are needed, they may be grown and monitored in sidearm flasks. We use nominal 500 mL screw-capped Nephelo flasks with 20 mm sidearms to permit direct correlation of OD_{580} of flask preparations with that of tubed cultures.

1. Place a 50 mm Teflon-coated magnetic stirring bar in the flask.
2. Prepare and autoclave 180 mL of the DTA base directly in the flask and add 20 mL of the sterile glucose and albumin mixture solution aseptically to the cooled medium.

3. Inoculate the medium with 2 mL of a culture (OD_{580} of 0.4) and incubate the flask at 37°C on a magnetic stirrer set to rotate at 180 rpm. Do not use a rotary platform shaker to stir flask cultures (*see* **Note 9**). Slight adjustments may be made in the volume of inoculum to accommodate for small deviations in OD_{580}, to yield a calculated intial OD_{580} of 0.004.

*3.1.3. Limitation of Aeration for Shiftdown to NRP Stages (see **Notes 10** and **11**)*

3.1.3.1. Configuration and Agitation of 0.5 HSR Tube Cultures

1. For small volumes of culture, use 20 mm screw-capped culture tubes (total capacity to the very top lip is 25.5 mL). Place an 8 mm long Teflon-coated magnetic stirring bar in each tube and autoclave.
2. Add 17.0 mL of DTA medium to each tube, leaving an air head space of 8.5 mL, corresponding to a 0.5 HSR.
3. Inoculate each tube with about 170 µL of working culture ($OD_{580} = 0.4$) to yield a calculated initial optical absorbance (OD_{580}) of 0.004 (which is too low to actually read directly) (*see* **Note 12**).
4. Close the tubes tightly with either a screw cap or a tightly fitting rubber vaccine cap (*see* **Note 13**). Use the latter if reagents are to be injected into the tubes during the course of the experiment.
5. If the experiment is to last longer than 21 d, seal the caps by quickly inverting them into Paraplast (premelted at 56°C) just deep enough to cover the cap and about 10 mm of the adjacent tube.
6. Place the tubes in plastic racks on the Biostir magnetic stirring table set at 120 rpm in a 37°C incubator.
7. Determine the OD_{580} daily, taking care not to agitate the tubes while transferring them to the spectrophotometer (*see* **Note 10**).
8. Plot growth curves with the optical measurements on a logarithmic scale to permit clear definition of the two deflection points, i.e., from aerobic growth into microaerophilic NRP stage 1, and then into anaerobic NRP stage 2 (**Fig. 1**).

3.1.3.2. Configuration and Agitation of 0.5 HSR Flask Cultures (*see* **Notes 10** and **14**)

1. Place a 50 mm stirring bar and 360 mL of DTA basal medium into a 500 mL Nephelo flask and autoclave. After cooling, add 40 mL of sterile glucose/albumin solution. The flasks have an actual total capacity, including sidearms and neck, of 600 mL; the 400 mL of medium leaves 200 mL of air space, which corresponds to 0.5 HSR.
2. Because of the large air-liquid interface in flasks, they must be stirred more slowly than 0.5 HSR cultures in tubes to avoid perturbation of the surface during incubation. Place the tightly capped flask cultures on a tissue culture magnetic stirrer set at 70 rpm and incubate at 37°C.
3. Tip some of the culture into the side arm to read OD_{580}. Do this gently to minimize agitation of the surface, both when tipping into the sidearm and when tip-

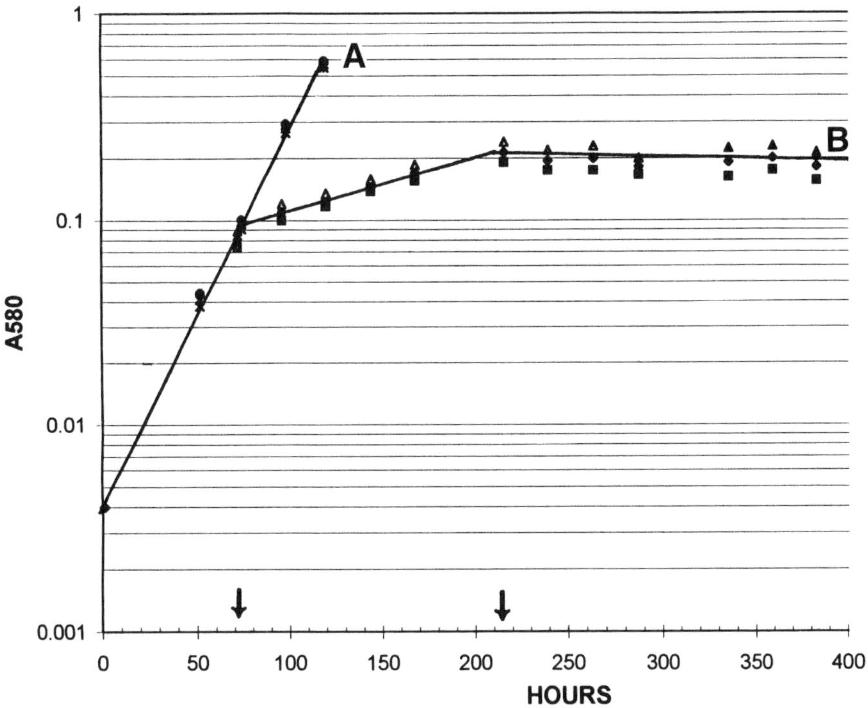

Fig. 1. Optical absorbance (OD_{580}) curves of *M. tuberculosis* grown under conditions of **(A)** vigorous aeration and **(B)** slow stirring in 0.5 HSR configuration. For the first 72 h of growth, there is sufficient dissolved oxygen in the 0.5 HSR tubes to permit logarithmic replication to occur at the same rate as occurs in the aerated tubes. After 72 h of incubation, sufficient depletion of dissolved oxygen has occurred in the 0.5 HSR tubes to cause an abrupt termination of replication in the 0.5 HSR tubes, but the optical absorbance continues to rise, albeit at a reduced rate, due to lipid synthesis; specific proteins are induced during this microaerophilic NRP stage 1. After the cultures have been incubated for over 200 h, the dissolved oxygen has been so severely depleted that the bacilli in the 0.5 HSR tubes enter anaerobic NRP stage 2 and the increase in OD_{580} stops.

ping fluid back from the sidearm to the main body of the flask (*see* **Note 15**). Flask cultures are usually harvested early enough that it is not necessary to dip the caps in Paraplast.

3.1.4. Initiation of Shiftup and Synchronized Replication from the NRP State

To permit bacilli in the NRP state to resume replication, it is necessary to reintroduce oxygen into the system. On recovery from the hypoxic condition, the bacilli exhibit synchronized replication.

1. Dilute 100 µL of an NRP stage 2 culture into 10 mL of DTA, and vortex to aerate the medium and disperse the cells
2. Immediately sample a small aliquot for plating (*see* **Subheading 3.1.5.**).
3. Dispense additional aliquots of the diluted culture into small tubes, and incubate at 37°C, in a stationary manner, i.e., without continuous agitation (*see* **Note 16**).
4. Remove a tube at 4–6 h intervals. Vortex vigorously, dilute and plate for colony counts (*see* **Subheading 3.1.5.**). Discard the remainder of the sample. Use a fresh sample for each sampling.

3.1.5. Determination of Colony Forming Units

1. Aseptically dispense 3.0 mL aliquots of molten complete DOA agar into each well of a sterile 12-well tissue culture plate. Allow the agar to set, and incubate for 48 h in a humidified incubator to confirm sterility. (If colonies are to be selected for genetic purposes, we have found it useful to incorporate 0.05% Tween-80 in the agar. This yields soft colonies that are more easily picked and emulsified in liquid medium with a toothpick or other fine tool.)
2. Dilute 100 µL of the well-mixed culture into 9.9 mL of DTA. Mix this 10^{-2} dilution vigorously; if available, a low energy sonicating cleaning bath may be used for a few seconds to help break clumps.
3. Transfer 100 µL of this dilution to a 900 µL DTA blank, mix, and continue the 10-fold dilution series up to the 10^{-6} dilution.
4. Because of the difficulty in recovering fluid with micropipet tips from a deep container, we prefer to carry out the dilution series in small, shallow vials as follows. Place 8 mm Teflon-coated magnetic stirring bars in a number of 2 mL short form screw-capped vials and autoclave. To avoid evaporation loss on standing, dispense 900 µL of the DTA diluent to each vial immediately before the dilutions are to be made. As each dilution is made, cap the vial and place on a magnetic stirrer for at least 10 s to mix before transferring an aliquot to the next vial of diluent.
5. Plate 20 µL aliquots of the 10^{-6} to 10^{-3} dilutions onto triplicate wells of agar in the 12-well plate. This dilution range should give satisfactory counts in most instances. In cases where bactericidal agents are being tested, it may be necessary to start plating at lower dilution.
6. Incubate the plates, with their well-fitting covers in place, in a humidified incubator at 36–37°C, and examine twice weekly for emergence of colonies, starting 14 d after inoculation (*see* **Note 17**).
7. Count colonies by inverting the plate without opening it, and examining it with transmitted light at 100X magnification on a dissecting microscope. If droplets of condensate on the culture plate lid cause too much light diffraction, briefly open the plate and wipe off the drops with sterile cotton swabs.

3.1.6. Cell Disruption

The bacilli may be disrupted for recovery of enzymes or antigens by treatment in the cuphorn attachment of a sonicator. The procedure to be described may be applied to product of one, or even a pool of cells from 10 or more tubed cultures.

1. Rapidly chill the cultures in an ice bath.
2. Centrifuge in sealed cups in a refrigerated centrifuge at 800*g* for 30 min.
3. Aspirate the supernatant without disturbing the sediment and centrifuge for 5 min to drain residual fluid from the walls, and aspirate.
4. Resuspend the bacilli in a single 10 mL aliquot of PBS-T, vortex and repeat the two stage centrifugation (30 min and 5 min).
5. Repeat the PBS-T two-stage wash procedure. The Tween in the buffer at this stage is necessary to keep the bacilli from clumping and trapping protein from the medium.
6. Discard supernatant and resuspend the cells in 2.0 mL of PBS without Tween or in DTT/Mg buffer (or other specialized buffer) in a round bottomed culture tube (*see* **Note 18**). This suspension should now be free of both residual protein from the culture medium and Tween-80 (presence of the latter may interfere with sonication efficiency).
7. Mount the tube in a clamp, with the bottom about 2–3 mm above the face of the cuphorn in a biological safety hood and sonicate at maximum output, recirculating ice water through the cup around the tube (*see* **Note 18**).
8. Distribute the sonicate among microcentrifuge tubes, centrifuge at 5000*g* to remove cell debris, and filter sterilize the supernatant through a 22 μm pore-sized, low protein-binding membrane filter.

3.2. Assay of Markers

3.2.1. Nucleic Acid Synthesis

Tritiated uracil may be added to the culture tube at the beginning of the experiment, or for pulse labeling it may be added by syringe and needle through a vaccine cap sealing a 0.5 HSR culture tube ***(16,24)***. If it is added by syringe to a 0.5 HSR culture, avoid any introduction of air bubbles into the tube.

1. Add ^{3}H-uracil to yield 1 μCi/mL of culture and incubate for the desired period of time.
2. Mix vigorously and filter 2–5 mL through a 25 mm, 0.45 μm pore size membrane.
3. Wash thoroughly with unlabeled uracil or water.
4. Dissolve the filter in 1 mL of 2-ethoxyethanol for 2 h.
5. Mix with scintillation fluid and count radiation. This will yield a measure of total label incorporated into nucleic acid.
6. Transfer a second 2–5 mL aliquot of the culture to a clean tube and add 0.1 vol of 3.0 *M* KOH.
7. Mix and incubate at 37°C for 24 h. Filter, wash, and process as described in **steps 2–5**. This will yield a measure of label incorporated into DNA. The difference between total bound label and DNA label corresponds to the ^{3}H incorporated into RNA (*see* **Note 5**).

3.2.2. α Crystallin Protein

The α crystallin chaperone protein may be visualized in extracts of tubercle bacilli in NRP stages by conventional electrophoresis in SDS–12% polyacrylamide gels, comparing its migration to that of defined molecular weight markers. It is generally referred to as a 16 kDa protein *(20)*, but there are small discrepancies in apparent molecular weight as determined in different laboratories, ranging up to 19 kDa *(27)*. Although its identity may be inferred from the absence of a corresponding protein band in extracts of actively growing aerated cultures (AG) cultures, to confirm that identity perform a Western blot using the specific monoclonal antibody.

3.2.3. Glyoxylate Reductive Aminase (16)

1. Determine the protein concentration of the bacillary extract by any standard protein assay method.
2. Add the following reagents to a UV-transparent microcuvet in the order specified: 400 µL of 0.1 *M* phosphate buffer pH 6.4, 200 µL of 2 *M* ammonium sulfate, 100 µL of 0.5 *M* glyoxylate substrate, and 100 µL of NADH solution.
3. Place the cuvet in a recording UV spectrophotometer set at a wave length of 340 nm and note the initial A_{340}.
4. Equilibrate for 5 min, start the recorder, and add aliquots of lysate and/or H_2O sufficient to include a range from 100 to 500 µg protein per sample and to bring the total volume of reagents in the cuvet to 1.0 mL. Stir with care to avoid bubbles and record the rate at which A_{340} declines. Based on initial concentration of 80 µ*M* NADH and the amount of protein in the test sample, calculate the specific activity of the enzyme extract as µmoles NADH oxidized/h/mg protein.

3.2.4. Nitrate Reduction (21)

This assay is based on measurement of the rate of production of nitrite ion in cultures containing sodium nitrate. For routine monitoring of the activity of nitrate reductase in whole cultures, $NaNO_3$ is included in the culture medium at concentrations of 2 and 10 m*M* (*see* **Notes 19–21**).

1. Dispense the following reagents in the order shown into 13 × 100 mm test tubes: 3.7 mL of 0.1 *M* HCl, 100 µL of 0.2% sulfanilamide stock, 10–200 µL of the bacterial suspension. Add water to bring total reaction volume to 4 mL.
2. Read and record A_{530} of mixture to establish a turbidity correction for samples taken from older dense cultures.
3. Add 100 µL of 0.1% NEDD, vortex, allow color to develop for 15 min at room temperature and immediately read A_{530}.
4. Prepare a standard curve using 10–200 µL of the 250 µ*M* nitrite standard.
5. Calculate concentration in original cell suspension using the standard curve.

3.2.5. Assay of Adenosine Triphosphate (ATP) (16)

1. Transfer 1.0 mL of each culture to be assayed to a 1.5 mL microcentrifuge tube and spin in a microfuge in a biological safety hood at approx 10,000*g* for 5 min.
2. Remove and discard supernatant and spin again to drain further traces of medium from wall.
3. Add 1.0 mL of HBT buffer and resuspend the cells using a Pasteur pipet.
4. Dispense aliquots of up to 100 µL of the cell suspensions, or of the ATP standard into 13 × 100 mm disposable glass culture tubes and make up the volume to 100 µL with plain HEPES buffer.
5. Add 30 µL of chloroform and place the uncapped tubes in a preheated (80°C) heating block located in a vented hood such that the air flows in across the tubes (*see* **Note 22**). After exactly 20 min, wash down the sides of each tube with exactly 4.9 mL of plain HEPES buffer and vortex.
6. Mix 100 µL of sample or ATP standard and 50 µL of plain HEPES buffer in a standard Turner Luminometer tube and place in the luminometer.
7. Add 50 µL of the luciferin–luciferase reagent, and record the light unit reading.
8. Prepare a standard curve from light readings produced by known amounts of ATP, and record the results as either ng/mL of original culture, as ng/mL/unit of OD_{580}, or as ng/CFU.

3.2.6. Susceptibility to Antimicrobial Agents

Inasmuch as no replication of tubercle bacilli occurs under microaerophilic or anaerobic conditions, there is no point to trying to study bacteriostatic effects of drugs during NRP stages 1 and 2. Studies must be confined to a search for bactericidal effects.

3.2.6.1. Drugs Without Bacteriostatic Effects During Aerobic Growth (Nitroimidazole Drugs)

In the case of nitroimidazole drugs, such as metronidazole, no bacteriostatic effects are seen during the early aerobic stages of growth, i.e., before the bacilli enter NRP-1, so these drugs may be added at the time the cultures are inoculated and their bactericidal effects assessed after the bacilli have spent time in anaerobic NRP stage 2, when the redox potential has dropped low enough to permit activation of the drug.

1. Inoculate multiple 0.5 HSR tubes, with and without drug, to an initial calculated OD_{580} of 0.004 (*see* **Subheading 3.1.3.1.**).
2. Incubate on the magnetic stirrer for 72 h.
3. Remove individual sets of cultures, one drug-free and the other(s) containing different concentrations of drug or different drugs that are being screened for activity each day until the cultures have been in NRP stage 2 for 96 h, based on the final plateau deflection of the turbidity curve.

4. On each sampling day, remove aliquots for colony counting to determine death rate (*see* **Subheading 3.1.5.**). Discard the opened 0.5 HSR tubes once they have been exposed to oxygen. Use an unopened set of these tubes for each day's reading.

3.2.6.2. Drugs with Bacteriostatic Effects During Aerobic Growth

For drugs that are inhibitory to actively growing bacilli, it will be necessary to add them aseptically to 0.5 HSR cultures after they have entered NRP stages 1 and 2. Since there may be differences in responses by bacilli in each of these two stages, separate sets must be used for testing effect of drugs added to NRP stage 1 and NRP stage 2 cultures, respectively.

1. Inoculate multiple 0.5 HSR tubes to an initial calculated OD_{580} of 0.004 and seal with rubber vaccine caps (*see* **Subheading 3.1.3.1.**).
2. Incubate until in either NRP1 or NRP2 stage (*see* **Subheading 3.1.3.1.**).
3. Prepare a concentration of the drug to be added such that 100 μL contains the desired amount (larger volumes may introduce significant amounts of dissolved oxygen). Inject into tube using needle. Take care not to introduce bubbles of air when introducing the needle (*see* **Note 23**).
4. Sample, dilute, and plate according to the same protocol shown above for the nitroimidazole drugs.

4. Notes

1. Although no attempt has been made to assess the role of all of the ingredients of DTA broth in the hypoxic shiftdown, the effect of addition or deletion of some ingredients can be predicted. Medium containing glycerol should not be used for the standard hypoxic shiftdown model as it is known to greatly accelerate the depletion of oxygen in the medium; this may lead to death and autolysis of bacilli before they can adapt to the hypoxic shock ***(13)***. A detergent such as Tween-80 must be present to prevent clumping of bacilli. This is critical for three reasons, (1) to permit accurate reading of optical absorbance, (2) to minimize settling of large clumps, and (3) because the centers of large clumps may not have access to as much oxygen as the cells at the surface of the clump, which could lead to shiftdown of some members of the population of apparently well-aerated cultures. A consequence of this latter effect was suggested by the detection of traces of the URB-1 (putative α crystallin) protein in extracts of bacilli that had been grown on the surface of detergent-free medium ***(18)***. A disadvantage to the presence of Tween-80 is the need to supplement the medium with albumin to bind toxic traces of oleate that may be released from this detergent. This requires that the cells be well washed be remove the exogenous albumin if one is to assay cell protein as a basis for specific activity of enzymes. The consequence of change of any ingredient of the medium must be monitored in terms of their effects on growth dynamics and on appearance of markers of hypoxic shifts before they are incorporated into routine procedure.

2. Alternatively prepare from Dubos Broth Base (Difco) and Dubos Medium Albumin (Difco) as described by the manufacturers. The ingredients in the liquid medium should not be changed for arbitrary reasons of convenience, but only within the context of specific experimental designs. All liquid culture experiments are conducted in DTA broth.
3. The main use of solid medium in this system is for the counting of colonies or selection of clones. A number of different solid media might be acceptable for these purposes, but they should not contain any of the inhibitory substances that are sometimes advocated to suppress contaminants when the media are used for clinical diagnostic purposes. We routinely use Dubos oleic albumin agar, which may also be prepared from Dubos Oleic Agar Base (Difco) and Oleic Albumin Complex (Difco).
4. Although we can specify solutions we have found useful for harvesting and washing tubercle bacilli and their disruption for recovery of antigens and other stable products, the composition of solutions in which to disrupt the bacilli for assay and recovery of enzymes or nucleic acids will depend on the specific product of interest. Therefore only a few solutions will be described here.
5. Tritiated thymidine is not satisfactory for labeling DNA that is synthesized by tubercle bacilli, because it is hydrolyzed by thymidine phosphorylase ***(24)***. If the doubly labeled [5,6-^{3}H]uracil is used, allowance in calculating yields must be made for the loss of one of the tritiums as some of the uracil is methylated to thymine, so that the specific activity of product incorporated into DNA will be only half that of the product incorporated into RNA ***(16)***.
6. Both free glyoxylic acid and its sodium salt are hygroscopic and unstable. Store the solids in tightly capped containers at –20°C. Upon removing the container from the freezer, allow it to come to room temperature before opening to prevent condensation of moisture in the bottle.
7. We prefer to use *M. tuberculosis* for study of the hypoxic shiftdown model, because it is the pathogen of greatest concern in worldwide mycobacterial disease. For reasons of speed and/or safety, two other species have been substituted in similar studies. *M. smegmatis* has been selected for some studies because of its very short generation time and its lack of pathogenicity. However, this species is far removed on the phylogenetic scale from *M. tuberculosis*, and it exhibits only limited similarity in its responses to hypoxic stress. It does not exhibit the well-defined two-stage optical or viability curves seen with the tubercle bacillus ***(29)*** nor the cell wall thickening ***(17)*** nor the induction of the glyoxylate reductive aminase ***(30)*** associated with the hypoxic shiftdown; it does, however, exhibit anaerobic susceptibility to metronidazole and a synchronous shiftup pattern upon reinitiation of aeration. The avirulent BCG vaccine strain of *M. bovis* is phylogenetically very closely related to *M. tuberculosis* and does exhibit a well-defined two-stage shiftdown curve ***(31)***, as does the virulent Ravenel strain of *M. bovis* (Wayne, L.G., unpublished observations). *M. bovis* BCG also shares with *M. tuberculosis* the cell wall thickening ***(17)*** and the induction of the α crystallin protein ***(17,31)*** and glyoxylate reducing enzyme ***(16,31)*** during shiftdown to

microaerophilic NRP stage 1, the anaerobic susceptibility to metronidazole on entry into NRP stage 2 ***(16,31)*** and the synchronous replication associated with aerobic shiftup from NRP stage 2 ***(16,24,31)***. On the other hand, neither the virulent nor the avirulent strains of *M. bovis* exhibit the low grade NAR activity during aerobic growth, nor the strong NAR activity associated with NRP stage 1 that are characteristic of *M. tuberculosis* (Wayne, L.G., unpublished observations). The latter observation indicates that the NAR activity is not critical to hypoxic survival of tubercle bacilli, but suggests that it may be one of a set of alternative mechanisms for anaerobic generation of energy that help provide flexibility of adaptation to stress conditions. Whether other markers of shiftdown exist that distinguish between these two species remains to be seen, but we believe that BCG, although a useful adjunct to the study of the NRP state, must not be allowed to substitute too extensively for *M. tuberculosis* in the study of that phenomenon.

8. Under these conditions, the bacilli should exhibit logarithmic growth at a constant rate until OD_{580} exceeds 0.50, corresponding to about 3×10^8 CFU/mL ***(14)***; after this a slight progressive decline in growth rate may be seen, although continuing incubation will yield more than twice that cell density. However, caution must be applied in interpreting physiologic properties of cultures at these higher densities because some oxygen depletion may be occurring, even if not enough to cause shiftdown to the NRP state.
9. The reason for the growth repression of tubercle bacilli in DTA when flasks are subjected to rotary agitation remains unknown; vigorous magnetic stirring is, by contrast, stimulatory to growth. It has been speculated that the effect may be related to a tidal sweep of fluid under rotary agitation, with displacement of cells at the three phase liquid-glass-air interface, and loss of bacilli from the liquid phase ***(28)***. It has been reported that glycerol in the medium reverses the repressive action of rotary incubation ***(32)***, but glycerol should not be used in the hypoxic studies for reasons indicated in **Note 1**.
10. The headspace ratio (HSR) and the mode and speed of stirring of cultures specified here were arrived at after careful comparison of variations in these parameters and should not be changed except for very specific experimental reasons. When too high an HSR is used (i.e., too much air), a clear division between NRP stages 1 and 2 is not seen. If the HSR is too low, the time the culture spends in microaerophilic NRP stage 1 is markedly diminished. A magnetic stirrer must be used to keep the cells suspended without perturbing the surface. If the cultures are agitated too vigorously with significant agitation of the surface, such as occurs with a rotary shaker, the medium undergoes too rapid an equilibration with the headspace gas, accelerating the loss of oxygen. The consequence is an abrupt transition into the anaerobic stage, essentially bypassing the inductions of microaerophilic NRP stage 1 that are needed to protect the bacilli under anaerobic conditions ***(16)***. Different models of slow-speed magnetic stirrers (i.e., tissue culture stirrers) may be used for 0.5 HSR tubed cultures. We specify the Wheaton Biostir here because the design and 2×2 configuration of the magnetic impellers permits as many as three plastic racks, 25×10.5 cm each, holding 40 culture

tubes each, to be placed on the platform, and the magnetic bars in all 120 tubes will be agitated. Other slow-speed magnetic stirrers have not yielded as consistent distribution of rotary forces, and positions in the rack must be left empty. If it is necessary to use such a stirrer, it is essential to determine if such "blind spots" exist, and avoid them. Care should also be taken to ensure that the stirrer does not generate excess heat in the tubes, requiring some insulation of the bottoms of the racks.

11. The problem of maintaining a uniformly dispersed suspension of bacilli in a culture while controlling the rate at which dissolved oxygen is depleted is solved by using slowly and gently stirred medium in sealed containers with a known initial volumetric ratio of head space air to liquid culture medium (head space ratio). Experience has shown that an HSR of 0.5 is optimal for producing cultures with well-defined transitions between the NRP stages ***(16)***. After trials of different mixing modalities, we have established that magnetic stirring can be adjusted such that the bacilli remain in uniform suspension, but without any perturbation of the surface of the medium; these conditions are essential for providing consistent shiftdown patterns of the cultures.
12. Alternatively, a bottle containing enough media for the entire experiment may be inoculated to the same calculated initial OD_{580} and dispensed in 17 mL aliquots to the tubes.
13. Although we initially used septa in screw caps to seal tubes into which reagents were to be introduced ***(16)***, we later found that they were more likely to leak and allow air into the tubes as a vacuum developed during the incubation; tight fitting vaccine caps were less likely to cause this problem.
14. Production of reproducible limited HSR growth curves that exhibit clear transitions into the two NRP stages with optimal inductions associated with the shiftdown requires that equilibration between head space gas and dissolved oxygen proceed at a slow and consistent pace, i.e., without perturbation of the surface of the culture medium. For this reason it is best to work with tubed cultures, as described above (**Subheading 3.1.3.1.**). Even if larger volumes are required, it is often best to prepare multiple tubes and pool their contents for harvest of organisms at appropriate times. Nevertheless, there may be occasions when such large volumes are needed that flask cultures must be used.
15. Although tubed cultures may be handled briefly without disturbing the culture surface, the contents of flasks with their large surface area are much more easily disturbed on handling. The very act of tipping the culture from body of flask to the sidearm for the necessary optical readings modifies the equilibration rate between mediumhead space gas (*see* **Note 8**). This handling must be done as gently as possible. In some critical cases it may be best to use multiple tubes rather than single flasks for most consistent product; 25 0.5 HSR tubes will yield about 400 mL, the equivalent of one flask, and the cultures may be pooled for large scale harvest.
16. An initial mix and dilution of the NRP stage 2 cells is necessary to permit maximum aeration and ensure distribution of comparable suspensions to each of the

tubes for subsequent sampling. However, continuous agitation during the first cycle of aerobic shift up will lead to erratic results, whereas allowing the dilute suspensions to stand in air-saturated medium without further agitation permits demonstration of synchronous replication. This effect cannot be ascribed to sensitivity of the NRP bacilli to excess oxygen, since the first dilution medium is already saturated with air, and the inoculum is too small to lead to any significant depletion of dissolved oxygen over the first few replication cycles. It is possible that there is something resembling a quorum sensing effect associated with a product that is initially secreted into the micromilieu of each cell, and is washed away by the agitation.

17. Some colonies arise from intact cells and others from damaged/repaired cells, so all do not appear at the same rate. Colonies stabilize earlier from actively growing cultures than from old cultures in NRP stage 2. Counting of colonies must be continued for up to 6 wk, or until the number of countable colonies in a well have been constant for a week, or until all wells show apparently diminishing counts due to spreading and fusion of colonies. The number of colonies counted in wells yielding between 10 and 50 colonies are used to calculate CFU/mL of original culture.
18. The suspension should become fairly transparent, although opalescent, after 5 to 15 min of treatment. With adequate circulation of ice water the contents of the tube will remain cool enough that enzymes are not harmed, although the area of glass at the top of the tube that is above the cooling bath may become quite warm. It is important to use a round bottomed tube rather than a conical bottomed one for sonication to ensure efficient energy transfer to the suspension.
19. To get a good picture of the comparative dynamics of nitrate reduction in AG vs 0.5 HSR cultures, samples should be taken daily from the second through the eighth day of incubation from cultures inoculated to correspond to an initial OD_{580} of 0.004. The AG cultures should reduce nitrate at a steady rate that reflects the increase in OD_{580} of the culture itself and is substrate (nitrate) concentration dependent, but slower than the late 0.5 HSR cultures. The 0.5 HSR preparations should show an abrupt increase in rate of reduction of the nitrate substrate to nitrite as the culture enters NRP stage 1 at 72 h, and a plateau when nitrite concentration reaches about 2 m*M* (after the culture has been in NRP stage 1 for an additional 72 h), even if nitrate substrate well in excess of 2 m*M* was originally present.
20. The volume of suspension to be assayed may be adjusted directly or by sample dilution in order to bring the final reading within the range of the standard curve. A 100 μL aliquot of 250 μm sodium nitrite should always be run in a separate tube as positive standard.
21. To monitor nitrite production in AG cultures, repeated samples may be taken aseptically from the same culture tube. However, since opening the tube would alter the degree of aeration of the limited oxygen 0.5 HSR model, a separate culture must be used for each sample to be assayed.
22. This assay for ATP is based on the method of Dhople *(33)*, but modified in our laboratory after evaluation of factors affecting stability and reproducibility. The

depth of the 13 mm holes in the 80°C aluminum heating block should be 45 mm. If a block is used that has deeper holes, sand should be poured into the holes to permit the top 55 mm of the open glass reaction tubes to protrude into the air. This configuration permits the $CHCl_3$ to be evaporated out of the mixture, eliminating interference with the luciferase activity, while allowing water that evaporates from the warm mixture to condense and drip back, preventing the sample from drying out. Keeping the sample wet reduces variability in the assay. The final dilution of treated sample with 4.9 mL of plain buffer reduces the concentration of Tween-80, or any trace of $CHCl_3$ that might be carried over, either of which could interfere with the luciferase reaction in the next stage. The combination of heat and $CHCl_3$ treatment will kill the bacilli in the tubes.

23. When cultures enter the hypoxic stages, significant amounts of oxygen have been absorbed from the head space, and a partial vacuum is created in the tubes ***(16)***. If practical, it is best to break this vacuum by introducing sterile nitrogen gas into the tube through the vaccine cap after the culture has entered the desired NRP stage when prolonged further incubation is needed.

References

1. Communicable Disease Center. *The Arden House Conference on Tuberculosis*, Washington, DC, U.S. Dept. of Health, Education and Welfare, Public Health Service publication **7,** 1961.
2. Wayne, L. G. (1994) Dormancy of *Mycobacterium tuberculosis* and latency of disease. *Eur. J. Clin. Microbiol. Infect. Dis.* **13,** 908–914.
3. Palmer, C. E., Shaw, L. W., and Comstock, G. W. (1958) Community trials of BCG vaccination. *Am. Rev. Tuberc. Pulm. Dis.* **77,** 877–907.
4. Rieder, H. L., Cauthen, G. M., Comstock, G. W., and Snider, D. E. (1989) Epidemiology of tuberculosis in the United States. *Epidemiol. Rev.* **11,** 79–98.
5. Wayne, L. G. (1960) The bacteriology of resected tuberculous pulmonary lesions. II. Observations on bacilli which are stainable but which cannot be cultured. *Am. Rev. Respir. Dis.* **82,** 370–377.
6. Wayne, L. G. and Salkin, D. (1956) The bacteriology of resected tuberculous pulmonary lesions. I. The effect of interval between reversal of infectiousness and subsequent surgery. *Am. Rev. Tuberc. Pulm. Dis.* **74,** 376–387.
7. Sever, J. L. and Youmans, G. P. (1957) Enumeration of viable tubercle bacilli from the organs of nonimmunized and immunized mice. *Am. Rev. Tuberc. Pulm. Dis.* **76,** 616–635.
8. Orme, I. M. (1988) A mouse model of the recrudescence of latent tuberculosis in the elderly. *Am. Rev. Respir. Dis.* **137,** 716–718.
9. McCune, R. M., Tompsett, R., and McDermott, W. (1956) The fate of *Mycobacterium tuberculosis* in mouse tissues as determined by the microbial enumeration technique. II. The conversion of tuberculosis infection to the latent state by the administration of pyrazinamide and a companion drug. *J. Exp. Med.* **104,** 763–802.
10. McCune, R. M. and Tompsett, R. (1956) The fate of *Mycobacterium tuberculosis* in mouse tissues as determined by the microbial enumeration technique. I. The persis-

tence of drug-susceptible tubercle bacilli in the tissues despite prolonged antimicrobial therapy. *J. Exp. Med.* **104,** 737–762.

11. McCune, R., Lee, S. H., Deuschle, K., and McDermott, W. (1957) Ineffectiveness of isoniazid in modifying the phenomenon of microbial persistence. *Am. Rev. Tuberc. Pulm. Dis.* **76,** 1106–1109.
12. Grosset, J. (1978) The sterilizing value of rifampicin and pyrazinamide in experimental short-course chemotherapy. *Bull. Int. Union Against Tuberculosis.* **53,** 5–12.
13. Wayne, L. G. and Diaz, G. A. (1967) Autolysis and secondary growth of *Mycobacterium tuberculosis* in submerged culture. *J. Bacteriol.* **93,** 1374–1381.
14. Wayne, L. G. (1976) Dynamics of submerged growth of *Mycobacterium tuberculosis* under aerobic and microaerophilic conditions. *Am. Rev. Respir. Dis.* **114,** 807–811.
15. Wayne, L. G. and Lin, K.-Y. (1982) Glyoxylate metabolism and adaptation of *Mycobacterium tuberculosis* to survival under anaerobic conditions. *Infect. Immun.* **37,** 1042–1049.
16. Wayne, L. G. and Hayes, L. G. (1996) An in vitro model for the sequential study of shiftdown of *Mycobacterium tuberculosis* through two stages of nonreplicating persistence. *Infect. Immun.* **64,** 2062–2069.
17. Cunningham, A. F. and Spreadbury, C. L. (1998) Mycobacterial stationary phase induced by low oxygen tension: Cell wall thickening and localization of the 16-kilodalton α-crystallin homolog. *J. Bacteriol.* **180,** 801–808.
18. Wayne, L. G. and Sramek, H. A. (1979) Antigenic differences between extracts of actively replicating and synchronized resting cells of *Mycobacterium tuberculosis. Infect. Immun.* **24,** 363–370.
19. Yuan, Y., Crane, D. D., and Barry, C. E.,III (1996) Stationary phase-associated protein expression in *Mycobacterium tuberculosis*: Function of the mycobacterial α-crystallin homolog. *J. Bacteriol.* **178,** 4484–4492.
20. Yuan, Y., Crane, D. D., Simpson, R. M., et al. (1998) The 16-Da α-crystallin (Acr) protein of *Mycobacterium tuberculosis* is required for growth in macrophages. *Proc. Natl. Acad. Sci. USA* **95,** 9578–9583.
21. Wayne, L. G. and Hayes, L. G. (1998) Nitrate reduction as a marker for hypoxic shiftdown of *Mycobacterium tuberculosis. Tuberc. Lung. Dis.* **79,** 127–132.
22. Goldman, D. S. and Wagner, M. J. (1962) Enzyme systems in the mycobacteria. XIII. Glycine dehydrogenase and the glyoxylic acid cycle. *Biochim. Biophys. Acta* **65,** 297–306.
23. Wayne, L. G. and Sramek, H. A. (1994) Metronidazole is bactericidal to dormant cells of *Mycobacterium tuberculosis. Antimicrob. Agents Chemother.* **38,** 2054–2058.
24. Wayne, L. G. (1977) Synchronized replication of *Mycobacterium tuberculosis. Infect. Immun.* 17,528–17,530.
25. Segal, W. (1984) Growth dynamics of in vivo and in vitro grown mycobacterial pathogens, in *The Mycobacteria—A Sourcebook* (Kubica, G. P. and Wayne, L. G., eds.), Marcel Dekker, New York, pp. 547–573.

26. Wilkinson, R. J., Wilkinson, K. A., De Smet, K. A. L., et al. (1998) Human T- and B-cell reactivity to the 16 kDa α-crystallin protein of *Mycobacterium tuberculosis. Scand. J. Immunol.* **48,** 403–409.
27. Lee, B.-Y., Hefta, S. A., and Brennan, P. J. (1992) Characterization of the major membrane protein of virulent *Mycobacterium tuberculosis. Infect. Immun.* **60,** 2066–2074.
28. Wayne, L. G. (1994) Cultivation of *Mycobacterium tuberculosis* for research purposes, in *Tuberculosis — Pathogenesis, Protection, and Control* (Bloom, B. R., ed.), ASM Press, Washington, pp. 73–84.
29. Dick, T., Lee, B. H., and Murugasu-Oei, B. (1998) Oxygen depletion induced dormancy in *Mycobacterium smegmatis. FEMS Microbiol. Lett.* **163,** 159–164.
30. Hutter, B. and Dick, T. (1998) Increased alanine dehydrogenase activity during dormancy in *Mycobacterium smegmatis. FEMS Microbiol. Lett.* **167,** 7–11.
31. Lim, A., Eleuterio, M., Hutter, B., Murugasu-Oei, B., and Dick, T. (1999) Oxygen depletion-induced dormancy in *Mycobacterium bovis* BCG. *J. Bacteriol.* **181,** 2252–2256.
32. Lyon, R. H., Lichstein, H. C., and Hall, W. H. (1961) Factors affecting the growth of *Mycobacterium tuberculosis* in aerobic and shake culture. *Am. Rev. Respir. Dis.* **83,** 255–260.
33. Dhople, A. M. and Hanks, J. H. (1973) Quantitative extraction of adenosine triphosphate from cultivable and host-grown microbes: calculation of adenosine triphosphate pools. *Appl. Microbiol.* **26,** 399–403.

17

Macrophage Virulence Assays

Pauline T. Lukey and Elizabeth U. Hooker

1. Introduction

1.1. Immunopathology of Tuberculosis

Mycobacterium tuberculosis is a facultative intracellular pathogen, which can survive and replicate within the host macrophage. It is transmitted via the aerosol route, which delivers the bacillus to the alveolus of the lungs. The initial phase of granuloma formation within the lung requires that the bacterium is ingested by alveolar macrophages. Intracellular replication begins and an inflammatory reaction, involving recruitment of mononuclear leukocytes to the site, is initiated. The resultant accumulation of mononuclear leukocytes (monocytes, macrophages, and lymphocytes) is known as a granuloma. The growth of the mycobacteria at this stage in the infection is largely intracellular and acid fast bacilli can be visualized within the macrophages of the granuloma *(1)*.

As the immune response continues and the granuloma increases in size, the macrophages at the center begin to die, probably due to a combination of virulence factors from the mycobacteria and deprivation of oxygen and nutrients, forming a central area of caseous necrosis. The mycobacteria are seen to survive and replicate extracellularly, within the necrotic center of the granuloma. However, as the caseum solidifies, the bacteria begin to disappear — they can no longer be visualized by Ziehl-Neelsen staining, nor can they be cultured by conventional methods *(1)*.

It is at this stage that a crossroads is reached, and the granuloma can either resolve or liquefy. Resolution of the granuloma involves the deposition of fibrin and collagen, which enclose the granuloma and contain the infection. Alternatively, for reasons that are as yet unknown, the caseum liquefies, the bacteria reappear and exponential growth of the bacteria recommences. The liquefied granuloma may rupture into a bronchus whereupon the bacteria are released

From: *Methods in Molecular Medicine*, vol. 54: *Mycobacterium Tuberculosis Protocols*
Edited by: T. Parish and N. G. Stoker © Humana Press Inc., Totowa, NJ

into the airway. From there they can disseminate and reseed the lung of the same host or, if aerosolized, infect a new host *(1)*.

Thus, one can see that a key stage in the life cycle of *M. tuberculosis* is spent within the human macrophage. It is likely that the metabolic requirements of survival within this hostile environment cause the bacillus to adapt to these stresses by inducing the expression of genes involved in virulence. Therefore, in order to study the "virulence" phenotype of *M. tuberculosis*, an in vitro model is required that will mimic this stage in its life cycle. Furthermore, the development of novel antimycobacterials, which will be effective against the bacillus during its intracellular phase, requires a robust in vitro model to test such agents.

1.2. Macrophage Models

In vitro models of macrophage infection by *Mycobacterium* spp have been used to assay virulence *(2–8)* and the intracellular activity of antimycobacterials *(9–12)*. However, the details of the models used vary almost as much as the conclusions reached. The species used as a source of macrophages varies and includes humans *(5,6,9,12)*, mice *(2,3)*, and rabbits *(10,11)*. The strain of *M. tuberculosis* used to infect the macrophages is another source of variability, e.g., *M. tuberculosis* H37Ra, H37Rv *(7,9)*, Erdman *(12)*, and clinical isolates *(5,9)*. Species of mycobacteria other than *M. tuberculosis* have also been tested, e.g., *M. bovis* BCG *(7)* and *M. avium (8)*. Other sources of variability include the use of frozen or actively growing bacilli, the multiplicity of infection, the time allowed for phagocytosis to occur, and death of the macrophages during the culture period. That *M. tuberculosis* is cytotoxic for macrophages is known *(3,10)*, the extent of the toxicity depends on all of the variables cited above. The result of macrophage cytotoxicity is that those macrophages that are most heavily infected die rapidly and become nonadherent. Therefore, it is essential that the contribution of dead nonadherent macrophages containing viable bacilli is included in the assay. However, detailed examination of the different methodologies reveals that these nonadherent, dead macrophages are sometimes discarded (e.g., *5*) and in some experiments they are included (e.g., *6*). Disregarding these nonadherent dead macrophages results in an underestimate of the total number of colony forming units of mycobacteria in these particular experiments.

Despite all of these discrepancies, the consensus is that *M. tuberculosis* can replicate by between two and three logs within macrophages over a period of 7–10 d in vitro *(2,4–6)* and that some antimycobacterials kill the intracellular mycobacteria, most notably rifampicin *(9)*. The confusion arises when comparisons are made between different strains in the different models. Paul et al. *(4)* concluded that *M. tuberculosis* H37Ra and H37Rv grow equally well within human macrophages, but that H37Ra grows less well than H37Rv in mouse macrophages. In contrast, Silver et al. ***(6)*** concluded that H37Rv increased by two logs in human monocytes and bronchoalveolar lavage macrophages but that H37Ra did not replicate at all in these macrophages. These discrepancies may be explained by certain methodological differences, e.g., Paul et al. ***(4)*** used actively growing *M. tuberculosis* H37Ra and H37Rv, whereas Silver et al. ***(6)*** used the same strains freshly thawed from the –70°C. In addition, Silver et al. ***(6)*** incorporated the dead nonadherent macrophages whereas Paul et al. ***(4)*** claim that no macrophage death is seen over a 6 d culture period, though it is not clear if dead macrophages are included at later time points.

In conclusion, one can understand the need for an in-depth understanding of the limitations of any model used to mimic a complex in vivo situation and an attempt must be made to minimize any potential sources of artefacts. The present authors feel that the following considerations should contribute to the validity of the model:

1. Human macrophages are a more relevant source of host cells than mice or rabbits.
2. Actively growing mycobacteria appear more virulent than those freshly thawed from storage at –80°C, even though the colony forming ability is not affected.
3. For long-term intracellular growth experiments, low multiplicities of infection that result in only very few macrophages being infected initially are preferable.
4. Viable mycobacteria can be obtained from heavily infected dead, nonadherent macrophages and these need to be included in the assay, especially at later time points.
5. *M. tuberculosis* H37Rv that has been growing in Middlebrook 7H9 supplemented with albumin-dextrose complex supplement (ADC) and Tween-80 will not grow in tissue culture medium containing serum over the assay period of 10 d — in fact, a decrease in colony forming units (CFU) is obtained.

Thus, we propose the following methodology, which should minimize the potential sources of variability seen in the literature. The in vitro macrophage model described is used to study intracellular replication of *M. tuberculosis* using colony forming units as readout. Two sources of macrophages are described, monocyte-derived macrophages (MDM) and the macrophage-like cells derived from a THP1 cell line ***(13)***. MDM have the advantage in that they are normal human macrophages (phagocytic, MHC class II positive) and should reflect the in vivo situation better than a cell line. However, an element of variability exists in using MDM, as each individual donor is different and very little additional information is available from the blood bank. Furthermore, the amount of blood available from an individual is limited and therefore the number of macrophages available for each experiment is also limited. THP1, on the other hand, can be expanded to reach vast numbers of cells and are more reproducible. The disadvantage is that they are not normal macrophages, they are aneuploid and may also express few MHC class II molecules on their surface. However, they are phagocytic and express the CR3 receptor, which is important for entry of *M. tuberculosis*. So, the choice of which source of macrophages to use depends largely on the type of experiment to be performed and the questions to be asked.

2. Materials

2.1. Human Macrophage Preparation

Two sources of human macrophages are described, that is, MDM and the human macrophage-like cell line THP1. Remember to work in a class II safety cabinet and use sterile technique for the tissue culture work.

1. Buffy coat from the blood bank (Colindale, UK) or THP1 cell line, American Type Culture (ATCC) number TIB 202 (ATCC, Rockville, MD).
2. Dulbecco's minimal essential medium with glutamine (DMEM) (Gibco-BRL, Paisley, UK).
3. Dulbecco's PBS (D-PBS) (Gibco-BRL).
4. Tissue culture flasks (75 cm^2 surface area) with vented caps.
5. Tissue culture flasks (225 cm^2 surface area) with vented caps.
6. Conical sterile 50 mL centrifuge tubes with screw caps.
7. Fetal calf serum (FCS).
8. Ficoll hypaque (Lymphoprep, Amersham Pharmacia Biotech, Little Chalfont, Bucks, UK).
9. Hemocytometer.
10. Inverted microscope.
11. Bench top centrifuge with swing buckets.
12. Phorbol ester (phorbol 12-myristate 13-acetate [PMA], Sigma). Only required for THP1 cell preparation. Make a stock solution of 1 mg/mL in DMSO. Aliquot and store at –20°C. **Caution:** Phorbol esters are tumor promoters; therefore, wear double gloves, work on a labmat, and neutralize all contaminated plastic in 10% bleach overnight prior to disposal.
13. Tissue culture plates with 24-wells (Falcon, Becton Dickinson, Cowley, Oxford).
14. 37°C, 5% CO_2, 95% humidity incubator.
15. Disposable plastic pipets and pipet aid.
16. Sodium dodecyl sulfate (SDS) solutions — 0.25% SDS and 0.025% SDS solutions in water.

3. Methods

3.1. Macrophage Preparation

3.1.1. Monocyte-Derived Macrophages

1. Make the buffy coat up to 100 mL with D-PBS in a 250 mL tissue culture flask (*see* **Note 1**).

2. Add 10 mL of lymphoprep to each of 4 × 50 mL centrifuge tubes.
3. Layer 25 mL of diluted buffy coat onto the lymphoprep (*see* **Note 2**).
4. Centrifuge at 400*g* for 30 min at room temperature with the brake OFF.
5. Remove the plasma only and retain separately for later use (*see* **Note 3**).
6. Remove the mononuclear leukocytes (MNL) without any red blood cell contamination (*see* **Note 4**).
7. Place the MNL layer from each gradient (approx 10 mL) into a clean 50 mL centrifuge tube.
8. Make up to 50 mL with D-PBS.
9. Centrifuge at 100*g* for 10 min (*see* **Note 5**).
10. Pour off the supernatant (*see* **Note 6**).
11. Resuspend the pellets by flicking the tube, pool, and make up to 50 mL with D-PBS.
12. Repeat **steps 9** and **10** twice more to ensure that all platelets have been removed by differential centrifugation.
13. Resuspend the pellet in 25 mL of DMEM without serum.
14. Count the number of cells using a hemocytometer (*see* **Note 7**).
15. Make the cells up to 5×10^6/mL in DMEM without serum (*see* **Note 8**).
16. Add 1 mL of cell suspension to each well of a 24-well plate.
17. Incubate in a CO_2 incubator for 30 min (*see* **Note 9**).
18. Remove the nonadherent lymphocytes (*see* **Note 10**) by adding 1 mL of D-PBS, pipeting up and down three times and removing any residual nonadherent cells.
19. Repeat **step 18** again.
20. Add 1 mL of DMEM with 10% autologous plasma (*see* **Note 11**).
21. Incubate the adherent cells in the 24-well plates in a CO_2 incubator for 7 d (*see* **Note 12**).
22. Remove any residual nonadherent cells again as in **steps 17** and **18**.
23. Add fresh medium (DMEM with 10% autologous plasma).
24. The macrophages are now ready for infection.

3.1.2. Preparation of THP1 Cell Line

The THP1 cell line requires propagation using standard tissue culture techniques of splitting and feeding. It is suggested that regular (every 6 mo) mycoplasma screening is carried out, as mycoplasma contamination can severely affect the reliability of this cell line and that passage number should be limited to 30.

1. On a Friday, add 5×10^6 THP1s (*see* **Note 7**) to 50 mL of DMEM with 10% FCS (*see* **Note 13**) in a 225 cm^2 flask.
2. Incubate the flask standing upright in a CO_2 incubator at 37°C for 3 d.
3. On the following Monday lie the flask down and incubate for a further 2 d (*see* **Note 14**).
4. On the following Wednesday, add 50 mL of fresh DMEM 10% FCS to the cells.
5. Incubate for a further 2 d.

6. On the following Friday, harvest the cells by gently tapping the flask to remove loosely adherent THP1s and recovering the 100 mL of medium containing the cells.
7. Pellet the cells at 200*g* for 10 min.
8. Discard the supernatant.
9. Resuspend the cell pellet (by flicking the tube) in 25 mL of fresh DMEM 10% FCS and count the cells (*see* **Note 7**).
10. Make the cells up to 5×10^5/mL in DMEM-10% FCS (*see* **Note 15**).
11. Add PMA to a final concentration of 5 ng/mL (*see* **Note 16**).
12. Add 1 mL of cell suspension (containing PMA) to each well of 24-well plates.
13. Incubate for 3 d in the CO_2 incubator (*see* **Note 17**).
14. Remove any residual nonadherent THP1s and PMA by washing with D-PBS as described for the MDM (**Subheading 3.1.2., steps 18** and **19**).
15. Add 1 mL of fresh DMEM-10% FCS to each well.
16. The macrophages are now ready for infection.

3.1.3. Infection of Macrophages

The macrophages are to be infected with a late log phase culture of *Mycobacterium tuberculosis* in Middlebrook 7H10 plus ADC and Tween-80. The passage number should be less than 5 and the OD_{550} should be in the region of 0.6–0.8 (*see* **Note 18**).

1. Transfer the macrophages to the ACDP3 laboratory and work in a class I/III safety cabinet (*see* **Note 19**).
2. Pellet 1 mL of late log phase culture of *M. tuberculosis* H37Rv at 2000*g* for 20 min (or 8000*g* for 5 min).
3. Discard supernatant.
4. Allow to stand for 10 min to allow aerosols to settle.
5. Resuspend pellet in 1 mL DMEM-10% FCS (for THP1 infection) or DMEM-10% autologous plasma (for MDM infection).
6. Dilute the bacteria 1:10 in the relevant tissue culture medium.
7. Add 100 μL of this to each well of the 24-well plate (*see* **Note 20**). Triplicate wells should be infected for each time point, e.g., for three time points infect nine wells.
8. Incubate the macrophages overnight at 37°C, 5% CO_2, and 95% humidity to allow phagocytosis to occur.
9. Plate serial dilutions of the bacterial suspension in order to determine an accurate bacterial count (*see* **Note 21**).
10. Remove nonphagocytosed mycobacteria and wash the macrophages three times with 1 mL of D-PBS. Amikacin has been used in some experiments to remove extracelluar mycobacteria ***(14)***; however, we feel that this adds unnecessary complications (*see* **Note 22**).
11. Add 1 mL of fresh tissue culture medium to each well.
12. The cells are now ready for intracellular growth to be determined.

3.1.4. Harvesting of Intracellular Mycobacterium tuberculosis

1. Remove the medium from triplicate wells and add to separate 15 mL centrifuge tubes marked A, B, and C each containing 100 µL of 0.25% SDS (*see* **Note 23**).
2. Add 1 mL of 0.025% SDS to each of the wells to lyse the adherent macrophages (*see* **Note 24**).
3. Remove the dissolved macrophages and combine them with the lysed nonadherent macrophages from their respective wells.
4. Wash the wells three times with 0.025% SDS and add to respective tubes (total volume of 5 mL).
5. Pellet the mycobacteria at 2000*g* for 20 min.
6. Discard supernatant.
7. Allow to stand for 10 min to allow aerosols to settle.
8. Resuspend the pellet in 1 mL MADCTW by gently flicking the sealed tube.
9. Plate serial dilutions to determine CFUs (*see* **Note 21**).
10. Place the rest of the macrophages back in the incubator.
11. These steps can be repeated at d 4 and 7 after the initial infection (*see* **Note 25**).

4. Notes

1. The buffy coat consists of concentrated white blood cells and platelets from 500 mL of donor blood. The volume is generally about 50 mL.
2. Use a 10 mL pipet and pipet aid. Hold the tube in one hand and tilt it slightly toward the pipet containing 10 mL of buffy coat. Touch the tip of the pipet onto the surface of the lymphoprep and withdraw the pipet up the side of the tube while gently and slowly dispensing the blood. Ensure that the blood forms a layer on the surface of the lymphoprep and does not mix with the lymphoprep.
3. After centrifugation the blood will separate into several layers. The bottom, most dense layer will be the red blood cells. Polymorphonuclear leukocytes (PMNL) will form a fuzzy layer directly on top of the red blood cells. The lymphoprep will form a clear layer on top of the PMNL. The MNL and the platelets will form a layer on top of the lymphoprep. The top, least dense layer will be the plasma, which has a yellow color.
4. MNL include lymphocytes and monocytes. Approximately 90% of the MNL are lymphocytes and 10% are monocytes.
5. Centrifugation at 100*g* is to separate the platelets from the MNL. The MNL will form a loose pellet whereas the platelets will largely remain in the supernatant.
6. The supernatant will appear cloudy because of the platelets but a visible pellet of MNL should be apparent.
7. The use of a hemocytometer is well described in the Sigma catalog. The procedure is as follows: place the coverslip on the hemocytometer and apply an aliquot of the cell suspension (approx 10 µL) by capillary action. Place the hemocytometer under the microscope and a grid will be seen over which the cells are distributed. The grid pattern is a 3 × 3 block pattern, i.e., nine blocks are visible (each of these large blocks is subdivided to aid counting). Count the number of cells in the

top left-hand square and the number in the bottom right-hand square. Determine the average and multiply by 10^4 to get number of cells/mL, e.g., number of cells in top left-hand square: 105; number of cells in bottom right-hand square: 112; average: 108×10^4 cells/mL (1.08×10^6 cells/mL). It may be necessary to dilute the sample if the cell number is too great. This must be incorporated into the calculation of the cell number, e.g., average × dilution factor × 10^4/mL.

8. On average approx 10^6 MNL should be obtained from 1 mL of human blood. In theory, approx 5×10^8 MNL should be obtained from a buffy coat of 500 mL blood and these should be resuspended in 100 mL to obtain 5×10^6 MNL/mL. In practice, the expected yield would be $2–3 \times 10^8$ MNL. As only 10% of MNL are monocytes, this translates into approx 3×10^7 monocytes from 500 mL blood.
9. This allows the monocytes to adhere to the tissue culture plastic.
10. The monocytes adhere very tightly to the plastic, so you can be quite robust with your pipeting. Use a 10 mL pipet and resuspend each mL of medium up and down three times before removing the medium.
11. The plasma removed from the top of the gradient is effectively 50% already, as it was diluted with D-PBS; so dilute it 1:5 with DMEM to get a 10% autologous plasma solution. If the plasma is cloudy, it may be contaminated with platelets. In this case, spin the plasma to pellet the platelets (500*g* 10 min) and filter through a 0.2 μm filter. Note that plasma cannot be interchanged between different donors because of incompatibility. If insufficient plasma is retrieved from the gradients it will be necessary to use human AB serum from male donors (available from Sigma). This latter option can be a problem due to variability between batches.
12. During the 7 d of adherence, the monocytes differentiate into macrophages.
13. The fetal calf serum must be heat inactivated at 56°C for 30 min. This is to inactivate complement and prevent it from lysing the cells. This can be performed in advance and the serum stored frozen at –20°C until used.
14. This increases the surface area and allows the cells to continue to replicate. Note that THP1 cells grow in suspension or are loosely adherent. A gentle tap will dislodge them.
15. This procedure should yield approx 10^8 THP1 cells/225 cm^2 flask. Therefore, you would need about 1.5 L of blood to obtain this number of monocytes.
16. PMA triggers the differentiation of THP1s into a macrophage-like morphology by directly activating protein kinase C. They become adherent and phagocytic and stop dividing. Remember that PMA is a tumor promoter and must be handled as described in **Subheading 2.**
17. This incubation period allows the cells time to differentiate into a macrophage-like phenotype.
18. Some workers use a stock of *M. tuberculosis*, frozen at –80°C and thawed prior to infecting the macrophages ***(6,12)***. However, we have found that this results in a lag phase where the bacteria adapt to 37°C, allowing the macrophages to gain some advantage. If an actively growing culture is used, no lag phase is observed and growth of the bacteria commences almost immediately.

19. All the subsequent steps should be performed in the ACDP3 suite, adhering to the local rules for working with *M. tuberculosis*.
20. This is a final dilution of the bacteria of 1:100. Approximately 5×10^5 macrophages are in each well, and a 1:100 dilution of a late log culture of *M. tuberculosis* should contain approx 10^7 CFU/mL. Therefore, we are adding 10^5 CFU/well, with a multiplicity of infection (MOI) of 1 bacterium/5 macrophages.
21. It is quite convenient to perform the serial dilutions in a 96-well microtiter plate. The starting culture (250 µL/well) is added to the first well of a row in triplicate. 225 µL of MADCTW is added to each subsequent well. Serial 1:10 dilutions are performed by transferring 25 µL from the first well into the next well and so on down the row. Remember to discard tips between each well. The highest dilution required is 10^{-5}. Aliquots of 50 µL plated onto 7H10 agar plates (plus OADC, Difco) in triplicate. After the spot has dried the wrap plates in foil, invert, incubate at 37°C for 3 wk and count the colonies.
22. This is to ensure that only intracellular mycobacteria are left in the well. In some cases amikacin can be added to specifically kill extracellular mycobacteria, as this antibiotic is reportedly unable to penetrate macrophages. This should be performed at 200 µg/mL for 1 h, followed by three wash steps. However, we have performed electron microscopy and confocal microscopy, which has convinced us that three washes are sufficient to remove extracellular mycobacteria for most purposes without the complication of adding antibiotics.
23. This step is not so important for the day 1 time point. However, as the infection progresses, macrophages will die and detach from the tissue culture plastic. These macrophages will contain live bacilli which must be incorporated into the calculation of the intracellular growth. The addition of SDS to the dead/dying nonadherent macrophages will lyse them and release the bacteria.
24. This can be monitored microscopically until all the macrophages have lysed. These low concentrations of SDS have no apparent effect on CFUs.
25. If longer time points are required it will be necessary to reduce the starting multiplicity of infection. At the MOI used in this example (approx 1 mycobacterium: 5 macrophages) all the macrophages will be dead by the end of the experiment (7 d after infection) and no further growth will be seen (*M. tuberculosis* will not grow in DMEM with serum, under the conditions described). Therefore, for a day 10 time point, a starting MOI of 1 mycobacterium to 50 macrophages will be required.

References

1. Canetti, G. (1955) *The Tubercle Bacillus in the Pulmonary Lesion of Man: Histobacteriology and its Bearing on the Therapy of Pulmonary Tuberculosis.* Springer Publishing Company, New York, NY.
2. Berthet, F. X., Lagranderie, M., Gounon, P., Laurentwinter, C., Ensergueix, D., Chavarot, P., Thouron, F., Maranghi, E., Pelicic, V., Portnoi, D., Marchal, G., and Gicquel, B. (1998) Attenuation of virulence by disruption of the *Mycobacterium tuberculosis erp* gene. *Science* **282,** 759–762.

3. McDonough, K. A. and Kress, Y. (1995) Cytotoxicity for lung epithelial cells is a virulence-associated phenotype of *Mycobacterium tuberculosis*. *Infect. Immun.* **63,** 4802–4811.
4. Paul, S., Laochumroonvorapong, P., and Kaplan, G. (1996) Comparable growth of virulent and avirulent *Mycobacterium tuberculosis* in human macrophages in vitro. *J. Infect. Dis.* **174,** 105–112.
5. Zhang, M., Gong, J. H., Lin, Y. G., and Barnes, P. F. (1998) Growth of virulent and avirulent *Mycobacterium tuberculosis* strains in human macrophages. *Infect. Immun.* **66,** 794–799.
6. Silver, R. F., Li, Q., and Ellner, J. J. (1998) Expression of virulence of *Mycobacterium tuberculosis* within human monocytes–virulence correlates with intracellular growth and induction of tumor necrosis factor alpha but not with evasion of lymphocyte-dependent monocyte effector functions. *Infect. Immun.* **66,** 1190–1199.
7. Bange, F. C., Brown, A. M., and Jacobs, W. R., Jr. (1996) Leucine auxotrophy restricts growth of *Mycobacterium bovis* BCG in macrophages. *Infect. Immun.* **64,** 1794–1799.
8. Bermudez, L. E., Parker, A., and Goodman, J. R. (1997) Growth within macrophages increases the efficiency of *Mycobacterium avium* in invading other macrophages by a complement receptor-independent pathway. *Infect. Immun.* **65,** 1916–1925.
9. Rastogi, N., Labrousse, V., and Goh, K. S. (1996) In vitro activities of fourteen antimicrobial agents against drug susceptible and resistant clinical isolates of *Mycobacterium tuberculosis* and comparative intracellular activities against the virulent H37Rv strain in human macrophages. *Curr. Microbiol.* . **33,** 167–175.
10. Mackaness, G. B. (1952) The action of drugs on intracellular tubercle bacilli. *J. Pathol. Bacteriol.* **64,** 429–446.
11. Mackaness, G. B. and Smith, N. (1952) The action of isoniazid (isonicotinic acid hydrazide) in intracellular tubercle bacilli. *Am. Rev. Tuberc.* **66,** 125–133.
12. Crowle, A. J., Sbarbaro, J. A., and May, M. H. (1988) Effects of isoniazid and of ceforanide against virulent tubercle bacilli in cultured human macrophages. *Tubercle* **69,** 15–25.
13. Auwerx, J. (1991) The human leukemia cell line, THP-1: a multifacetted model for the study of monocyte-macrophage differentiation. *Experientia* **47,** 22–31.
14. Fischer, L. J., Quinn, F. D., White, E. H., and King, C. H. (1996) Intracellular growth and cytotoxicity of *Mycobacterium haemophilum* in a human epithelial cell line (HEC-1-b). *Infect. Immunol.* **64,** 269–276.

18

Analysis of *Mycobacterium*-Infected Macrophages by Immunoelectron Microscopy and Cell Fractionation

Wandy Beatty and David G. Russell

1. Introduction

The ability of pathogenic *Mycobacterium* to establish and maintain an infection in a host is dependent on their capacity to survive within phagocytes *(1–3)*. Studies conducted on macrophage infections in culture have provided considerable insight into the mechanisms developed by these bacteria to ensure their survival. However, macrophages in culture are considerably more permissive than the phagocyte in its correct tissue environment and one has to be aware that the capacity of the macrophage to function as both an antigen-presenting cell (inducing or sustaining a cellular immune response) and an immune effector cell (mediating an antimicrobial response following activation with cytokines) places certain provisos on interpretation of in vitro infection experiments *(4,5)*. Despite this obvious caveat, our appreciation of the complex interplay between *Mycobacterium* spp. of varying degrees of virulence [*M. tuberculosis*, *M. bovis* (BCG) and *M. avium*] and their host macrophage has benefited considerably from the recent application of modern cell biological techniques to studies of infected cells in culture.

The techniques described in this chapter reflect the combination of structural, *in situ* analysis with biochemical characterization of isolated cellular fractions. In our view, it is important that both these avenues are pursued in parallel because they are complementary and provide important "checks and balances" for each other. Immunoelectron microscopy is an outstanding method for fine structural localization of molecules for which you have adequate antibodies and provides an invaluable indication of the heterogeneity of any given vacuole

From: *Methods in Molecular Medicine*, vol. 54: *Mycobacterium Tuberculosis Protocols*
Edited by: T. Parish and N. G. Stoker © Humana Press Inc., Totowa, NJ

population. However, it is limited in two important areas: the sample size is finite and only known molecules can be detected. In contrast, cell fractionation, isolation, and characterization of *Mycobacterium*-containing vacuoles provides a "true" average of vacuolar contents; it can provide information about novel molecules and is a more amenable method of quantifying vacuolar constituents. The drawbacks are the controls that need to be conducted to determine the purity of the vacuolar preparation. These can be quite complex depending on the possible source of any contaminant.

The final method described, density gradient electrophoresis, was developed in its current form by Pieters and colleagues ***(6)*** for analysis of endosomal/lysosomal differentiation and major histocompatibility antigens (MHC) class II molecule maturation. We have been using it for the isolation of membranous vesicles from infected macrophages to allow us to study the nature of trafficking pathways followed by *Mycobacterium*-derived molecules released by the intracellular bacilli. This technique has proven particularly useful for following bacterial cell wall lipids.

2. Materials

All the following protocols are optimized for murine bone-marrow macrophages, which are used in preference to macrophage-like cell lines because they preserve more of the characteristics of tissue-derived macrophages (*see* **Note 1**).

2.1. Immunoelectron Microscopy Materials (modified from ref. 7)

1. Infected macrophages (*see* **Note 1**).
2. PIPES/Mg buffer: 200 m*M* PIPES, 0.5 m*M* $MgCl_2$, pH 7.0.
3. Fixative: 4% paraformaldehyde in PIPES/Mg buffer, boil on a heated stir plate until dissolved, cool on ice, and filter through a 0.4 µm pore filter-sterilizing unit. Store the fixative at 4°C for up to 5 d.
4. 10% gelatin: dissolve gelatin (225 bloom from calf skin; Aldrich, St. Louis, MO) in hot PIPES/Mg buffer. Dispense into 500 µL aliquots and store at –20°C.
5. Polyvinyl pyrrolidone (PVP)/sucrose solution: 1.86 *M* sucrose, 20% PVP in PIPES/Mg buffer. To prepare, add 63.67 g of sucrose to 20 mL of 1 *M* PIPES, 2.5 m*M* $MgCl_2$, pH 7.0. Make the volume up to 80 mL with water and heat the solution until the sucrose is dissolved. Place 20 g of PVP in a 150 mL glass beaker, add approx 5 mL of the sucrose solution and mix into a paste with a glass rod. Add the sucrose solution gradually until a smooth mixture is achieved. Increase the volume to 100 mL, cover the mixture with Parafilm, and stir overnight. This facilitates removal of all the air bubbles. Dispense the clear, yellow PVP/sucrose solution into 1 mL aliquots and store at –20°C.
6. Block buffer: 5% fetal calf serum, 5% goat serum in PIPES/Mg buffer. Filter prior to use.

7. 2.3 *M* sucrose in 200 m*M* PIPES, 0.5 m*M* $MgCl_2$, pH 7.0.
8. Primary and secondary antibody (*see* **Note 2**).
9. Stain: 2% PVA, 0.3% uranyl acetate in water.
10. Aluminum stud.
11. Research and Manufacturing Company MT7/CR21 cryoultramicrotome (Tucson, AR).
12. 1 mm diameter wire loops.
13. Formvar-carbon coated grids (Electron Microscopy Sciences, Philadelphia, PA).
14. 24-well plates.
15. Terasaki plate.

2.2. Phagosome Isolation Materials (modified from ref. 8)

1. Homogenization buffer (1X): 250 m*M* (8.6% w/v) sucrose, 0.5 m*M* ethylene glycol tetraacetic acid (EGTA), 0.5 m*M* EDTA, 0.05% w/v gelatin (teleost gelatin, Sigma, St. Louis, MO), 20 m*M* HEPES, pH 6.8. Prepare as a 5X working strength stock solution to facilitate easier preparation of Ficoll and sucrose solutions.
2. 50% and 12% w/v sucrose solutions in homogenization buffer. Prepare by dissolving 50 g (or 12 g) of sucrose in 20 mL of 5X homogenization buffer and make up to 100 mL with H_2O.
3. Discontinuous sucrose gradient: layer 2 mL of 12% sucrose (in homogenization buffer) over 2 mL of 50% sucrose (in homogenization buffer) in a siliconized 15 mL centrifuge tube.
4. Protease inhibitors. Store each of the following as 100X stock solutions at –20°C: tosylamide phenylethyl chloromethylketone (TLCK) 10 mg/mL, pepstatin A 5 mg/mL, leupeptin 5 mg/mL, and E64 5 mg/mL. Add to the homogenization buffer prior to use; the final concentrations are TLCK 100 µg/mL, pepstatin A 50 µg/mL, leupeptin 50 µg/mL, and E64 50 µg/mL.
5. Ficoll solution: 10% low molecular weight Ficoll (70,000 kDa) in homogenization buffer.
6. Cell scrapers (Sarstedt, Newton, NC).
7. Plasticware, all polyproplylene (Sarstedt): 50 mL conical screw cap centrifuge tubes, 15 mL conical screw cap centrifuge tubes,1.5 mL screw cap microfuge tubes. Siliconize all plasticware by rinsing with Sigmacote (Sigma) and drying.
8. Custom-made floating ballbearing homogenizer with Luer lock syringe attachments
9. 47-mm 5-µm pore Nucleopore filter (Millipore, Bedford, MA).

2.3. Density Gradient Electrophoresis Materials (Modified from ref. 9)

2.3.1. Density Gradient Electrophoresis

1. Source of infected macrophages (*see* **Note 1**).
2. Phosphate-buffered saline (PBS): 136 m*M* NaCl, 2.5 m*M* KCl, 10 m*M* Na_2HPO_4, 1.8 m*M* KH_2PO_4, pH 7.0.

3. Homogenization buffer (*see* **Subheading 2.2., item 1**).
4. Cell scrapers.
5. Custom-made floating ballbearing homogenizer with Luer lock syringe attachments.
6. Ultracentrifuge.
7. Gradient apparatus.
8. Step gradient solutions: prepare 12% sucrose and 30% sucrose solutions in homogenization buffer.
9. Density gradient electrophoresis (DGE) buffer: 250 m*M* sucrose, 1 m*M* ethylenediaminetetracetic acid (EDTA), 0.5 m*M* EGTA, 10 m*M* triethanolamine, pH to 7.4 with acetic acid.
10. Dialysis membrane: 6–8000 molecular weight cutoff.
11. Ficoll solutions: make up 12% (10 mL per gradient), 10% (200 mL per gradient) and 8% (6 mL per gradient) Ficoll (70,000 kDa) solutions in DGE buffer.
12. Tuberculin syringes: 1 mL, 25-gage needle.
13. 70 µm mesh nylon bolt cloth (Becton Dickinson, Franklin Lakes, NJ).

2.3.2. Enzyme Assays for Verification of Cellular Fractions (Modified from **ref. 10**)

1. 4-Methylumbelliferyl-2-acetamido-2-deoxy-β-D-glucopyranoside (Sigma): 4 m*M* in dH_2O.
2. 0.4 *M* sodium acetate, pH 4.4.
3. 10% Triton X-100.
4. 96-well plates.
5. Stop solution: 1 *M* glycine, 1 *M* Na_2CO_3.
6. 4-Methylumbelliferyl-α-D-mannopyranoside (Sigma): 4 m*M* in dH_2O.
7. PBS (*see* **Subheading 2.3.1., item 2**).
8. Na-thymidine 5'-monophosphate, p-nitrophenylester (Sigma): 10 m*M* in dH_2O.
9. 0.1 *M* Tris-HCl, pH 9.0.

3. Methods

3.1. Immunoelectron Microscopy Methods

The following section describes the mechanics of immunoelectron microscopy but does not mention which antibodies are used; this is discussed in **Note 2** and in the pertinent references. Infected cultures of bone marrow-derived macrophages (BMMO) in T25 tissue culture flasks are processed as follows:

1. Fix cells with 5 mL of cold fixative in the flask.
2. Leave on a rocking table for 30 min (this is better kept cold if possible).
3. Pour off the medium, add 1 mL of fresh fixative, then **gently** scrape the cells free from the flask and transfer to a 1.5 mL microfuge tube.
4. Leave for a further 30 min on the rocking table.
5. Pellet the cells by centrifugation at 1000*g* for 5–10 s.

6. Wash the cells in the PIPES/mg buffer, pellet again, and remove all the buffer.
7. Keep the cells at room temperature. Resuspend the cell pellet in 50 μL of warm 10% gelatin and quickly centrifuge the cells at 2000*g* to pellet them before the gelatin sets.
8. Place the gelatin pellets on ice for 10 min to set the gelatin.
9. Cut the tip off the tube with a razor blade, and place directly in 1 mL fixative for 15 min.
10. Remove the gelatin-containing tip and place in 1 mL of 20% polyvinylpyrrolidone/sucrose solution.
11. Leave the tube on a rocking table overnight at 4°C or for 1–2 h at room temperature.
12. Gently remove the gelatin tip from the tube, trim the block with a razor blade, and place on the roughened tip of an aluminum stud.
13. Freeze by plunging directly into liquid nitrogen. The block can then be cut or stored in liquid nitrogen until needed.
14. Section in a cryoultramicrotome operating at –95°C and separate the sections using an eyelash. Lift off the knife with a 1 mm diameter wire loop holding a drop of 2.3 *M* sucrose solution.
15. Gently thaw to allow stretching of the sections prior to touching onto freshly glow discharged, formvar-carbon coated grids. Float the grids off the sucrose droplet by placing on the surface of PIPES/mg buffer.
16. Block the frozen sections for 20 min in block buffer in a 24-well plate.
17. Place the grids and sections face down in the primary antibody (diluted in block buffer) in 15 μL in the wells of a Terasaki plate for 30–60 min at room temperature or overnight at 4°C (*see* **Note 2**).
18. Carry out double labeling by mixing different species of primary and relevant secondary antibody.
19. Wash the grids in 2 mL of block buffer in a 24-well plate on a rocking table for 10 min at room temperature.
20. Place the grids in second antibody and incubate as above for the primary antibody.
21. Wash grids in a 24-well plate once with 2 mL of block buffer for 10 min, once with PIPES/mg buffer for 10 min, followed by two 5 min washes in double-distilled H_2O.
22. Stain and embed the grids in the PVA/uranyl acetate stain solution by placing the grids face down on a drop of stain on Parafilm on ice for 10 min. Lift the grid off with a wire loop, and drain the excess stain from the loop.
23. Air-dry the grid and examine by electron microscopy.

3.2. Phagosome Isolation Methods

The procedure detailed below will allow isolation of a cellular fraction that is enriched for *Mycobacterium*-containing vacuoles. The purity of the preparation will be highly variable between labs and experiments. Methods for assaying purity are discussed in **Note 3**. The protocol described will work for *M.*

tuberculosis, *M. avium*, or *M. bovis* (BCG) infections although the level of containment obviously differs.

1. Incubate monolayers of bone marrow-derived macrophages with mycobacteria as required. For isolation of early vacuoles use a 20:1 multiplicity of infection in minimal volume (3–4 mL) in two T75 flasks. A confluent T75 flask contains approx 5×10^6 cells.
2. Scrape the contents of two flasks using a cell scraper, into 10 mL of homogenization buffer with protease inhibitors.
3. Pellet the cells by centrifugation at 300*g* for 10 min at 4°C and resuspend in 1 mL of fresh homogenization buffer with protease inhibitors.
4. Lyse the cells (*see* **Note 4**) in a floating ballbearing homogenizer with Luer lock syringe attachments. The rate of lysis is variable because of the influence of cell density, so monitor lysis under the microscope every 5 passages above 10 passes. The lysate should ideally have intact nuclei that have sharp, phase-bright edges indicating that the cells are lysed and the perinuclear mass, which tends to associate with the nucleus, has been dispersed.
5. Following lysis, run two post nuclear spins at 100*g* for 6 min at 4°C to pellet intact cells and nuclei. Take samples from the pellet and the supernatant and examine them by microscopy to ensure that the supernatant is virtually clear of nuclei, and the pellet does not contain all the bacterial vacuoles.
6. Run the supernatant containing the bacterial phagosomes, under gravity, through a 47-mm 5-μm pore nucleopore filter and chase through with 5 mL of homogenization buffer (*see* **Note 5**).
7. Layer the filtered lysate carefully onto a discontinuous sucrose gradient. Centrifuge the gradients at 800*g* for 40 min at 4°C. Ensure that the brake is off on the centrifuge.
8. Harvest the 12/50% sucrose interface (approx 1.5 mL), dilute to 4 mL with homogenization buffer, and layer onto a 10% Ficoll cushion (2 mL) in a siliconized 15 mL centrifuge tube.
9. Centrifuge at 1400*g* for 40 min at 4°C.
10. Collect the bacterial vacuoles as a loose pellet at the tip of the centrifuge tube.

3.3. Density Gradient Electrophoresis Methods

We have found cell fractionation by density gradient electrophoresis to be an invaluable method for studying mycobacterial lipids that are released into the host cell and traffic with the membranes of that cell. Some of the methods that are used to label the bacteria and their constituents are discussed in **Note 6** and **ref. *16***.

3.3.1. Density Gradient Electrophoresis

1. Prepare macrophage cultures in T160 flasks (one confluent T160 flask/gradient).
2. Wash with cold PBS and place the cell monolayer on ice. Rinse cell monolayer with cold homogenization buffer.

3. Add 6 mL of homogenization buffer to each flask and scrape monolayers with cell scraper to remove cells. Collect cells in a 15 mL centrifuge tube and wash the flask with an additional 4 mL of homogenization buffer.
4. Centrifuge the cell suspension (10 mL total) at 300*g* for 10 min at 4°C and discard the supernatant.
5. Resuspend the pellet in 1 mL of homogenization buffer and lyse cells as described in **Subheading 3.2., step 4**.
6. Centrifuge the lysate at 100*g* for 6 min to remove nuclei. Retain the supernatant on ice, subject the pellet to an additional five passes through the syringe or floating ballbearing homogenizer and repeat the postnuclear spin. Collect and combine supernatants.
7. Prepare a step gradient of 2 mL of 12% sucrose (in homogenization buffer) over 2 mL of 30% sucrose (in homogenization buffer). Layer the supernatants onto the step gradient and centrifuge for 800*g* for 60 min at 4°C. The bacteria and large cell debris enter the 30% sucrose phase and tend to pellet at the base of the gradient.
8. Collect the supernatant from both the 12% phase and the 12/30% interface of the gradient. These fractions contain the macrophage-derived vesicles. Spin in an ultracentrifuge at 100,000*g* for 45 min at 4°C (*see* **Note 7**).
9. Set up the density gradients in the cold room. Secure the DGE columns in the upper buffer chamber of the DGE apparatus. Seal the base of the columns with prewet dialysis membrane and hold in place with a rubber O-ring.
10. Fill the lower chamber with DGE buffer and place the upper chamber containing columns onto lower chamber (*see* **Fig. 1**).
11. Put 10 mL of 12% Ficoll in the bottom of each column and carefully layer the sample (in 200 µL of 10% Ficoll in homogenization buffer) onto the 12% Ficoll cushion using tuberculin syringe.
12. With a two-chamber gradient maker, overlay a continuous gradient of 8% to 0% Ficoll on top of the sample (the chambers contain 6 mL DGE buffer and 6 mL 8% Ficoll to make 12 mL gradient). Carefully run the gradient solution down the side of the DGE column to avoid disrupting the sample or gradient itself.
13. Create a meniscus with DGE buffer at top of column and place a piece of Nitex cloth on top of column. This reduces disruption of gradient when filling upper buffer chamber. (Nitex will float and is removed after upper buffer chamber is filled.)
14. Fill the reservoir chamber and connect to the upper chamber, which fills back into the lower chamber and returns to the reservoir. Circulate the buffer between the chambers using a peristaltic pump.
15. Connect the anode (+ve) terminal of the power pack to the upper electrode of the DGE apparatus and run at 15 mA constant current (starts at approx 100 V) for four gradients.
16. After approx 2 h, three distinct bands should be evident. The upper band is comprised of late endosomes and lysosomes, the middle contains intermediate endocytic compartments, Golgi, and ER, and the lower band contains early endosomes and plasma membrane.

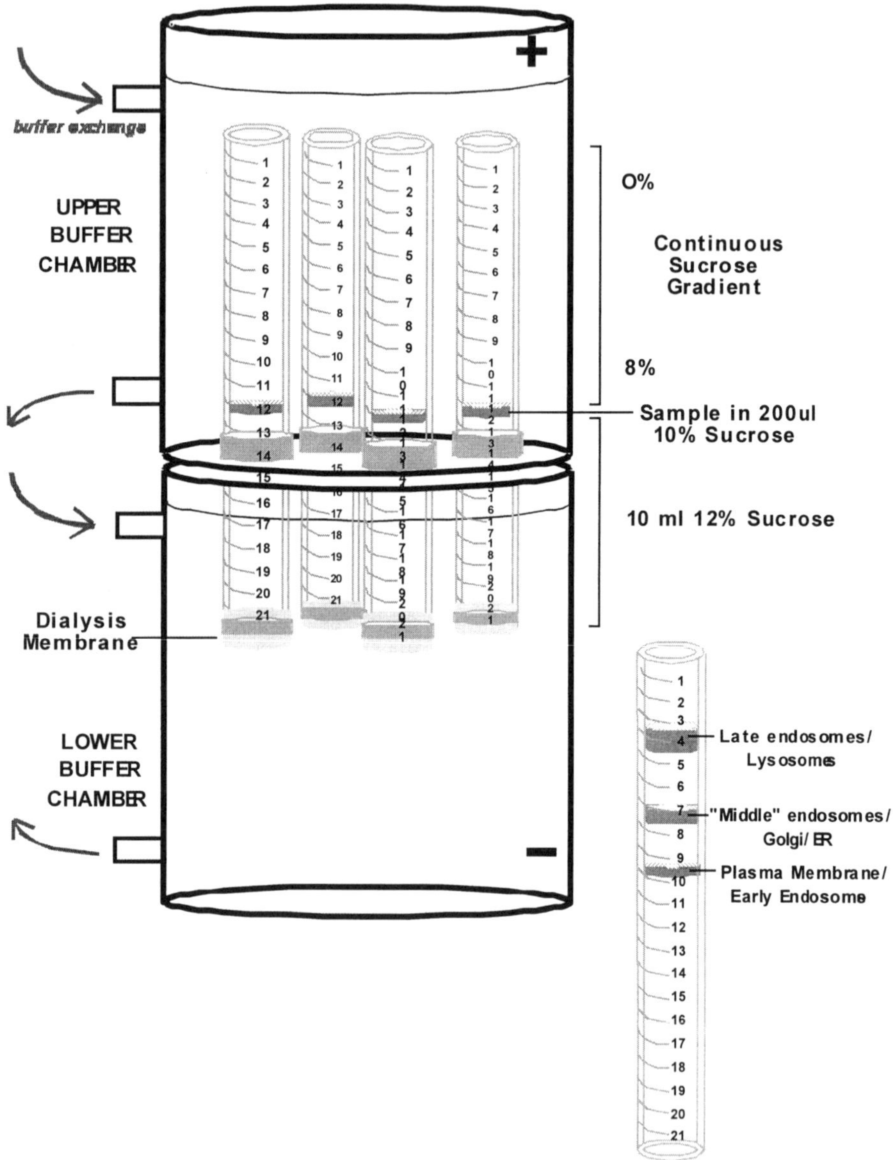

Fig 1. A diagram of the density gradient apparatus demonstrating the distribution of the sample and solutions, and the cycling of the buffer.

17. Harvest fractions from the entire gradient from the top of the column by siphon. Concentrate the vesicular material in the fractions by ultracentrifugation at 100,000*g* for 45 min at 4°C.

18. Characterize the subcellular fractions by analysis of enzymatic activity analysis of known biochemical markers by Western blot or immunoelectron microscopy.

3.3.2. Enzyme Assays for Verification of Cellular Fractions

3.3.2.1. β-Hexaminidase

β-Hexaminidase (lysosomal marker) is detected using 4-methylumbelliferyl-2-acetamido-2-deoxy-β-D-glucopyranoside as a substrate (*see* **Note 8**).

1. Prepare the reaction mixture by combining 2.5 mL of substrate, 2.5 mL of 0.4 *M* sodium acetate pH 4.4, 125 µL of 10% Triton X–100, and 4.6 mL of dH_2O.
2. Warm the solution to 37°C.
3. Add 50 µL of each DGE fraction and 150 µL of reaction mixture to the wells of a 96-well plate and incubate at 37°C for 1 h.
4. Stop the assay with 50 µL of stop buffer.
5. Read the reaction spectrophotometrically at excitation 364/emission 448.

3.3.2.2. α-Mannosidase II

α-Mannosidase II (Golgi marker) is detected using 4-methylumbelliferyl-α-D-mannopyranoside as a substrate (*see* **Note 9**).

1. Prepare reaction mixture containing 5 mL of substrate, 5 mL of PBS, 250 µL of 10% Triton X-100, and 9.75 mL of dH_2O.
2. Warm the solution to 37°C.
3. Add 50 µL of each DGE fraction and 150 µL of reaction mixture to the wells of a 96-well plate and incubate at 37°C for 1 h.
4. Stop the assay with 50 µL of stop buffer.
5. Read the reaction spectrophotometrically at excitation 364/emission 448.

3.3.2.3. Alkaline Phosphodiesterase

Alkaline phosphodiesterase (plasma membrane marker) is detected using Na-thymidine 5'-monophosphate, p-nitrophenylester as a substrate (*see* **Note 10**).

1. Prepare the reaction mixture by combining 2 mL of substrate, 2 mL of 0.1 *M* Tris-HCl, pH 9.0, and 4 mL of dH2O.
2. Add 50 µL of each DGE fraction and 150 µL of reaction mixture to wells of a 96-well plate.
3. Incubate at 37°C for 2 h or until yellow color is evident in positive samples.
4. Stop the assay with 50 µL of stop buffer.
5. Read absorbance at 410 nm.

4. Notes

1. Macrophages. Because macrophages are plastic cells that respond to their environment, there is no ideal substitute for the tissue macrophage. Macrophage-like cells lines such as J774 are frequently used as alternates but they have several

distinct shortcomings: They divide faster than *M. tuberculosis*, they lack certain important trafficking receptors such as the cation-independent mannose 6-phosphate receptor, which is responsible for delivery of lysosomal hydrolases, and finally, they are considerably less responsive to macrophage-activating cytokines than primary macrophages. We have opted for bone marrow-macrophages as a compromise, we can amplify the cells in culture but they stop growing upon removal of the L-cell-conditioned medium. They express the "correct" complement of lysosomal constituents and can be activated to kill mycobacteria by exposure to macrophage-activating cytokines ***(4)***.

2. We have included the methods we used for immunoelectron microscopy but have not detailed any markers or antibodies. These are described in depth in the papers concerning the mycobacteria-containing vacuoles (*see* **refs. *4,8,11,12***). However, we use the rat monoclonal anti-LAMP1 (lysosome associated glycoprotein 1) 1D4B as a standard reagent. LAMP1 is present through the endosomal/lysosomal network of these macrophages and is highly abundant in the lysosome. For endosomal trafficking studies we incubate infected macrophages with 1 mg/mL either biotinylated dextran 10 kDa (detected with streptavidin/rabbit anti-streptavidin or mouse antistreptavidin) or fluoresceinated dextran 10 kDa (detected with rabbit antifluorescein). We use Jackson Immunoresearch lab gold-conjugated second antibodies exclusively.
3. Phagosome isolation. We have described methods for enrichment of mycobacteria-containing phagosomes; however, there are two additional issues that need to be dealt with: (1) What should one use as a vacuole for comparison and (2) how does one control for the purity of the vacuole preparation? With respect to the first issue: we use IgG-coated Dynabeads that can be isolated by magnetic selection as described previously ***(8,13)***. These particles have provided a reasonable comparison indicating how the maturation of phagosomes formed around inert bodies proceed. Second, the issue of purity. We have used electron microscopy to examine the cleanliness of our phagosome preparations; however, this is inadequate because it is subjective, and does not allow quantitation or identification of contaminants. We have developed a more rigorous approach to assaying contamination based on a cross-over contamination assay. This assay allows one to assess contamination in radiolabeled preparations or in preparations where infected cells have been fed endocytic tracers. To evaluate the purity of isolated vacuoles, four T75 flasks of macrophages are prepared, two of which are metabolically labeled with ^{35}S methionine overnight. Particles are added to one labeled and one unlabeled flask. The cells from all four flasks are scraped and combined for processing as follows. The labeled cells with particles are combined with unlabeled cells with no particles, and the unlabeled cells with particles are combined with the labeled cells with no particles. After the isolation procedures are complete an equivalent aliquot from the two samples is measured for radioactivity. The % contamination is calculated as cpm from particles in unlabeled cells/cpm. from particles in labeled cell + cpm from particles in unlabeled cells × 100. In the protocols given the levels of contamination varies between 3–8%.

Two-dimensional polyacrylamide gel electrophoresis (2D-PAGE) analysis of labeled proteins copurified with phagosomes from unlabeled cells indicated that there was no selection for specific contaminating proteins. In trafficking experiments involving transferrin or cholera toxin trafficking, the tracer is used in place of the radioactivity.

4. For BCG and *M. avium*: passage the suspension 20–30 times through a tuberculin syringe with 25-gage needle placed in a glass Corex tube on ice. Extreme care is taken (1) to avoid inoculating oneself, (2) to avoid accumulating air bubbles and froth, and (3) to minimize aerosol generation. Cover the Corex tube with Parafilm and push the syringe through it to ensure that aerosol spread of bacteria is avoided.
5. This step helps yield extremely pure bacterial phagosomes; however, it does cause extensive loss of material. For some trafficking studies where we know that we do not have a contamination problem with the marker of interest we omit this filter step.
6. When analyzing subcellular organelles for the presence of bacterial-derived constituents, it is necessary to confirm that the subcellular preparation is free of bacteria. The method for separation of bacteria from subcellular organelles on a sucrose gradient (described in **Subheading 3.**) was developed using macrophages infected with mycobacteria labeled with fluorescein isothiocyanate (FITC)-carbazide or mycobacteria expressing the green fluorescent protein (GFP). Following separation on a sucrose step gradient (*see* **Subheading 3.3.**) fractions are carefully removed from the top of the gradient and analyzed by fluorescent microscopy for the presence of labeled bacteria. Bacteria are present in the lower region of the gradient allowing for isolation of subcellular organelles (remain in upper region) free of bacteria. This can be confirmed by Western blot analysis of the gradient using antibodies specific to GFP or to mycobacterial constituents that are not released from the bacteria. With the exception of enzymatic assays, we have not detailed the markers or antibodies used for characterization of subcellular organelles separated by DGE. These have been described in detail elsewhere and thus will only be summarized briefly. Compartments belonging to the endosomal system have been identified by allowing cells to endocytose horseradish peroxidase (HRP). Using BMMO we have found that internalization of HRP for 4 min labels early endosomes. A 4 min pulse followed by a 10 min chase labels an intermediate endocytic compartment. A 30 min chase will load late endosomal and lysosomal compartments with HRP. The presence of HRP in the DGE subcellular fractions can be determined spectrophotometrically using O-dianisidine as a substrate or by spotting fractions onto nitrocellulose followed by enhanced chemiluminescence (ECL) analysis (Super Signal, Pierce, Rockford, IL). Recycling endosomes can be identified by using labeled transferrin ***(14)***.
7. For improved separation, treat with trypsin prior to centrifuging. Add 25 μg of trypsin per mg of protein in the vesicular fraction and incubate for 5 min at 37°C. Place on ice immediately and add 100 μg protein soybean inhibitor per mg of total protein. Centrifuge at 100,000*g* for 45 min at 4°C and **very gently** resuspend the pellet in 200 μL of 10% Ficoll in DGE buffer using a tuberculin syringe.

8. In addition to β-hexaminidase, lysosomes can be identified by the presence of β-galactosidase (using 4-methylumbelliferyl-β-D-galactopyranoside as a substrate) ***(10)***, or using antibodies specific to LAMP1 or the lysosomal form of cathepsin D ***(15)***.
9. Golgi can be identified by the presence of α-mannosidase (described above) as well as galactosyl transferase (using ^{3}H-UDP-galactose and ovalbumin as an acceptor) ***(6)***. The endoplasmic reticulum (ER) can be identified by briefly pulsing cells with ^{35}S-methonine or ^{35}S-cysteine ***(6)***.
10. Plasma membrane contains alkaline phosphodiesterase, but can also be identified by iodination or biotinylation of the surface. In addition, antibodies to numerous markers of subcellular compartments can be used for Western blot characterization of DGE subcellular fractions.

Acknowledgments

Work was supported by the following US Public Health Service grants, AI 43702, AI 33348HL 55936. DGR is a recipient of the Burroughs Wellcome Award in Molecular Parasitology.

References

1. Clemens, D. L. (1997) *Mycobacterium tuberculosis*: bringing down the wall. *Trends Microbiol.* **5,** 383–385.
2. Deretic, V., Via, L. E., Fratti, R. A., and Deretic, D. (1997) Mycobacterial phagosome maturation, rab proteins, and intracellular trafficking. *Electrophoresis* **18,** 2542–2547.
3. Russell, D. G., Sturgill-Koszycki, S., Vanheyningen, T., Collins, H., and Schaible, U. E. (1997) Why intracellular parasitism need not be a degrading experience for Mycobacterium. *Philos. Trans. R. Soc. Lond. B. Biol. Sci.* **352,** 1303–1310.
4. Schaible, U. E., Sturgill-Koszycki, S., Schlesinger, P. H., and Russell, D. G. (1998) Cytokine activation leads to acidification and increases maturation of *Mycobacterium avium*-containing phagosomes in murine macrophages. *J. Immunol.* **160,** 1290–1296.
5. Via, L. E., Fratti, R. A., McFalone, M., Pagan-Ramos, E., Deretic, D., and Deretic, V. (1998) Effects of cytokines on mycobacterial phagosome maturation. *J. Cell. Sci.* **111,** 897–905.
6. Tulp, A., Verwoerd, D., and Pieters, J. (1993) Application of an improved density gradient electrophoresis apparatus to the separation of proteins, cells and subcellular organelles. *Electrophoresis* **14,** 1295–1301.
7. Russell, D. G. (1994) Immunoelectron microscopy of endosomal trafficking in macrophages infected with microbial pathogens. *Methods Cell. Biol.* **45,** 277–288.
8. Sturgill-Koszycki, S., Schaible, U. E., and Russell, D. G. (1996) Mycobacterium-containing phagosomes are accessible to early endosomes and reflect a transitional state in normal phagosome biogenesis. *EMBO J.* **15,** 6960–6968.
9. Engering, A., Lefkovits, I., and Pieters, J. (1997) Analysis of subcellular organelles involved in major histocompatibility complex (MHC) class II-restricted antigen presentation by electrophoresis. *Electrophoresis* **18,** 2523–2530.

10. Storrie, B. and Madden, E. A. (1990) Isolation of subcellular organelles. *Methods Enzymol.* **182,** 203–225.
11. Russell, D. G., Dant, J., and Sturgill-Koszycki, S. (1996) *Mycobacterium avium*- and *Mycobacterium tuberculosis*-containing vacuoles are dynamic, fusion-competent vesicles that are accessible to glycosphingolipids from the host cell plasmalemma. *J. Immunol.* **156,** 4764–4773.
12. Xu, S., Cooper, A., Sturgill-Koszycki, S., van Heyningen, T., Chatterjee, D., Orme, I., Allen, P., and Russell, D. G. (1994) Intracellular trafficking in *Mycobacterium tuberculosis* and *Mycobacterium avium*-infected macrophages. *J. Immunol.* **153,** 2568–2578.
13. Chakraborty, P., Sturgill-Koszycki, S., and Russell, D. G. (1994) Isolation and characterization of pathogen-containing phagosomes. *Methods Cell. Biol.* **45,** 261–276.
14. Tulp, A., Verwoerd, D., Benham, A., and Neefjes, J. (1997) High-resolution density gradient electrophoresis of proteins and subcellular organelles. *Electrophoresis* **18,** 2509–2515.
15. Ullrich, H. J., Beatty, W. B., Russell, D. G. (1999) Direct delivery of procathepsin D to phagosomes: implications for phagosome biogenesis and parasitism by Mycobacterium. *Eur. J. Cell. Biol.* **78,** 739–748.
16. Beatty, W. B., Rhoades, E. R., Ullrich, H. J., Chatterjee, D., and Russell, D. G. (2000) Trafficking and release of mycobacterial from infected macrophages. *Traffic* **1,** 235–247.

19

Real Time PCR Using Molecular Beacons

A New Tool to Identify Point Mutations and to Analyze Gene Expression in Mycobacterium tuberculosis

Riccardo Manganelli, Sanjay Tyagi, and Issar Smith

1. Introduction

1.1. Molecular Beacons

Molecular beacons are a novel family of hybridization probes, which emit fluorescence upon interaction with their target. They are hairpin-shaped oligonucleotides with a central part complementary to the target, flanked by two 5–6 base pair (bp) inverted repeats, which can form a stable stem. A fluorescent moiety is covalently linked to the 5' end of the molecule, whereas the quenching moiety, 4-(4'-dimethylaminophenylazo)benzoic acid (DABCYL), is covalently linked to the 3' end. The stem keeps the two moieties in close proximity to each other, causing the fluorescence of the fluorophore to be quenched by energy transfer. When molecular beacons bind to their target, they undergo a conformational change that results in the restoration of fluorescence of the internally quenched fluorophore *(1)* (**Fig. 1**). Molecular beacons are extremely specific, and can clearly discriminate between targets differing only by a single nucleotide *(2,3)*. When present in a PCR reaction where their target is the amplification product, molecular beacons can form a stable hybrid with the amplicon during the annealing step. The intensity of fluorescence at the annealing step in each amplification cycle is a direct measure of amplicon concentration *(2,4)* (**Fig. 2**). Another interesting feature of molecular beacons is that they can be coupled to a variety of differently colored fluorophores. This allows multiplex PCR reactions where different DNA fragments can be amplified and detected simultaneously in the same tube *(2,3)*.

From: *Methods in Molecular Medicine,* vol. 54: *Mycobacterium Tuberculosis Protocols*
Edited by: T. Parish and N. G. Stoker © Humana Press Inc., Totowa, NJ

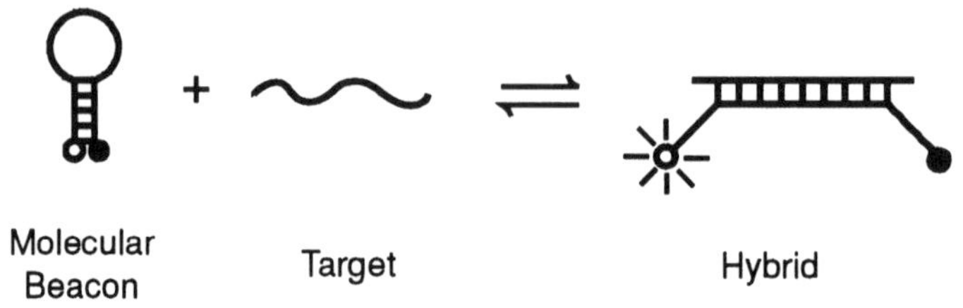

Fig. 1. Operation of molecular beacons. On their own, these molecules are nonfluorescent, because the stem hybrid keeps the fluorophore (○) close to the quencher (●). When the probe sequence in the loop hybridizes to its target, forming a rigid double helix, a conformational reorganization occurs that separates the quencher from the fluorophore, restoring fluorescence *(1)*.

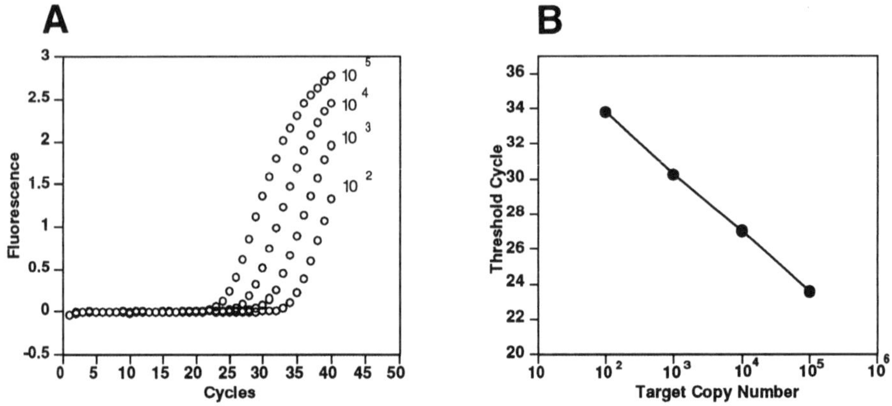

Fig. 2. Real time measurement of amplicon synthesis during PCR using molecular beacons. **(A)** Four PCR reactions were initiated with a different number of template molecules (indicated). The concentration of amplicons present after each cycle of amplification was determined by measuring fluorescence during the last few seconds of the annealing step. **(B)** Inverted relationship between the threshold cycle (the cycle at which the fluorescent signal becomes detectable above the background) and the logarithm of the initial number of template molecules. In this example, the target is *M. tuberculosis* H37Rv chromosomal DNA. The primers-molecular beacon set used in the reaction was specific for *sigA* (reprinted from **ref. *4***).

1.2. Detection of Point Mutations

The emergence of multidrug-resistance (MDR) *Mycobacterium tuberculosis* represents a major problem in tuberculosis treatment. Conventional testing for antibiotic susceptibility takes from 2–8 wk, during which time the patient's health can deteriorate dramatically **(5)**. Since almost all MDR *M. tuberculosis* strains are resistant to rifampin, resistance to this antibiotic has been proposed as a marker for MDR tuberculosis **(6)**. Rifampin resistance is usually associated with mutations in an 81-bp region of the *rpoB* gene **(6)**. Analysis of this region of *rpoB* has been used to predict rifampin susceptibility of clinical strains using sequence analysis **(7,8)**, single-strand conformational polymorphism analysis **(6)**, heteroduplex analysis **(9)**, and RNA/RNA mismatch assays **(10)**. All of these techniques are significantly faster than the conventional culture-based techniques for drug sensitivity, but are still time consuming and require sophisticated technical expertise. Piatek et al. **(11)** recently developed a very easy and effective method for the sequence analysis of the 81-bp region of the *rpoB* gene using a set of five overlapping molecular beacons, each capable of distinguishing various single point mutations. The 81-bp fragment of *rpoB* was amplified in five parallel PCR reactions, each of which contained a molecular beacon specific for about 20 bp of the amplicon. Each molecular beacon was designed to hybridize only to the wild-type sequence. The absence of fluorescence in one or more reactions indicated the presence of one or more mutations. Each of the five reactions also contained primers and a molecular beacon specific for the amplification and the detection of a fragment of the mycobacterial 16S rRNA as a positive control. The molecular beacon for 16S rRNA was coupled with tetramethylrhodamine (TET) and the molecular beacon for *rpoB* was coupled with fluorescein (FAM) so that the two reactions could be distinguished. A sixth reaction was carried out with primers and molecular beacon specific for the insertion element IS*6110* to confirm that the DNA of the sample was from *M. tuberculosis*.

This technique can be easily adapted for the detection of other mutations known to result in drug resistance in *M. tuberculosis* (for example, mutations in *katG* and *inhA* conferring resistance to isoniazid) and for the identification of mycobacteria in clinical samples.

In this chapter, we describe how to design and characterize a molecular beacon capable of discriminating between two targets differing only in a single nucleotide and we also describe a protocol to perform the assay.

1.3. Gene Expression in M. tuberculosis

M. tuberculosis must adapt to a changing and challenging environment during infection; moreover, it has been proposed to be able, under certain circumstances, to enter a "persistent" state **(12)**. This suggests that the regulation of gene expression plays a major role in its pathogenicity as it is expected that different genes would be induced or repressed during different stages of the infection process.

Several methods have been used to monitor gene epression in *M. tuberculosis*: fusion with reporter genes such as *lacZ* or *gfp*, RNAse protection assays, differential display PCR, Northern blot analysis, customized amplification libraries, and reverse transcriptase-PCR (RT-PCR) ***(13,14)***. The limited number of mycobacteria that can be recovered from samples such as infected tissue or macrophages makes PCR-based techniques the methods of choice for quantitative measurements of gene expression. We recently developed a quantitative RT-PCR assay coupled with molecular beacons that enabled us to study the differential expression of 10 genes in cultures of *M. tuberculosis* exposed to various stresses ***(4)***. The method relies upon the use of a constitutively expressed gene (*sigA*) as an internal control to correct for variability in the efficiency of the reverse transcription reaction as well as for differences in RNA concentrations from sample to sample. A standard reverse transcription reaction is followed by a quantitative PCR with molecular beacons. The use of molecular beacons to detect and measure the reaction product enhances both the sensitivity and the specificity of the PCR reaction. Moreover, by following the PCR reaction in real time, the investigator can easily recognize the onset of the linear phase of the reaction, which permits accurate quantitation.

In this chapter, we describe this RT-PCR technique as well as a method for the preparation of mycobacterial DNA and RNA from infected human macrophages. The method is designed to provide seven identical sets of seven samples collected at various times during an infection of 72 h. These seven samples consist of two samples of extracellular bacteria and five samples of intracellular bacteria (T_1, T_6, T_{24}, T_{48}, and T_{72}). The RNA can be used to study the differential gene expression during growth in macrophages, whereas the DNA can be used to measure the growth of the intracellular bacteria.

2. Materials

2.1. Synthesis of Molecular Beacons

Molecular beacons are synthesized from oligonucleotides containing terminal aminosulfhydryl functional groups by coupling them to activated dyes. The detailed procedures are available on the worldwide web at http://www.molecular-beacons.org. They can also be obtained from a number of oligonucleotide synthesis companies such as Research Genetics (Muntsville, AL), Midland Certified Reagents (Midland, TX), Life Technologies (Gaithersburg, MD), Biosearch Technologies (Novato, CA), Stratagene (La Jolla, CA), and TriLink BioTechnologies (San Diego, CA) in the United States and Eurogentec (Herstal, Belgium), Oswel (Southampton, UK), and TIB Molbiol (Berlin, Germany) in Europe.

2.2. Media for M. tuberculosis

1. Middlebrook 7H9 liquid medium (Difco, Detroit, MI) supplemented with 10% bovine serum albumin, dextrose, and sodium chloride (ADC), 0.2% glycerol, and 0.05% Tween-80.
2. Middlebrook 7H10 solid medium (Difco) supplemented with 10% ADC, 0.2% glycerol, and 0.05% Tween-80.

2.3. Cell Cultures

1. RPMI 1640 medium (Life Technologies) with 2 m*M* L-glutamine adjusted to 1.5 g/L sodium bicarbonate (Life Technologies), 4.5 g/L glucose (Life Technologies), 10 m*M* HEPES (Life Technologies), and 1.0 m*M* sodium pyruvate (Life Technologies), supplemented with 5×10^{-5} *M* 2-mercaptoethanol (Life Technologies) and fetal bovine serum, 10% (HyClone, Logan, UT).
2. Phorbol 12-myristate 13-acetate (PMA) (Sigma-Aldrich, St. Louis, MO) (*see* **Note 1**).
3. Phosphate-buffered saline, pH 7.2 (PBS) (Life Technologies).
4. Tissue culture flasks (Becton Dickinson, Lincon Park, NJ).
5. 24-well plates (Becton Dickinson).
6. Trypan Blue solution (0.4%) (Sigma-Aldrich).
7. Inverted microscope.
8. CO_2 incubator.

2.4. Extraction of Nucleic Acids

1. TRI Reagent (Molecular Research Center, Cincinnati, OH).
2. 1-Bromo-3-chloropropane (BCP) (Molecular Research Center).
3. Polyacryl Carrier (Molecular Research Center).
4. TRI reagent/carrier solution: TRI reagent + 1/100 vol polyacryl carrier.
5. 0.1-mm sterile zirconia/silica beads (Biospec Products, Bartlesville, OK).
6. 2-mL screw cap microcentrifuge tubes with O-rings (Fisher Scientific, Pittsburgh, PA).
7. 0.5% w/v sodium dodecyl sulfate (SDS)
8. BeadBeater (Biospec Products).
9. Isopropanol.
10. 75% ethanol.
11. 0.1 *M* sodium citrate in 10% ethanol.
12. 10 m*M* Tris-HCl, pH 7.5.
13. Diethylpyrocarbonate (DEPC)-treated H_2O.

2.5. Reverse Transcription

1. Gene-specific reverse primers.
2. AMV reverse transcriptase (USB, Cleveland, OH) (*see* **Note 2**).
3. 5X AMV RT buffer (provided with the enzyme).
4. dNTP solution (1.0 m*M* each) (Promega, Madison, WI).

2.6. PCR with Molecular Beacons

1. Applied Biosystem 7700 Prism spectrofluorometric thermal cycler (Perkin-Elmer, Norwalk, CT) (*see* **Note 3**).
2. Ampli*Taq* Gold DNA Polymerase (Perkin-Elmer) (*see* **Note 4**).
3. TaqMan Buffer A without $MgCl_2$ (provided with the enzyme) (*see* **Note 5**).
4. 25 m*M* $MgCl_2$ (provided with the enzyme).
5. Optical micro tubes (Perkin-Elmer).
6. dNTP solution (2.5 m*M* each) (Promega).
7. Primers:
   sigA: 5'-GAGATCGGCCAGGTCTACGGCGTG-3'
5'-CTGACATGGGGGCCCGCTACGTTG-3' *(4)*
   IS*6110*: 5'-CTAACCGGCTGTGGGTAG-3'
5'-GTCTTTCAGGTCGAGTAC-3' *(11)*
   16S rRNA: 5'-GAGATACTCGAGTGGCGAAC-3'
5'-GGCCGGCTACCCGTCGTC-3' *(11)*
8. Molecular beacons (arm sequences are underlined):
   sigA: FAM-5'-GCGAGAGTTGCGCCATCCGACTCGC-3'-DABCYL *(4)*
   IS*6110*: FAM-5'-GCACCGAGGTGGCCATCGTGGAAGCGGGTGC-3'-DABCYL *(11)*
   16S rRNA: TET–5'-CGAGCATAGGACCACGGGATGCAGCTCG-3'-DABCYL

3. Methods

3.1. How to Design a Molecular Beacon

In order to detect synthesis of products during PCR, molecular beacons should be designed so that they are able to hybridize to their targets at annealing temperatures used for PCR, whereas in the absence of the target, the molecular beacons remain closed and nonfluorescent. This can be ensured by choosing the length of the probe and arm sequences appropriately. In order to discriminate amplicons that differ from each other only by a nucleotide, the length of the probe sequence should be such that it would dissociate from its perfectly complementary target at temperatures 7–10°C higher than the annealing temperature of the PCR. The melting temperature of the probe target-hybrid can be predicted with the percent GC rule (*see* **Note 6**) using the probe sequence without the stem. In practice, lengths of the probe sequences usually range from 15–30 nucleotides.

After selecting a probe sequence, two complementary arm sequences should be added on either side of the probe sequence. In order to ensure that the molecular beacons remain closed in the absence of the target, the length, sequence, and GC content of the stem should be chosen such that the melting temperature of the stem is 7–10°C higher than the detection temperature (annealing temperature). The melting temperature of the stem can not be predicted by the percent GC rule since the stem forms by an intramolecular hybridization event. Instead, a DNA folding program (such as Zuker folding program available on the Internet, at http://www.ibc.wustl.edu/~zuker/) should be utilized to estimate the free energy of formation of the stem hybrid, from which its melting temperature can be predicted. Usually the stems are 5–7 nucleotides long. In general, GC-rich stems of 5, 6, and 7 bp will melt at between 55°C and 60°C, 60°C and 65°C, and 65°C and 70°C, respectively.

It is important that the conformation of free molecular beacons is the intended hairpin, rather than other structures that do not place the fluorophore in the immediate vicinity of the quencher or form extremely long stems. The former will cause high background signals and the latter will slow the molecular beacon denaturation and reduce its ability to bind its target. A folding of the selected sequence by the Zuker DNA folding program will reveal such problems. If the alternative structures are a result of the choice of the stem sequence, the stem sequence can be altered, whereas if the alternative structures arise from the probe sequence itself, the frame of the probe can be moved along the target to obtain probe sequences that are not self-complementary.

As with PCR primers in general, the sequence of the molecular beacon should be checked against those of the primers to make sure there are no areas of complementarity that may cause the molecular beacon to bind to primers and increase background. The primers used in PCR experiments with molecular beacons should be designed to produce a relatively short amplicon, in general less than 150 bp. The rationale of choosing a short amplicon is that the molecular beacon is an internal probe which must compete with the opposite strand of the amplicon for binding to its complementary target. Having a shorter amplicon allows the molecular beacon to compete more efficiently for binding to its target and, therefore, produces better results during molecular beacon PCR experiments.

3.2. Characterization of Molecular Beacons

Following the design and synthesis, the melting characteriztics of the molecular beacon in PCR buffer conditions should be verified experimentally to ensure that the molecular beacon is functioning as expected. This also allows determination of the appropriate annealing temperature for subsequent PCR experiments.

1. Prepare three tubes containing 200 n*M* molecular beacon, 4 m*M* $MgCl_2$, and 10 m*M* Tris-HCl, pH 8.0, in a volume of 50 µL.
2. Add an oligonucleotide perfectly complementary to the molecular beacon (without the self-complementary arms) to one of the tubes and an oligonucleotide differing from the first one in only one position to another tube, at a final concentration of 400 n*M*.

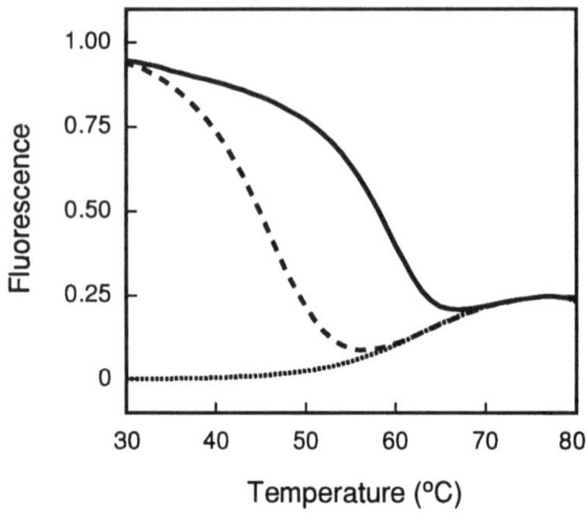

Fig. 3. Thermal denaturation profiles of a molecular beacon (dotted line), of its hybrid with a perfectly complementary target (continuous line) and of its hybrid with a mismatched target (dashed line).

3. Determine the fluorescence of each solution as a function of temperature using the spectrofluorometric thermal cycler. Decrease the temperature of the tubes from 80°C to 30°C in 1°C steps, with each step lasting 1 min, while monitoring the fluorescence during each step.

Figure 3 illustrates a typical molecular beacon melting profile. The dotted line represents the fluorescence obtained with the molecular beacon alone, the continuous line represents the fluorescence of its hybrid with a perfectly complementary target, and the dashed line represents the fluorescence of its hybrid with a target that is mismatched by a single nucleotide. An annealing temperature should be chosen at which the molecular beacon will bind efficiently to its perfectly complementary target but not to the mismatched target, and at which the molecular beacon will adopt a stem-loop conformation if the target is not present. Therefore, in the example illustrated in **Fig. 3** the annealing temperature should be 55°C (the center of the window of discrimination).

3.3. Detection of Point Mutations

1. Design a FAM-coupled molecular beacon homologous to the region that is subjected to search for point mutations. It must be able to discriminate between the wild-type sequence and one with a single mismatch (*see* **Subheading 3.2.** and **Note 7**).
2. Subject the sample to a multiplex PCR reaction containing the primers-molecular beacon set specific for 16S rRNA (whose molecular beacon is coupled with TET),

and the primers-molecular beacon set specific for the target sequence subjected to search for point mutations (whose molecular beacon is coupled with FAM). Also perform a PCR reaction with the primers-molecular beacon set for the insertion sequence IS*6110*.

3. Set up each PCR reaction in final volume of 25 µL to contain 1X TaqMan Buffer A, 4 m*M* $MgCl_2$, 0.25 m*M* each dNTP, 1.75 U Ampli*Taq* Gold polymerase, 0.5 µ*M* of each primer, 0.3 µ*M* of the appropriate molecular beacon, and 1.75 µL of template (1–5 ng of chromosomal DNA).
4. Perform the reactions in the Applied Biosystem 7700 Prism spectrofluorometric thermal cycler (which is able to differentiate between fluorescence emitted from the two different fluorophores). After 10 min at 94°C to activate the enzyme, perform 40 cycles with the following conditions: 94°C denaturation for 30 s; annealing for 1 min at a suitable temperature for the particular primers-beacon sets (*see* **Subheading 3.2.**); 72°C extension for 30 s. Measure fluorescence during the annealing steps.
5. If the wild-type sequence is present, fluorescence from both FAM (molecular beacon specific for the wild-type sequence) and TET (molecular beacon for 16S rRNA) should be detected. If a mutation is present in the region of interest, only fluorescence from TET will be detected. If no fluorescence from TET is detected, the analysis will be considered to be indeterminate. Samples in which no fluorescence will be detected in the reaction with the primers-molecular beacon set for the insertion sequence IS*6110* will be considered as negative for the presence of *M. tuberculosis* DNA.

3.4. Infection of Macrophages

1. Resuspend 6×10^7 THP-1 cells in 80 mL of warm RPMI with 50 n*M* PMA—final cell concentration 7.5×10^5/mL (*see* **Note 8**).
2. Seed three 24-well tissue culture plates with 1 mL/well.
3. Incubate at 37°C for 24 h.
4. Dilute a sample of *M. tuberculosis* H37Rv growing exponentially in warm RPMI and another sample in warm 7H9 up to a concentration of 3.7×10^5 cfu/mL.
5. Replace the media of 55 wells with the RPMI inoculated with mycobacteria (infected macrophages). Replace the media of the other wells with uninoculated RPMI (uninfected control macrophages).
6. Simultaneously seed 7 wells of a 24-well tissue culture plate not containing macrophages with 1 mL of inoculated RPMI, and 7 wells with 1 mL of inoculated 7H9.
7. Incubate the plates at 37°C for 1h.
8. Remove the media from all wells containing macrophages, wash them twice with warm PBS, and add fresh media.
9. At the same time transfer the inoculated media from the plate not containing macrophages (**step 6**) to 1.5 mL microcentrifuge tubes, chill on ice for 3 min and centrifuge at 5000*g* for 5 min at 4°C. Remove the supernatant, resuspend each pellet in 300 µL of TRI Reagent/+ 1/100 vol of polyacryl carrier, transfer to a

2-mL screw cap micro centrifuge tube with O-rings and freeze on dry ice. Store at –70°C (*see* **Note 9**).

10. At each time point (1; 6; 24, 48,72 h):
    a. Remove media from two wells containing infected macrophages, lyse the cells by adding 1 mL 0.05% SDS and plate the bacteria at appropriate dilutions on 7H10 plates for cfu determination.
    b. Remove media from two wells, one containing infected, the other uninfected macrophages and stain with 20 µL of Trypan-Blue for analysis of macrophage viability (*see* **Note 10**).
    c. Treating one well at a time, remove the media from 7 wells containing infected macrophages, lyse the cells of each well by adding 300 µL of cold TRI Reagent/carrier, transfer the lysate immediately to a 2-mL screw cap microcentrifuge tube with O-rings and freeze on dry ice (*see* **Note 11**).
    d. Store at –70°C.

3.5. RNA Extraction

1. Add 150 µL of zirconia/silica beads to the frozen lysate (from **Subheading 3.4.**).
2. Place the tubes with the frozen samples in the BeadBeater and subject to 2 × 1 min pulses with a 2 min rest on ice.
3. Transfer the sample to a clean tube.
4. Add 100 µL of TRI reagent/carrier to the original tube to wash the beads and add it to the previously transferred sample.
5. Incubate the sample at room temperature for 10 min.
6. Spin for 10 min at 12,000*g* at 4° C.
7. Transfer the supernatant to a clean tube (save the pellet for DNA extraction).
8. Add 30 µL of BCP and shake vigorously for 15 s (do not vortex).
9. Incubate 10 min at room temperature and then spin at 12,000*g* for 15 min at 4°C.
10. Transfer the upper phase to a new tube (save the lower phase for DNA extraction) (*see* **Note 12**).
11. Add 150 µL of isopropanol.
12. Incubate 5 min at room temperature and then spin at 12,000*g* for 8 min at 4°C.
13. Remove supernatant and add 300 µL of 75% ethanol (*see* **Note 13**).
14. Mix and then spin at 7500*g* for 5 min at 4°C.
15. Remove the supernatant and air dry the pellet 3–5 min.
16. Dissolve in 30 µL DEPC-treated H_2O.
17. Add 300 µL of TRI reagent/carrier and repeat from **steps 8–15**.
18. Dissolve in 12 µL DEPC-treated H_2O.
19. Store at –70°C.

3.6. DNA Extraction

1. Resuspend the pellet from **step 7** of **Subheading 3.5.** with the lower phase collected during **step 10** of **Subheading 3.5.**
2. Add 200 µL 95% ethanol, mix by inverting and incubate for 5 min at room temperature to allow the DNA to precipitate.

3. Spin at 2000*g* for 5 min at 4°C.
4. Remove supernatant and wash the pellet twice with 300 mL of 0.1 *M* sodium citrate in 10% ethanol. For each wash, incubate the pellet with the solution for 5 min at room temperature and spin at 3,000*g* for 5 min at 4°C (*see* **Note 14**).
5. Wash the DNA pellet with 500 µL of 75% ethanol, and spin at 2000*g* for 5 min at 4°C.
6. Remove the supernatant and air dry the pellet 5 min at room temperature.
7. Dissolve the pellet in 100 µL of 10 m*M* Tris (pH 7.5) (*see* **Note 15**).
8. Remove cell debris by centrifuging at 12,000*g* for 10 min.

3.7. Reverse Transcription (see Note 16)

1. In a PCR tube add 2.5 pmol of each antisense primer (up to four different primers plus the primer for *sigA*), 2 µL of 5X AMV RT buffer and 2 µL of RNA sample, in a final volume of 10 µL (*see* **Note 17**).
2. Denature in a thermocycler at 95°C for 1 min 30 s. Carry out the annealing between the RNA and the antisense primers for 3 min at 65°C followed by 3 min at 57°C (*see* **Note 18**). Place the tube on ice.
3. Add 3.5 µL of annealing mixture to 1.1 µL of dNTP solution (1 m*M* each), 0.4 mL of 5X AMV RT buffer and 8 U of AMV in a final volume of 5.5 µL (*see* **Note 19**).
4. Incubate 30 min at 47°C (*see* **Note 20**), inactivate the enzyme for 1 min at 95°C and place the tube on ice.
5. Dilute with 70 µL of H_2O (*see* **Note 21**).
6. Prepare identical samples not treated with AMV as a control to monitor the amount of DNA carryover during RNA purification (mock reverse transcription).

3.8. Quantitative PCR with Molecular Beacons (see Note 22)

1. Each reaction (25 µL) consists of 1X TaqMan Buffer A, 4 m*M* $MgCl_2$, 0.25 m*M* each dNTP, 1.75 U Ampli*Taq* Gold polymerase, 0.5 µ*M* of each primer, 0.3 µ*M* of the appropriate molecular beacon, and 1.75 µL of template, which could be cDNA (when measuring gene expression) or DNA (when measuring the growth of the intracellular bacteria).
2. Perform the reactions in the Applied Biosystem 7700 Prism spectrofluorometric thermal cycler. After 10 min at 94°C to activate the enzyme, perform the following two sets of cycles. First set (15 cycles): touchdown with the annealing temperature decreasing 0.5°C per cycle starting from 65°C. 94°C denaturation; 72°C extension (all steps 30 s long). Second set (25 cycles): 94°C denaturation for 30 s; 57°C annealing for 1 min; 72°C extension for 30 s. Measure the fluorescence during the annealing steps of the second sets of cycles (*see* **Note 23**).
3. In order to obtain a standard curve for each primers-beacon set, run four different PCR reactions in parallel with the uncharacterized samples, using as template 10-fold dilutions of known amounts of H37Rv chromosomal DNA (10^2, 10^3, 10^4, and 10^5 copies).

3.9. Data Analysis

1. Plot the threshold cycles obtained from amplification of the DNA standard as a function of the logarithm of the number of target molecules. This curve is described by the equation $n = a + b \log(x)$, where n is the number of target copies, x is the threshold cycle obtained amplifying n target copies, a is the intercept and b is the slope of the resulting curve. Solve the equation in order to calculate the constants a and b specific of each primers-beacon set (*see* **Note 24**).
2. Using the constants calculated from above, solve the equation for the number of target copies present in the uncharacterized samples.
3. When the uncharacterized sample consists of cDNA, subtract the values obtained amplifying the mock reverse transcriptions from those obtained amplifying the reverse transcription (*see* **Note 25**).
4. For each gene analyzed, calculate the ratio between the amount of cDNA in the samples from intracellular mycobacteriathat in the samples from extracellular mycobacteria, normalizing for the amount of *sigA* cDNA: (*geneX* $\text{cDNA}^{\text{intracellular}}$/*sigA* $\text{cDNA}^{\text{intracellular}}$)/(*geneX* $\text{cDNA}^{\text{extracellular}}$/*sigA* $\text{cDNA}^{\text{extracellular}}$). This value represents the ratio of the amount of mRNA of a given gene found in intracellular bacteria to that found in extracellular bacteria, normalized to *sigA* mRNA.

4. Notes

1. Resuspend PMA in H_2O at a concentration of 1.5 m*M* and keep frozen at –70°C in small aliquots.
2. We have been using AMV reverse transcriptase, since it works well at 47°C, which is desirable when dealing with nucleic acids with a high GC content. However a number of companies have recently advertised new recombinant reverse transcriptases designed for quantitative RT-PCR which, according to the producer, are highly efficient with GC-rich templates (Omniscript RT, Quiagen, Hilden, Germany; ThermoScript, Life Technologies).
3. Two other instruments that can perform PCR and monitor fluorescence have become available: Icycler (Biorad, Hercules, CA) and Lightcycler (Roche Diagnostic, Nutley, NJ)
4. Ampli*Taq* Gold DNA polymerase is completely inactive until it is activated at 94°C. This is very useful because it minimizes false priming without requiring a hot start.
5. This buffer contains the dye 6-carboxy-X-rhodamine (6-rox). The fluorescence of this dye is used by the spectrophotometric thermal cycler as a normalization reference.
6. T_m (in degrees Celsius) = $81.5 + 16.6 \times \log [Na^+] + 0.41 \times (\%GC) - 675/\text{length}$. For the calculation set the Na^+ concentration to 1 *M*.
7. When the sequence of the mutant allele is not known, or as in the case of *rpoB* in *M. tuberculosis*, many different mutations can result in drug resistance, the most reliable method consists of performing two different PCR reactions in the same tube. The first PCR product will be the DNA fragment being studied, whose

molecular beacon will be coupled to FAM and will be specific for the wild-type sequence. The second PCR product will be a fragment of the gene encoding 16S rRNA; the molecular beacon specific for it will be coupled to TET and it will represent the positive control for the amplification.

When the sequence of all the different alleles to discriminate is known, it is possible to perform a single PCR reaction amplifying the fragment containing the region which includes the differences among the various alleles. Molecular beacons specific for each allele, coupled with different fluorophores, will be included in the PCR reaction. The color of the fluorescence resulting from the hybridization of the molecular beacons to their targets will reveal which allele is present in the sample ***(15)***. This technique, using rRNA as target sequence, could be extremely valuable in tests for identification of pathogenic mycobacteria in clinical specimens.

8. THP-1 is a human monocytic cell line. THP-1 cells grow in a nonadherent fashion until induced with PMA; at this point they differentiate into macrophages, stop cell division and adhere to tissue culture flasks ***(16)***. It is very important that THP-1 cells not be passaged continuously. In our experience cell cultures passaged less than 45 d differentiate stably after 24 h induction with 50 n*M* PMA and can be maintained after infection with *M. tuberculosis* for at least another week. During this time, intracellular bacteria double almost once a day. It is important to avoid high concentrations of PMA: we noticed that cells differentiated for longer than 24 h or with concentrations of PMA higher than 50 n*M* die when infected with *M. tuberculosis*. If cells are subcultured for more than 45 d, higher concentrations of PMA or longer times of induction are needed in order to obtain stable differentiation and often cells become nonadherent after several days of incubation.
9. The RNA from bacteria incubated in 7H9 represents the standard for calculation of differential gene expression during growth in macrophages. The RNA from bacteria incubated in RPMI will be used to determine if exposure to RPMI prior to uptake by macrophages alters the expression of the studied genes.
10. Do not allow the macrophages to dry before adding the dye, and observe them under the microscope immediately. If the cells are allowed to dry, they will die quickly. Dead cells stain blue, live cells remain colorless. Usually about 95% of the macrophages remain viable until the end of the experiment and little, if any, difference can be noted between viability of infected and uninfected cells.
11. Treating one well at a time reduces the time required between collection and freezing of the sample. This is important since bacterial RNA has a very short half-life and could be degraded during the manipulation of the sample. TRI Reagent solubilizes most bacteria and eucaryotic tissues almost immediately and is designed to stabilize the RNA, but it does not lyse mycobacteria.
12. It is extremely important to avoid touching the interface with the pipet-tip, since this contains the DNA.
13. Usually the pellet is almost invisible after the isopropanol precipitation, since it is very transparent. However, after the wash in 75% ethanol, it will be more visible.

14. Be careful when removing the supernatant, since the pellet might be very loose.
15. It is very important to use Tris buffer to resuspend this pellet, since it is almost insoluble in H_2O.
16. Reverse transcription of all the studied genes and the control (*sigA*) is carried out in the same tube. This is necessary in order to correct for tube to tube variability in reverse transcription as well as for differences in the amounts of total RNA in the different samples.
17. Prepare one annealing reaction for each of the 7 RNA samples (5 intracellular time points and two extracellular controls). To minimize sample to sample variability prepare a master-mix with all the antisense primers and aliquot it into 7 tubes before adding the templates.
18. For a higher degree of reproducibility perform annealing in a thermal cycler. Optimal annealing temperature should be determined empirically for each primer, but the use of many primers at the same time makes this impractical. We designed all our primers so that 57°C was a suitable annealing temperature.
19. Prepare a master-mix with all the reagents, aliquot it into 7 tubes, and then add the templates. Be very careful to mix the master-mix well after adding the enzyme, since the presence of glycerol makes the solution particularly difficult to disperse evenly.
20. Since slight variations in the temperature could affect the efficiency of the reverse transcriptase it is advisable to perform the incubation in a thermal cycler.
21. It is necessary to dilute the reverse transcriptase reaction, since it can inhibit the PCR reaction.
22. Due to the extreme sensitivity of PCR it is very important to avoid any kind of external DNA contamination which can invalidate the results. The use of molecular beacons decreases the risk of template contamination since there is no need to run the PCR product on an agarose gel (the most frequent source of contamination). Nonetheless, it is preferable to perform all the manipulations in a controlled environment (preferably a laminar flow hood) which can be UV-irradiated. It is also important to have a set of pipetors dedicated solely to PCR and to use aerosol barrier tips when pipeting samples containing nucleic acids in order to avoid contamination of the pipettors.
23. The use of a touchdown reduces the probability for nonspecific PCR products, which could compete with the specific amplicon and thus modify the kinetics of the reaction. Although an optimal annealing temperature should be determined for each primers-beacon set, the use of many different sets at the same time makes this impractical. We designed all our primers and beacons so that 57°C would be a suitable annealing temperature.
24. The values of the constants can be easily calculated using most graphic software packages such as DeltaGraph (DeltaPoint, Monterey, Ca) or KaleidaGraph (Abelbeck Software, Reading, PA).
25. Usually, the amount of DNA that copurifies with the RNA is not significant, thus making the subtraction superfluous. Nonetheless, it is advisable to perform the control to check the performance of the reverse transcriptase and because in the

case of genes expressed at very low level, levels of DNA contamination may become significant.

Acknowledgments

We thank Jeanie Dubnau, Ben Gold, Salvatore Marras, Roberta Provvedi, Marcela Rodriguez, and Shaun Walters for valuable discussions. This work was supported by NIH Grant AI 44856 (awarded to I.S.) and by NIH Grant HL-43521 (awarded to Fred Russel Kramer).

References

1. Tyagi, S. and Kramer, F. R. (1996) Molecular beacons: probes that fluoresce upon hybridization. *Nat. Biotechnol.* **14,** 303–308.
2. Tyagi, S., Bratu, D. P., and Kramer, F. R. (1998) Multicolor molecular beacons for allele discrimination. *Nat. Biotechnol.* **16,** 49–53.
3. Marras, S. A. E., Kramer, F. S., and Tyagi, S. (1999) Multiplex detection of single-nucleotide variations using molecular beacons. *Genet. Anal.* **14,** 151–156.
4. Manganelli, R., Dubnau, E., Tyagi, S., Kramer, F. R., and Smith, I. (1999) Differential expression of 10 sigma factor genes in *Mycobacterium tuberculosis*. *Mol. Microbiol.* **31,** 715–724.
5. Pablos-Mendez, A., Sterling, T. R., and Frieden, T. R. (1996) The relationship between delayed or incomplete treatment and all-cause mortality in patients with tuberculosis. *JAMA* **276,** 1223–1228.
6. Telenti, A., Imboden, P., Marchesi, F., Lowrie, D., Cole, S., Colston, M. J. et al. (1993) Detection of rifampin-resistance mutations in *Mycobacterium tuberculosis*. *Lancet* **341,** 647–650.
7. Musser, J. M. (1995) Antimicrobial agents resistance in mycobacteria: molecular genetic insights. *Clin. Microbiol. Rev.* **8,** 496–514.
8. Pozzi, G., Meloni, M., Iona, E., Orrú, G., Thoresen, P. F., Ricci, M. L., Oggioni, M. R., Fattorini, L., and Orefici, G. (1999) *rpoB* mutations in multidrug-resistant strains of *Mycobacterium tuberculosis* isolated in Italy. *J. Clin. Microbiol.* **37,** 1197–1199.
9. Williams, D. L., Waguespack, C., Eisenach, K., Crawford, J. T., Portaels, F., Salfinger, M., et al. (1994) Characterization of rifampin resistance in pathogenic mycobacteria. *Antimicrob. Agents Chemother.* **38,** 2380–2386.
10. Nash, K. A., Gaytan, A., and Inderlied, C. B. (1997) Detection of rifampin resistance in *Mycobacterium tuberculosis* by use of a rapid, simple, and specific RNA/RNA mismatch assay. *J. Infect. Dis.* **176,** 533–536.
11. Piatek, A. S., Tyagi, S., Pol, A. C., Telenti, A., Miller, L. P., Kramer, F. R., and Alland, D. (1998) Molecular beacon sequence analysis for detecting drug resistance in *Mycobacterium tuberculosis*. *Nat. Biotechnol.* **16,** 359–363.
12. Wayne, L. G. (1994) Dormancy of *Mycobacterium tuberculosis* and latency of disease. *Eur. J. Clin. Microbiol. Infect.* **13,** 908–914.
13. Timm, J., Gomez, M., and Smith, I. (1998) Gene expression and regulation, in Mycobacteria: Molecular Biology and Virulence (Ratledge, C., and Dale, J. W. esd.), Blackwell Science, Oxford, UK, in press.

14. Dubnau, J. and Smith, I. (2000) New method for identification of *Mycobacterium tuberculosis* virulence genes (to be published).
15. Kostrikis, L. G., Tyagi, S., Mhlanga, M., Ho, D. D., and Kramer, F. R. (1998) Spectral genotyping of human alleles. *Science* **279,** 1228–1229.
16. Tsuchiya, S., Kobayashi, Y., Goto, Y., Okumura, H., Nakze, S., Konno, T., and Tada, K. (1982) Induction of maturation in cultured human monocytic leukemia cells by a phorbol diester. *Cancer Res.* **42,** 1530–1536.

20

Electronic Access to *Mycobacterium tuberculosis* Sequence Data

Julian Parkhill

1. Introduction

The complete genome sequence of the well studied laboratory strain of *Mycobacterium tuberculosis* (H37Rv) has been published by the Sanger Centre *(1)*, and this information will soon be complemented by the completion of a recent clinical isolate of *M. tuberculosis* (CDC1551/CSU93) by The Institute for Genomic Research *(2)*. In addition to these sequences, projects for the genomic sequencing of *Mycobacterium bovis* ***(3)***, *Mycobacterium leprae* ***(4)***, and *Mycobacterium avium* ***(5)*** are underway. A vast wealth of basic information about the fundamental genetic makeup of the *Mycobacteria* is already available, and this mine of essential data is set to expand still further. This information is obviously of great benefit to researchers in the field, but the sheer volume of data often makes it inaccessible. This chapter aims to briefly describe the principal methods of access currently available, and the benefits of each.

2. Accessing *M. tuberculosis* Sequences Through the World Wide Web (WWW)

Several WWW sites exist that are either specific for, or allow access to, *M. tuberculosis* genomic data. The most obvious is the Sanger Centre site *(6)*. At present the ability to customize data retrieval on this web site is fairly limited, but it does remain the primary source of the H37Rv data. The Sanger Centre site allows direct download by FTP of the complete sequence data, along with the annotation. This can be loaded into a sequence viewer, such as Artemis *(7)* for easy browsing. In addition to this, the BLAST server attached to the *M. tuberculosis* web page allows searching of the *M. tuberculosis* DNA sequence with DNA or protein sequences, and of the set of *M. tuberculosis* predicted

From: *Methods in Molecular Medicine*, vol. 54: *Mycobacterium Tuberculosis Protocols*
Edited by: T. Parish and N. G. Stoker © Humana Press Inc., Totowa, NJ

proteins, again with either DNA or protein sequences. The search of the protein sequences has the added advantage of allowing direct access, via hyperlinks, to the annotation for any of the proteins retrieved by the search. The individual annotations for each protein can also be retrieved directly using the Rv gene designation. The Sanger Centre site also allows access to the hierarchical list of genes, either as a flat file, or as a set of expandable tables, and to the individual sequences of the cosmids used to sequence the genome.

The TIGR *M. tuberculosis* website *(2)* provides similar information on the incomplete (CDC1551/CSU93) sequence, including access to annotation and sequence data by genome position or gene name, and will of course remain the primary source for genome information on this strain.

The website provided by the other partner in the *M. tuberculosis* H37Rv genome sequencing project, TubercuList *(8)* at the Institut Pasteur is considerably more complex, and will repay a thorough exploration. In addition to basic BLAST and FASTA searches against the genome data, the site allows searching by gene name, position on the chromosome, functional category, and a free text search of the annotation. The Tuberculist server provides interactive graphical maps of the TB genome, allowing the user to zoom in on specific regions, move around the map, and access the annotation for any particular gene. From the gene-specific annotation individual sequences (protein or DNA) can be downloaded. Tuberculist also provides links to automatically generated protein family clusters from individual genes.

In addition to these genome-specific websites, information about the *M. tuberculosis* genome can also be obtained from the public databases; this has the advantage that other information can be accessed, in addition to the genomic sequence and annotation. A simple example of this is the Sequence Retrieval System (SRS): There are many sites running SRS servers, but perhaps the most accessible is at EBI *(9)*. SRS allows text-based searching and retrieval of sequences from the major databases, either individually or in any combination, using simple or complex searches. For example, a search of the SWISSPROT, SWISSNEW, SPTREMBL, REMTREMBL, and TREMBLNEW databases with Organism: Mycobacterium* and GeneSymbol: dnaA will retrieve the sequences of 10 DnaA proteins from various mycobacteria including *M. avium*, *M. bovis*, *M. bovis* BCG, *M. leprae*, *M. smegmatis*, and *M. tuberculosis* H37Rv. SRS searches will thus allow very complex and specific mining of data from a wide variety of sources.

Text searching with SRS, and sequence similarity searching at EBI and similar websites will only give access to data submitted to the public databases (EMBL/GenBank/DDBJ). Most bacterial genome sequencing centers do not submit sequence data to these databases until after the annotation is complete, and the sequence is published in the scientific literature. Access to unfinished sequences for similarity searching is usually available at the website of the specific sequencing center. However, similarity searches can be performed simultaneously on almost all current finished and unfinished microbial sequences at the NCBI BLAST website *(10)*. At present this includes *M. avium*, *M. bovis*, *M. leprae*, *M. tuberculosis* H37Rv and CSU93. Care should be taken when using this information, as the sequence data is unfinished and is likely to contain errors.

Also available at NCBI is the excellent Entrez Genomes system *(11)*. Like Tuberculist, Entrez Genomes allows complex graphical exploration of individual published bacterial genomes. The section covering *M. tuberculosis* H37Rv *(12)* initially displays the complete circular map which, like that on the Tuberculist site, can be zoomed in to give a scrollable gene-level view of the genome. Clicking on an individual gene (or searching by the gene name) brings up a page containing precomputed BLAST searches of that protein against the public protein databases, and allows immediate searches to be launched using FASTA or BLAST against NCBI's database of unfinished microbial genome sequences. Links are also available from the individual proteins through to other Entrez services, such as the PubMed literature database, and the Entrez protein or nucleic acid servers which in turn will give access to related proteins, DNA sequences, and literature from the entirety of the public databases. The underlying complexity of the Entrez system is enormous, but it is fairly easy to master, and will repay the time spent investigating it.

3. Use of Artemis to View the *M. tuberculosis* Genome on Your Own Computer

Artemis *(7)* is a sequence viewer and annotation tool developed by the Sanger Centre for the analysis of genomic sequences. Artemis is written in Java, and will run on most platforms including Apple Macintosh, PC/Windows, and Unix (including Linux). Artemis will read and write EMBL and GenBank format files, and display the features in the context of the sequence and its six-frame translation. The entire sequence and annotation of *M. tuberculosis* H37Rv can be retrieved from the Sanger Centre website in a format suitable for loading into Artemis (other genomes can be downloaded from NCBI's Entrez Genomes pages). Viewing the sequence and annotation in Artemis allows the investigator to find genes of interest using free-text or sequence searches and view them in context of the surrounding genes and DNA. The sequence and features can be readily scrolled and zoomed into the level of the nucleotide sequence itself and out to the entire genome. Properties of the sequence, such as G+C content, frame-specific G+C content, G/C bias and codon preference can be plotted against the sequence and zoomed and scrolled in tandem with it. Hydrophobicity and hydrophilicity plots can be generated for individual protein sequences. Users of Artemis on Unix-based machines can automatically run searches and analysis on individual genes or sets of genes, and view the results through the Artemis interface. The results of any number of other analyses can be converted to Artemis format and overlaid on the sequence. Artemis can thus be used at a very basic level, to view the sequence and features within a biologically relevant context, or can be expanded by the user to allow in-depth analysis of the *M. tuberculosis*, or any other, sequence.

References

1. Cole S. T., Brosch R., Parkhill J., Garnier T., Churcher C., Harris D., Gordon S. V., Eiglmeier K., Gas S., Barry C. E. III., Tekaia F., Badcock K., Basham D., Brown D., Chillingworth T., Connor R., Davies R., Devlin K., Feltwell T., Gentles S., Hamlin N., Holroyd S., Hornsby T., Jagels K., Krogh A., McLean J., Moule S., Murphy L., Oliver K., Osborne J., Quail M. A., Rajandream, M-A., Rogers J., Rutter S., Seeger K., Skelton J., Squares S., Squares R., Sulston J. E., Taylor K., Whitehead S., and Barrell, B. G. (1998) Deciphering the biology of *Mycobacterium tuberculosis* from the complete genome sequence. *Nature* **393,** 537–544.
2. http://www.tigr.org/tdb/CMR/gmt/htmls/SplashPage.html
3. http://www.sanger.ac.uk/Projects/M_bovis
4. http://www.sanger.ac.uk/Projects/M_leprae
5. http://www.tigr.org/tdb/mdb/mdb.html
6. http://www.sanger.ac.uk/Projects/M_tuberculosis
7. http://www.sanger.ac.uk/Software/Artemis/
8. http://bioweb.Pasteur.fr/GenoList/TubercuList/
9. http://srs.ebi.ac.uk/
10. http://www.ncbi.nlm.nih.gov/BLAST/unfinishedgenome.html
11. http://www.ncbi.nlm.nih.gov:80/entrez/query.fcgi?db=Genome
12. http://www.ncbi.nlm.nih.gov/cgi-bin/Entrez/framik?db=Genomeandgi=135

21

Proteomics

Joanna C. Betts and Marjorie A. Smith

1. Introduction

The term "proteomics" describes the technologies collectively used to define the *prote*in complement of the gen*ome* or "proteome" ***(1,2)***. The recent growth of this discipline is reflected in the many review articles available ***(3–7)***. In addition to describing all the proteins encoded by the genome, the proteome also provides information on protein expression under defined conditions or at a particular point in time, the occurrence of posttranslational modifications, and the distribution of proteins within the cell. Proteomics, most commonly, combines the technique of two-dimensional polyacrylamide gel electrophoresis (2D-PAGE), developed simultaneously but independently by O'Farrell ***(8)*** and Klose ***(9)*** in 1975, with image analysis, protein mass spectrometry, and database searching to assign protein identities to spots from 2D gels. Recent advances in the sensitivity and accuracy of protein mass spectrometry ***(3,10–12)***, coupled with availability of the complete genome sequence of two strains of *Mycobacterium tuberculosis* (***13***, http://www.tigr.org/), have facilitated the study of the proteome of this organism. Under defined growth conditions, this may help to elucidate the mechanism of *M. tuberculosis* survival within the host.

Several recent studies of the proteome of *M. tuberculosis* have been reported. These cover the analysis of both total cell lysates ***(14,15)*** and culture filtrate proteins ***(16,17)***. The response of *M. tuberculosis* to different environmental conditions such as those mimicking the host environment has also been performed using 2D gels ***(18–21)***. In addition, 2D gel databases of *M. tuberculosis* have recently been published on the internet; *M. tuberculosis* and *M. bovis* BCG databases from the Max Planck Institute, Berlin (http://www.mpiib-berlin.mpg.de/2D-PAGE/) and a *M. tuberculosis* culture filtrate database from

From: *Methods in Molecular Medicine*, vol. 54: *Mycobacterium Tuberculosis Protocols*
Edited by: T. Parish and N. G. Stoker © Humana Press Inc., Totowa, NJ

the Statens Serum Institute, Denmark (http://www.ssi.dk/en/forskning/tbimmun/tbhjemme.htm).

1.1. Two-Dimensional Gel Electrophoresis

There have been numerous publications and developments in 2D gel electrophoresis since O'Farrell and Klose first devised the technique *(8,9)*, although the principle remains the same. Proteins are first separated according to their isoelectric point (pI) by isoelectric focusing (IEF) and secondly according to their molecular mass by sodium dodecyl sulfate polyacrylamide gel electrophoresis (SDS-PAGE) *(22)*. Originally, the first dimension separation was performed in polyacrylamide gels cast in narrow tubes containing carrier ampholytes. A recent modification is the introduction of immobilized pH gradients (IPG) *(23)* on plastic-backed strips. These have the advantages of giving a more reproducible separation since the fixed pH gradient does not drift, extending the basic pH limit of IEF, and allowing increased sample loading capacity *(24)*. The high reproducibility of IPGs extends to interlaboratory comparisons *(25,26)*, making them useful for the development of 2D protein databases. However, rod gels are still used effectively by a number of labs *(27–29)*. The second dimension polyacrylamide slab gels are prepared as either single-concentration or gradient-polyacrylamide gels, which can be optimized to separate proteins over a specific molecular weight range. Many proteome map databases are now accessible via the World Wide Web *(30)*. These include the SWISS–2DPAGE database *(31,32)* (http://www.expasy.ch/ch2d/2d-index.html) and HSC-2DPAGE *(33,34)* (http://www.harefield.nthames. nhs.uk/nhli/protein/index.html).

1.2. Visualization

Many of the methods for detection of proteins in 2D polyacrylamide gels have been reviewed recently *(35,36)*. The most commonly employed techniques include Coomassie Brilliant Blue R250 and silver staining, silver being the more sensitive, detecting as little as 2–5 ng of protein *(37,38)*. A modified silver stain method has recently been shown to be compatible with in-gel proteolytic cleavage and mass spectrometry *(39)*, but has the disadvantage of being less sensitive than longer staining protocols. *M. tuberculosis* protein spots on 2D gels have often been visualized by autoradiography or phosphorimage analysis following in vivo radiolabeling with radioisotopes such as [^{35}S]methionine or [^{35}S]cysteine *(18–20)*. Phosphorimage analysis has the advantage of giving improved dynamic range, which is an important consideration in the quantitative analysis of protein synthesis *(40,41)*, but only allows the detection of recently synthesized, thiol-containing proteins.

1.3. Image Analysis

Effective image analysis relies upon highly reproducible 2D gels with low background staining. There are several different systems available for the digitization of gel images, ranging from charge coupled device (CCD) cameras, laser densitometers, and phosphorimagers to flat-bed scanners. Software packages for the analysis of 2D gels are capable of spot detection, background subtraction, spot matching, and quantitative analysis of the data produced. Commonly used software packages include Phoretix–2D (Nonlinear Dynamics, Newcastle, UK) and Melanie II (Bio-Rad, Hemel Hempstead, Herts, UK) *(42)*.

1.4. Protein Identification by Mass Spectrometry

Matrix-assisted laser desorption-ionization-time-of-flight (MALDI-TOF) mass spectrometry (MS) is most often employed as the initial technique in a hierarchical approach to protein identification *(3)*. Prior to analysis, proteins are proteolytically cleaved within gel pieces usually using trypsin *(39,43)*. The resulting MALDI mass spectrum consists of a series of highly accurate peptide masses, which provide a peptide mass "fingerprint" of the protein of interest. These peptide masses are then used to search against a computer-generated list formed from the simulated digest of a protein database with the same enzyme *(44–48)*. Protein hits are ranked according to the agreement between their measured and calculated peptide mass maps. In the case of proteins from completely sequenced genomes such as *M. tuberculosis*, these data alone may be sufficient for complete identification *(49)*. If, however, identification is not achieved at this stage, it becomes necessary to generate some amino acid sequence data. Techniques used for this purpose include nanoelectrospray tandem mass spectrometry *(50)* and liquid chromatography coupled to electrospray tandem mass spectrometry *(51)*. Several database search strategies exist for the identification of proteins based on tandem mass spectrometry analyses *(52)*. The most commonly applied techniques include the "peptide sequence tag" approach *(53)*, which combines partial amino acid sequence with mass information, and the SEQUEST algorithm *(51)*, which involves searching uninterpreted peptide fragmentation data against predicted spectra for peptides derived from database entries. Electrospray tandem mass spectrometry is also a particularly useful technique for the analysis of posttranslational modifications *(54,55)*.

The methods described in this chapter focus on the two-dimensional separation of *M. tuberculosis* proteins using the IPG strip technology in the first dimension, followed by conventional vertical SDS-PAGE with silver stain visualization. It is not meant as a definitive guide to 2D electrophoresis, for which there are various other sources of information available (*56,57*; http://

www.expasy.ch/ch2d/protocols/). Protein spot analysis by MALDI mass spectrometry is also covered. Optimal sample preparation plays a pivotal role in successful 2D analysis.

2. Materials (*see* Note 1)

2.1. IPG Strip Rehydration

1. IPG strip rehydration solution (50 mL): Dissolve 8 *M* urea (24 g), 2% (w/v) 3-[(3-cholamidopropyl)-dimethylammonio]-1-propanesulphonate (CHAPS) (1 g), 10 m*M* dithiothreitol (DTT) (80 mg), trace amount of bromophenol blue in water. Make solution up to 49 mL and aliquot into 0.98 mL aliquots. Store at –20°C. Add 2% (v/v) IPG buffer (20 µL) to each aliquot just prior to use and mix (*see* **Note 2**).
2. IPG strips (Amersham Pharmacia Biotech, Little Chalfont, Bucks, UK) (*see* **Note 3**).
3. Immobiline DryStrip Reswelling tray (Amersham Pharmacia Biotech).
4. DryStrip cover fluid (Amersham Pharmacia Biotech) (*see* **Note 4**).

2.2. First Dimension: Isoelectric Focusing (IEF)

1. IEF sample loading buffer (50 mL): 8 *M* urea (27 g), 4% (w/v) CHAPS (2 g), 40 m*M* Tris base (210 mg), 65 m*M* DTT (0.5 g), trace amount of bromophenol blue. Store in 1 mL aliquots at –20°C (*see* **Note 5**).
2. Multiphor II electrophoresis unit (Amersham Pharmacia Biotech) (*see* **Note 6**).
3. MultiTemp III Thermostatic circulator (Amersham Pharmacia Biotech).
4. EPS 3501 XL power supply (Amersham Pharmacia Biotech) (*see* **Note 7**).
5. Immobiline DryStrip kit (Amersham Pharmacia Biotech) (*see* **Note 8**).
6. DryStrip cover fluid (Amersham Pharmacia Biotech).
7. 25 × 200 mm culture tubes (*see* **Note 9**).

2.3. Second Dimension: Polyacrylamide Gel Electrophoresis (PAGE)

2.3.1. IPG Strip Equilibration

1. 1.5 *M* Tris-HCl, pH 8.8 (72.66 g/400 mL) (*see* **Note 10**).
2. IPG strip equilibration buffer 1 (40 mL): 0.375 *M* Tris-HCl, pH 8.8 (10 mL 1.5 *M* Tris-HCl, pH 8.8), 6 *M* urea (14.4 g), 30% (v/v) glycerol (12 mL), 2% (w/v) SDS (0.8 g). Add 2% (w/v) DTT (0.8 g) just prior to use (*see* **Note 11**).
3. IPG strip equilibration buffer 2 (40 mL): 0.375 *M* Tris-HCl, pH 8.8 (10 mL 1.5 *M* Tris-HCl, pH 8.8), 6 *M* urea (14.4 g), 30% (v/v) glycerol (12 mL), 2% (w/v) SDS (0.8 g). Add 2.5% (w/v) iodoacetamide (1 g) just prior to use (*see* **Note 11**).

2.3.2. Polyacrylamide Gel Preparation

1. 30% (v/v) acrylamide/0.8% (w/v) piperazine diacrylamide (PDA) stock solution: Dissolve 8 g PDA (Bio-Rad) in 750 mL acrylamide (40% (w/v) solution,

Amersham Pharmacia Biotech) and make up to 1 L with water. Store at 4°C (*see* **Note 12**).

2. 12% (w/v) acrylamide gel (720 mL): 1.5 *M* Tris-HCl, pH 8.8 (180.48 mL), 30% (w/v) acrylamide/0.8% (w/v) PDA (288 mL), 5 m*M* sodium thiosulfate (2.84 mL 20% (w/v) solution), water (243 mL). Mix, degas, then add 0.05% (v/v) TEMED (369 µL) and 0.08% (w/v) ammonium persulfate (APS) (5.54 mL of 10% (w/v) solution) with stirring (*see* **Note 13**).
3. Water saturated butan-1-ol.
4. Multigel casting chamber (Bio-Rad) (*see* **Note 14**).

2.3.3. Second Dimension SDS-PAGE

1. Vertical gel electrophoresis equipment (Bio-Rad) (*see* **Note 14**).
2. Power supply.
3. MultiTemp III Thermostatic circulator (Amersham Pharmacia Biotech).
4. Cathode buffer (1 L): 192 *M* glycine (14.4 g), pH 8.3 with Tris base, 0.1% (w/v) SDS (1 g) (*see* **Note 15**).
5. 2X anode buffer (2L): 0.375 *M* base (181.65 g), pH to 8.8 with acetic acid (*see* **Note 15**).
6. Agarose overlay: 0.5% (w/v) agarose in cathode buffer, trace bromophenol blue (*see* **Note 16**).
7. Nalgene staining boxes (Sigma, Poole, Dorset, UK).

2.4. Visualization: Silver Staining

*2.4.1. Hochstrasser Method (*see **Note 17***)*

1. 40% (v/v) ethanol, 10% (v/v) acetic acid.
2. 5% (v/v) ethanol, 5% (v/v) acetic acid.
3. 0.5 *M* sodium acetate (42.3 g/L), 1% (v/v) glutaraldehyde (20 mL/L of 50% (v/v) solution).
4. 0.05% (w/v) (0.5 g/L) naphthalene disulfonic acid disodium salt.
5. Silver stain (1 L): dissolve 8 g silver nitrate in 40 mL water, add to 213 mL water, 13.3 mL ammonium hydroxide, 2 mL 10 *M* NaOH slowly with stirring (*see* **Note 18**). Make up to 1 L with water.
6. Developer (1 L): 0.005% (w/v) citric acid (1 mL of 5% (w/v) solution), 0.1% (v/v) formaldehyde (2.7 mL of 37% (v/v) solution).
7. Stop solution (1 L): 5% (w/v) Tris base (50 g), 2% (v/v) acetic acid (20 mL).
8. 35% (v/v) ethanol, 5% (v/v) glycerol.

*2.4.2. Silver Stain for Subsequent Mass Spectrometry (*see **Note 17***)*

1. 50% (v/v) methanol, 5% (v/v) acetic acid.
2. 50% (v/v) methanol.
3. 0.02% (w/v) sodium thiosulfate (200 mg/L)
4. 0.1% (w/v) silver nitrate (1 g/L)- chilled (*see* **Note 19**).
5. Developer (1 L): 0.015% (v/v) formaldehyde (400 mL of 37% (v/v) solution) in 2% (w/v) sodium carbonate (20 g).

6. 5% (v/v) acetic acid.
7. 1% (v/v) acetic acid.

2.5. Image Analysis (see Subheading 1.4.)

1. CCD camera, densitometer, phosphorimager or flat-bed scanner.
2. Image analysis software.

2.6. Sample Preparation for Mass Spectrometry (see Note 20)

1. 100 m*M* ammonium bicarbonate (0.3953 g/50 mL).
2. Acetonitrile.
3. DTT solution: 1.5 mg/mL in 100 m*M* ammonium bicarbonate.
4. Iodoacetamide solution: 12 mg/mL in 100 m*M* ammonium bicarbonate.
5. Digestion buffer (1 mL): 50 m*M* ammonium bicarbonate (500 µL of 100 m*M* ammonium bicarbonate), 5 m*M* calcium chloride (50 µL of 100 m*M* solution) (*see* **Note 21**), water (450 µL).
6. Trypsin (unmodified, Boehringer sequencing grade, Boehringer Mannheim, Lewes, East Sussex, UK) 15 µg in 15 µL 0.01% (v/v) TFA. Store at –20°C. Add 100 µL of digestion buffer just prior to use (*see* **Note 22**).

2.7. Protein Identification: MALDI Mass Spectrometry

1. MALDI-TOF instrument with delayed extraction source (*see* **Note 23**).
2. Matrix solution: saturated solution of α-cyano-4-hydroxycinnamic acid in acetone mixed in a 4:1 ratio with a 10 g/L solution of nitrocellulose in acetone/isopropanol (1:1) (*see* **Note 24**).
3. Wash solution: 5% (v/v) formic acid.

3. Methods

3.1. IPG Strip Rehydration (see Note 25)

1. Just prior to use, defrost the rehydration solution and add the appropriate IPG buffer (*see* **Note 2**).
2. Ensure that the reswelling tray is level and pipet the appropriate amount of rehydration solution into each slot (*see* **Note 26**).
3. Remove the protective cover from the IPG strip. Position the IPG strip gel side down and pointed end of strip against the sloped end of the slot.
4. Overlay each strip with 2 to 3 mL of IPG cover fluid (*see* **Note 27**).
5. Slide the lid on the tray and allow the strip to rehydrate at room temperature for a minimum of 10 h. Overnight is recommended.

3.2. First Dimension: Isoelectric Focusing (IEF) (see Note 25)

1. Set the temperature on the MultiTemp III circulator to 17°C.
2. Pipet approx 10 mL of IPG cover fluid onto the cooling plate of the Multiphor II.
3. Assemble the Immobiline DryStrip tray and DryStrip aligner with the grooved side upward. Position onto the cooling plate so that the anode (positive) electrode

connection is positioned at the top of the plate by the cooling tubes. Connect the red and black electrode leads.

4. Cut two IEF electrode strips to a length of approx 110 mm. Place them on a clean, flat surface (e.g., glass plate) and soak each with 0.5 mL distilled water. Blot to remove excess water (*see* **Note 28**).
5. Remove an IPG strip from its slot in the reswelling tray using forceps. Transfer the strip to a groove on the DryStrip aligner with the pointed (acidic) end at the anode.
6. Repeat with all strips, placing into adjacent grooves and ensuring that the anodic gel edges are aligned.
7. Place the moistened electrode strips across each end of the IPG strips so that they are partially in contact with the gel surface of the IPG strips.
8. Align each electrode over the corresponding electrode strip and press down to ensure contact.
9. Position the sample cup bar just above the cathodic (negative) electrode so that the spacer just touches the electrode. Position sample cups on the bar so that they are aligned with the strips but not touching the gel. Press the cups down gently, ensuring good contact with the IPG strips.
10. In order to check that the cups are positioned correctly, pipet IPG cover fluid into each cup and check for leakage. Carefully reposition cups if they do leak and test again.
11. Pour IPG cover fluid into the tray to completely cover the strips and sample cups.
12. Pipet the samples (max 100 µL) into each cup (*see* **Note 29**).
13. Connect leads to power supply. Run the isoelectric focusing protocol as follows: Phase 1 (300 V, 10 mA, 10 W, 2 h), phase 2 (1000 V, 10 mA, 10 W, 1 h), phase 3 (3500 V, 10 mA, 10 W, 22 h) (*see* **Note 30**).
14. After IEF, proceed to the second dimension separation or store strips at –20°C (*see* **Note 9**).

3.3. Second Dimension: Polyacrylamide Gel Electrophoresis (PAGE)

3.3.1. IPG Strip Equilibration

1. The IPG strips should be placed in individual tubes with the support backing toward the tube wall.
2. Add the DTT-containing equilibration buffer 1 to each tube (10 mL per 18 cm strip).
3. Place tube on its side on a rocker and equilibrate for 15 min.
4. Remove the DTT solution and replace with the iodoacetamide-containing equilibration buffer 2. Equilibrate for 15 min as previously.

3.3.2. Preparation of Acrylamide Gels (see **Note 31**)

1. Prepare desired percentage acrylamide gel solution and cast gels as required. Gels should be overlaid with water saturated butan-1-ol solution (*see* **Note 32**).

2. After allowing a minimum of 1–2 h for polymerization, the overlay solution should be removed and the gel surface washed with distilled water.
3. Gels can be stored, wrapped in cling-film at 4°C for a maximum of 1 wk.

3.3.3. Running the Second Dimension

1. Set cooling temperature to 10°C (*see* **Note 33**).
2. Following strip equilibration, remove the iodoacetamide solution. Cut the IPG strip to size (*see* **Note 34**) and position between the glass plates onto the surface of the second dimension gel making sure that the plastic backing is against one of the glass plates. With a thin spatula, gently push the IPG strip so that it is in contact with the second dimension gel along its complete length. Ensure that no air bubbles are trapped between the strip and second dimension gel.
3. Overlay the strip with 0.5% agarose solution in cathode buffer (*see* **Note 16**).
4. Fill the lower reservoir with anode buffer and the upper reservoir with cathode buffer (*see* **Note 35**).
5. Run gels at constant current and stop when the dye front is approx 1–2 mm from the bottom of the gel (*see* **Note 36**).

3.4. Visualization: Silver Staining

3.4.1. Hochstrasser Method

1. Wash gels in water for 5 min.
2. Fix gels in 40% (v/v) ethanol, 10% (v/v) acetic acid for 1 h.
3. Soak gels in 5% (v/v) ethanol, 5% (v/v) acetic acid for 3 h or overnight (*see* **Note 37**)
4. Wash in water for 5 min.
5. Soak in 0.5 *M* sodium acetate, 1% (v/v) glutaraldehyde for 30 min.
6. Wash in water for 3 × 10 min.
7. Soak in 0.05% (w/v) naphthalene sulfonic acid for 2 × 30 min.
8. Rinse in water for 4 × 15 min. During this step prepare the silver stain.
9. Stain for 25 min.
10. Wash in water for 4 × 4 min.
11. Develop in 0.005% (w/v) citric acid, 0.1% (v/v) formaldehyde.
12. Stop in 5% (w/v) Tris base, 2% (v/v) acetic acid before the background starts to color and gels overstain (*see* **Note 38**). Pour a small amount of stop solution into developing gel to stop reaction. Discard this solution and then soak in stop solution for approx 1h.
13. Store gels in 35% (v/v) ethanol, 5% (v/v) glycerol.

3.4.2. Silver Stain for Subsequent Mass Spectrometry (see **Note 39**)

1. Fix gels in 50% (v/v) methanol, 5% (v/v) acetic acid for 1 h.
2. Soak gels in 50% (v/v) methanol overnight.
3. Wash with water for 3 × 10 min.
4. Sensitize by incubation in 0.02% (w/v) sodium thiosulfate for 2 × 15 min.

5. Rinse in chilled water for 3 × 10 min.
6. Submerge gels in chilled 0.1% (w/v) silver nitrate solution and incubate for 1–1.5 h at 4°C with shaking.
7. Discard the silver nitrate solution.
8. Rinse gels with water for 2 × 1 min.
9. Develop in 0.015% (v/v) formaldehyde in 2% (w/v) sodium carbonate.
10. Discard the developer after it turns yellow and replace with a fresh portion.
11. Discard the developer and wash gel with 5% (v/v) acetic acid.
12. Store silver-stained gel in 1% (v/v) acetic acid at 4°C.

3.5. Image Analysis (see Subheading 1.4.)

1. Scan gels using digitization equipment available.
2. Analyze protein spot patterns using software package of choice or by eye.

3.6. Sample Preparation from Polyacrylamide Gels for Mass Spectrometry

3.6.1. Protein Band/Spot Excision

1. Excise protein spot from the gel with scalpel, cutting as close to the edge as possible.
2. Cut into small pieces (approx 2 × 2 mm) and transfer into a 0.5 mL Eppendorf tube.

3.6.2. Reduction and Alkylation

1. Wash gel particles with 100–150 μL water for 5 min. Spin down the gel pieces and remove liquid (*see* **Note 40**).
2. Add acetonitrile to approx 3–4 times the volume of the gel pieces and leave for 10–15 min until gel pieces have shrunk (*see* **Note 41**). Dry the gel pieces in a vacuum centrifuge.
3. Swell pieces in DTT solution by adding enough liquid to cover the gel pieces and incubate for 30 min at 56°C.
4. Spin down the gel particles and remove excess liquid. Shrink the gel pieces with acetonitrile.
5. Replace the acetonitrile with iodoacetamide solution. Incubate for 20 min at room temperature in the dark.
6. Remove the iodoacetamide solution. Wash gel particles with 150–200 μL 100 m*M* ammonium bicarbonate for 15 min.
7. Spin down gel particles and remove all liquid. Shrink the gel pieces with acetonitrile.
8. Spin down gel particles and remove all liquid. Dry the gel pieces in a vacuum centrifuge.

3.6.3. Washing of Gel Pieces (Coomassie-Stained Gels Only)

1. If gel pieces are still blue, rehydrate in 100–150 μL 100 m*M* ammonium bicarbonate and after 15 min, add an equal volume of acetonitrile.
2. Shake for 15–20 min, then spin down and remove all liquid.

3. Shrink the gel pieces with acetonitrile. Repeat above steps until particles are colorless.
4. Dry the gel pieces in a vacuum centrifuge.

3.6.4. In-Gel Digestion with Trypsin

1. Rehydrate the gel particles in the digestion buffer containing trypsin on ice for 30–45 min. After 15–20 min check samples and add more buffer if all liquid has been absorbed by the gel pieces.
2. Remove any remaining supernatant. Add 5–25 μL of the digestion buffer without trypsin to cover gel pieces and keep them wet during enzyme cleavage.
3. Leave samples at 37°C overnight.

3.7. Protein Identification: MALDI Mass Spectrometry

1. After overnight incubation, spin down droplets condensed on tube lid.
2. Spot 0.6 μL matrix material onto MALDI sample target.
3. Take a 0.5 μL aliquot of the digest mixture and load into a 0.5 μL droplet of 5% (v/v) formic acid previously applied to the matrix.
4. Air-dry at room temperature and wash with 1 μL 5% (v/v) formic acid prior to insertion into the instrument.
5. Acquire mass spectrum (*see* **Note 42**).
6. Search peptide mass list against protein database (*see* **Note 43**).

4. Notes

1. It is important to adopt clean laboratory working practices to reduce the risk of contaminants such as keratin, which may result in spurious protein spots and also contaminate mass spectra. Gloves must always be worn and equipment washed and rinsed well with distilled water. The highest quality reagents and purest water available should always be used.
2. The optimal rehydration solution will depend on the specific protein solubility of the sample. Urea solubilizes and denatures proteins. The urea concentration can be increased to 9 or 9.8 *M* if necessary to aid solubilization. Detergent is used to solubilize hydrophobic proteins and prevent protein aggregation. Only nonionic and zwitterionic detergents may be used. Triton X–100 or NP–40 may be used in place of CHAPS. Reducing agents are required to break disulfide bonds and allow complete unfolding of proteins. Dithioerythritol (DTE) or 2-mercaptoethanol may be used in place of DTT. However, higher concentrations of 2-mercaptoethanol are required and impurities may result in artifacts ***(58)***. The IPG buffer is a carrier ampholyte mixture which aids separation and sample solubility. IPG buffers specific for each pH range are available. Bromophenol blue acts as a tracking dye and can be used to monitor progress of IEF.
3. IPG strips are available from Amersham Pharmacia Biotech in a number of lengths and pH ranges. We have found pH 4.0–7.0 (linear) and pH 3.0–10.0 (nonlinear) to be the most useful for separation of *M. tuberculosis* proteins (**Fig. 1**). We routinely use 18 cm strips on 20 × 20 cm large format second dimension gels.

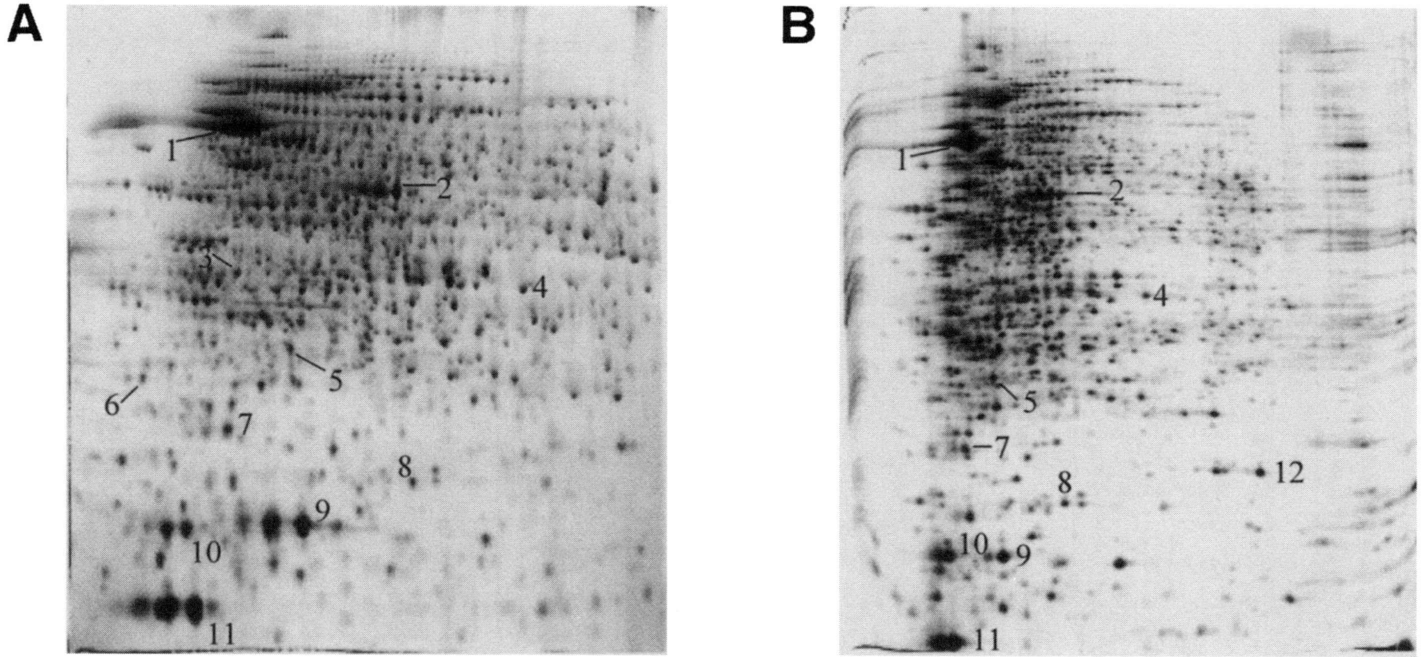

Fig. 1. Silver-stained 2D gels of *M. tuberculosis* H37Rv. Proteins were extracted from a late-log phase culture of *M. tuberculosis*. First dimension separation was performed using 18 cm IPG strips. Proteins were then separated on 12% polyacrylamide gels in the second dimension. Some protein spots which have been identified by MALDI mass spectrometry are labeled (1–12) and their identities listed in **Table 1**. **(A)** pH 4–7 separation. **(B)** pH 3–10 nonlinear separation.

Table 1
Proteins Identified by MALDI Mass Spectrometry of Spots Excised from 2D Gels of *M. tuberculosis*

Spot[a]	Protein	Rv no.	Accession no.	MW (kDa)	pI
1	GroEL-2	Rv0440	P06806	56.6	4.69
2	EF-TU	Rv0685	P31501	43.6	5.13
3	Antigen 84	Rv2145c	P46816	28.3	4.57
4	35 kDa antigen	Rv2744c	P31511	29.3	5.58
5	22.7 kDa protein	Rv1626	006143	22.7	4.93
6	AhpC	Rv2428	Q57348	21.6	4.17
7	20.4 kDa protein	Rv3841	P96237	20.4	4.48
8	18.6 kDa protein	Rv2140c	006235	18.6	5.28
9	16 kDa antigen	Rv2031c	P30223	16.1	4.74
10	50s ribosomal protein	Rv0652	P37381	13.4	4.33
11	GroES	Rv3418c	P09621	10.8	4.35
12	AhpD	Rv2429	Q57353	18.8	6.60

[a]Numbers correspond to spot labeling on **Fig. 1**.

4. Dow Corning 200 silicone fluid can also be used in place of the DryStrip cover fluid.
5. The sample buffer should always include the denaturing agent urea at a concentration of at least 8 *M*. Thiourea is often used in addition to urea to aid the solubility of membrane proteins ***(59–62)***. The zwitterionic detergent CHAPS helps to ensure complete sample solubilization and prevents aggregation. If the mycobacterial proteins have been extracted in the presence of SDS, this must be diluted out with sample buffer containing an excess of a zwitterionic or nonionic detergent. SDS forms negatively charged complexes with proteins which will not focus properly during IEF. The final concentration of SDS must be 0.25% or lower and the ratio of the excess detergent to SDS should be at least 8:1.
6. The protocol described uses the Multiphor II electrophoresis unit and Immobiline DryStrip kit. An alternative would be to use the IPGphor electrophoresis system which enables strip rehydration and focusing to be performed in one step. Power supply and temperature control are built into the latter.
7. The power supply used must provide a minimum of 3500 V and be able to run at low current. The IPG gels have very low conductivity and therefore the current is often in the low μA range. The low-current shut-off must be bypassed by turning the current check option off.
8. The Immobiline DryStrip kit includes DryStrip tray, DryStrip aligner, electrodes, sample cup bar, sample cups, and electrode strips.
9. Culture tubes (25 × 20 mm) are useful for the storage of IPG strips after IEF. Plastic document wallets can also be used to store multiple strips. Strips should

be stored at –20°C, or for longer term storage, at –80°C. The culture tubes are also useful to hold individual strips during the equilibration procedure.

10. Tris-HCl should be made fresh on day of use. This solution is also used to make the polyacrylamide gels.
11. The equilibration step saturates the IPG strip with the SDS buffer system required for second dimension separation. The Tris maintains the correct pH for electrophoresis. Both urea and glycerol reduce the effects of electroendosmosis and improve transfer of proteins into the second dimension gel. SDS is required to denature proteins and form negatively-charged protein-SDS complexes. The amount of SDS bound to a protein, and hence the additional negative charge is directly proportional to the mass of the protein and therefore allows separation of proteins according to their molecular mass. DTT maintains proteins in a reduced, denatured state. Iodoacetamide is introduced in a second equilibration step. This alkylates thiol groups on proteins, preventing their reoxidation during electrophoresis and thus reduces streaking and other artefacts. 40 mL of equilibration solution is sufficient for four IPG strips (10 mL per strip).
12. Piperazine diacrylamide (PDA) is a crosslinker, which gives a reduction in diamine silver stain background, increased resolution, and higher gel strength ***(63,64)***.
13. Gels are not polymerized in the presence of SDS. This helps prevent micelles containing acrylamide monomer forming and therefore increases the homogeneity of pore size and reduces the concentration of unpolymerized monomer in the polyacrylamide. The SDS in the cathode buffer is sufficient to maintain the necessary negative charge on the proteins. A 12% single percentage gel gives good resolution of *M. tuberculosis* cellular proteins from approx 10–120 kDa (**Fig. 1**). The percentage acrylamide can be increased or decreased depending on the mass range required. Gradient gels can also be used, giving a wider overall separation range but are more difficult to cast. Volumes given produce 720 mL of solution which is sufficient to cast 12 gels (20 × 20 cm, 1.5 mm thick) using the Bio-Rad multicasting chamber. It is most convenient to cast multiple gels within a multicasting chamber and this also aids gel reproducibility. Either 1.0 or 1.5 mm gels can be cast. Thicker gels are more easy to handle and give higher protein capacity. Thinner gels generally stain and destain more quickly and give less background.
14. Both Bio-Rad and Hoeffer supply vertical electrophoresis systems suitable for 2D electrophoresis. Different gel size formats are available as are systems capable of running several gel simultaneously. We routinely use 20 × 20 cm gels. Multigel casting chambers are also available from the equipment suppliers.
15. This buffer system improves spot resolution ***(65)***. Anode and cathode buffers are best used fresh and should not be stored for more than 1 wk. pH cathode buffer with Tris and then add SDS as this can interfere with the pH electrode.
16. Agarose overlay is optional but does help to keep the IPG strip in position, preventing it from moving or floating in the cathode buffer. The combination of the IPG strip and agarose avoids the need for a stacking gel. The agarose should be fully melted during IPG strip equilibration and allowed to cool to approx 56°C

before use. Slowly pipet enough to seal the strip and allow to solidify. Bromophenol blue is used to track the progress of electrophoresis and if agarose is not used this should be included in the final equilibration step.

17. The ammoniacal silver-stain method developed by Hochstrasser (http://www.expasy.ch/ch2d/protocols/) is extremely sensitive and should be used in order to visualize the maximum number of proteins for initial proteome comparison. Unfortunately, the glutaraldehyde step may result in covalent modification of proteins, thus leaving them unamenable to mass spectrometry. An alternative staining method should therefore be used when it is intended to analyze protein spots by mass spectrometry (**Subheadings 2.4.2.** and **3.4.2.**) *(39)*. This stain is generally less sensitive which is why it is preferable to first visualize gels using the ammoniacal stain, then rerun gels for sequencing of spots. 1 L of solution is sufficient to stain four large format gels.
18. It is important to ensure that the silver-stain solution remains clear. When the silver nitrate is added, a brown precipitate appears which disappears on stirring.
19. The use of chilled solutions minimizes protein oxidation and is therefore advantageous for subsequent mass spectrometry. Both the silver nitrate solution and distilled water used for washing the gels should be placed at 4°C prior to commencing the staining procedure.
20. Solutions for the reduction, alkylation, and proteolysis of protein spots prior to mass spectrometry should be made fresh on day of use to avoid contamination.
21. Calcium chloride is included in the digestion buffer to limit trypsin autolysis.
22. Trypsin is the most commonly used protease since it generates peptides in the 800–2500 Dalton mass range which is optimal for both MALDI and electrospray mass spectrometry. The advantage of using unmodified trypsin is that autolytic peptides present in mass spectra can be matched to the trypsinogen sequences in the database. Other proteases may also be employed for the in-gel digestion procedure if desired.
23. MALDI-TOF instrument manufacturers include Micromass (Manchester, UK), Perseptive Biosystems (Framingham, MA) and Bruker (Bremen, Germany). The delayed extraction ion source provides a high degree of peak resolution and improved signal-to-noise ratio, resulting in greatly improved mass accuracy and hence improved database search specificity *(66)*.
24. α-Cyano-4-hydroxycinnamic acid is routinely used for the fast evaporation matrix deposition method described here *(67,68)*. Sinapinic acid, ferulic acid, and 2,4,6-trihydroxyacetophenone may also be used. The addition of nitrocellulose results in improved performance and tolerance to contaminants.
25. Detailed experimental protocols for 2D electrophoresis using Amersham Pharmacia Biotech IPG strips are provided in their brochure *(56)*.
26. The amount of rehydration solution to be used varies with the IPG strip length. For 18 cm strips 350 μL should be used. It is important that the reswelling tray is level in order to ensure even reswelling of strips.
27. The cover fluid is necessary to prevent urea crystallization and evaporation.

28. It is important that the electrode strips are damp but not wet as excess water can cause streaking.
29. To avoid protein precipitation, it is best to load a maximum of 60–100 µg protein per 100 µL. For spot identification by mass spectrometry it is often advantageous to increase sample loading. This may be achieved either by including the sample in the rehydration solution ***(69)*** or by loading the sample repeatedly during IEF.
30. The low initial voltage reduces sample aggregation and aids entry of proteins into the IPG strip. Optimal focusing conditions vary with the nature and amount of sample loaded. As the IEF proceeds, the bromophenol blue dye will move toward the anode and should give a sharp line.
31. Polyacrylamide gels can also be purchased precast in a variety of formats from several suppliers including Amersham Pharmacia Biotech, Bio-Rad, and Novex.
32. Overlaying with water-saturated butanol reduces gel exposure to oxygen which inhibits polymerization and helps to create a flat gel surface.
33. Temperature should be controlled using a thermostatic circulator as this improves gel reproducibility and reduces gel distortion due to heating.
34. For some second dimension gels, it may be necessary to cut the IPG strips to length. In this case, the pointed plastic backing only should be cut from the anode end and any extra should be cut from the cathode end of the strip.
35. For the Bio-Rad X-Cell II system approx 3.5 L of anode buffer and 400 mL of cathode buffer is required.
36. The current per gel will vary according to gel thickness and the system used. We use 1.5 mm thick gels and run at a current of 40 mA per gel as recommended by Hochstrasser (http://www.expasy.ch/ch2d/protocols/). Running time is approx 4–5 h.
37. Since this is a lengthy silver-stain method, it is most convenient to leave the gels to soak overnight at this stage.
38. The stop solution should be prepared in advance as the development can proceed rapidly.
39. This silver-stain protocol is an in-house modified version of that published by Shevchenko et al. ***(39)*** and has been optimized for the staining of 2D gels.
40. Gel loader pipets are the most convenient to use to avoid inadvertent removal of gel pieces while removing solutions.
41. After shrinking with acetonitrile gel pieces become white and stick together.
42. The highest degree of peptide mass accuracy is achieved by internal mass calibration using the matrix ion peak at *m/z* 1060.10 and trypsin autolysis ions at *m/z* 2163.06 and *m/z* 2289.15. In cases where these ions are not apparent, spectra may be calibrated externally or internally by the addition of peptide standards.
43. Proteins are identified by peptide mass fingerprinting ***(44–48)***. Several database search programs are available as stand-alone packages or via the internet. These include PeptideSearch (http://www.mann.embl-heidelberg.de/), ProFound (http://prowl.rockefeller.edu/cgi-bin/ProFound), ProteinProspector (http://falcon.ludwig.ucl.ac.uk/mshome3.2.htm), and Mascot (http://www.matrixscience.com/cgi/index.pl?page=/home.html). Generally, a sequence coverage of 15% or better

is required to give an unambiguous identification. A mass accuracy of 50 ppm should also be achieved. In some cases an unambiguous identification may not be obtained, for example, in the case of small basic or hydrophobic proteins and for low level proteins. In this case, the sample should be taken for further analysis by electrospray tandem mass spectrometry ***(50,51)***.

Acknowledgment

Many thanks to Hannah Wilson for all her work on the silver-stain protocol optimization.

References

1. Wasinger, V. C., Cordwell, S. J., Cerpa-Poljak, A., Yan, J. X., Gooley, A. A., Wilkins, M. R., Duncan, M. W., Harris, R., Williams, K. L., and Humphery-Smith, I. (1995) Progress with gene-product mapping of the Mollicutes: *Mycoplasma genitalium. Electrophoresis* **16,** 1090–1094.
2. Wilkins, M. R., Pasquali, C., Appel, R. D., Ou, K., Golaz, O., Sanchez, J. C., Yan, J. X., Gooley, A. A., Hughes, G., Humphery-Smith, I., Williams, K. L., and Hochstrasser, D. F. (1996) From proteins to proteomes: large scale protein identification by two-dimensional electrophoresis and amino acid analysis. *Biotechnology* **14,** 61–65.
3. Humphery-Smith, I., Cordwell, S. J., and Blackstock, W. P. (1997) Proteome research: Complementarity and limitations with respect to the RNA and DNA-worlds. *Electrophoresis* **18,** 1217–1242.
4. Pennington, S. R., Wilkins, M. R., Hochstrasser, D. H., and Dunn, M. J. (1997) Proteome analysis: from protein characterisation to biological function. *Trends Cell* Biol. **7,** 168–173.
5. Wilkins, M. R., Williams, K. L., Appel, R. D., and Hochstrasser, D. H., eds. (1997) *Proteome Research: New Frontiers in Functional Genomics*. Springer-Verlag.
6. Cash, P. (1998) Characterisation of bacterial proteomes by two-dimensional electrophoresis. *Anal. Chim. Acta.* **372,** 121–145.
7. Klose, J. (1999) Genotypes and phenotypes. *Electrophoresis* **20,** 643–652.
8. O'Farrell, P. H. (1975) High resolution two-dimensional electrophoresis of proteins. *J. Biol. Chem.* **250,** 4007–4021.
9. Klose, J. (1975) Protein mapping by combined isoelectric focusing and electrophoresis of mouse tissues. A novel approach to testing for induced point mutations in mammals. *Humangenetik* **26,** 231–243.
10. Jungblut, P. and Thiede, B. (1997) Protein identification from 2-DE gels by MALDI mass spectrometry. *Mass Spec. Rev.* **16,** 145–162.
11. Roepstorff, P. (1997) Mass spectrometry in protein studies from genome to function. *Curr. Opin. Biotechnol.* **8,** 6–13.
12. Yates, J. R., III (1998) Mass spectrometry and the age of the proteome. *J. Mass Spectrom.* **33,** 1–19.
13. Cole, S. T., Brosch, R., Parkhill, J., Garnier, T., Churcher, C., Harris, D., Gordon, S. V., Eiglmeier, K., Gas, S., Barry, C. E. III, Tekaia, F., Badcock, K., Basham, D.,

Brown, D., Chillingworth, T., Connor, R., Davies, R., Devlin, K., Feltwell, T., Gentles, S., Hamlin, N., Holroyd, S., Hornsby, T., Jagels, K., Krogh, A., McLean, J., Moule, S., Murphy, L., Oliver, K., Osborne, J., Quail, M. A., Rajandream, M.-A., Rojers, J., Rutter, S., Seeger, K., Skelton, J., Squares, R., Squares, S., Sulston, J. E., Taylor, K., Whitehead, S., and Barrell, B. G. (1998) Deciphering the biology of *Mycobacterium tuberculosis* from the complete genome sequence. *Nature* **393,** 537–544.

14. Urquhart, B. L., Atsalos, T. E., Roach, D., Basseal, D. J., Bjellqvist, B., Britton, W. L., and Humphery-Smith, I. (1997) "Proteomic contigs" of *Mycobacterium tuberculosis* and *Mycobacterium bovis* (BCG) using novel immobilised pH gradients. *Electrophoresis* **18,** 1384–1392.
15. Urquhart, B. L., Cordwell, S. J., and Humphery-Smith, I. (1998) Comparison of predicted and observed properties of proteins encoded in the genome of *Mycobacterium tuberculosis* H37Rv. *Biochem. Biophys. Res. Commun.* **253,** 70–79.
16. Sonnenberg, M. G. and Belisle, J. T. (1997) Definition of *Mycobacterium tuberculosis* culture filtrate proteins by two-dimensional polyacrylamide gel electrophoresis, N-terminal amino acid sequencing, and electrospray mass spectrometry. *Infect. Immun.* **65,** 4515–4524.
17. Weldingh, K., Rosenkrands, I., Jacobsen, S., Rasmussen, P. B., Elhay, M. J., and Andersen, P. (1998) Two-dimensional electrophoresis for analysis of *Mycobacterium tuberculosis* culture filtrate and purification and characterisation of six novel proteins. *Infect. Immun.* **66,** 3492–3500.
18. Lee, B. Y. and Horwitz, M. A. (1995) Identification of macrophage and stress-induced proteins of *Mycobacterium tuberculosis*. *J. Clin. Invest.* **96,** 245–249.
19. Garbe, T. R., Hibler, N. S., and Deretic, V. (1996) Response of *Mycobacterium tuberculosis* to reactive oxygen and nitrogen intermediates. *Mol. Med.* **2,** 134–142.
20. Garbe, T. R., Hibler, N. S., and Deretic, V. (1999) Response to reactive nitrogen intermediates in *Mycobacterium tuberculosis*: Induction of the 16-kilodalton α-crystallin homolog by exposure to nitric oxide donors. *Infect. Immun.* **67,** 460–465.
21. Wong, D. K., Lee, B. Y., Horwitz, M. A., and Gibson, B. W. (1999) Identification of fur, aconitase, and other proteins expressed by *Mycobacterium tuberculosis* under conditions of low and high concentrations of iron by combined two-dimensional gel electrophoresis and mass spectrometry. *Infect. Immun.* **67,** 327–336.
22. Laemmli, U. K. (1970) Cleavage of structural proteins during assembly of the head of bacteriophage T4. *Nature* **227,** 680–685.
23. Bjellqvist, B., Ek, K., Righetti, P. G., Gianazza, E., Westermeier, R., and Postel, W. (1982) Isoelectric focusing in immobilized pH gradients: principle, methodology, and some applications. *J. Biochem. Biophys. Methods* **6,** 317–339.
24. Görg, A., Postel, W., and Gunther, S. (1988) The current state of two-dimensional electrophoresis with immobilized pH gradients. *Electrophoresis* **9,** 531–546.
25. Corbett, J. M., Dunn, M. J., Posch, A., and Gorg, A. (1994) Positional reproducibility of protein spots in two-dimensional polyacrylamide gel electrophoresis using immobilised pH gradient isoelectric focusing in the first dimension: an interlaboratory comparison. *Electrophoresis* **15,** 1205–1211.

26. Blomberg, A., Blomberg, L., Norbeck, J., Fey, S. J., Larsen, P. M., Larsen, M., Roepstorff, P., Degand, H., Boutry, M., Posch, A., and Gorg, A. (1995) Interlaboratory reproducibility of yeast protein patterns analysed by immobilized pH gradient two-dimensional gel electrophoresis. *Electrophoresis* **16,** 1935–1945.
27. Jungblut, P. R., Otto, A., Favor, J., Lowe, M., Muller, E.-C., Kastner, M., Sperling, K., and Klose, J. (1998) Identification of mouse crystallins in 2D protein patterns by sequencing and mass spectrometry. Application to cataract mutants. *FEBS Lett.* **435,** 131–137.
28. Tietz, P., de Groen, P. C., Anderson, N. L., Sims, C., Esquer-Blasco, R., Meheus, L., Raymackers, J., Dauwe, M., and LaRusso, N. F. (1998) Cholangiocyte-specific rat liver proteins identified by establishment of a two-dimensional gel protein database. *Electrophoresis* **19,** 3207–3212.
29. Klose, J. (1999) Large-gel 2-D electrophoresis. *Methods Mol. Biol.* **112,** 147–172.
30. Appel, R. D., Bairoch, A., and Hochstrasser, D. F. (1999) 2-D databases on the World Wide Web. *Methods Mol. Biol.* **112,** 383–391.
31. Appel, R. D., Sanchez, J. C., Bairoch, A., Golaz, O., Miu, M., Vargas, J. R., and Hochstrasser, D. F. (1993) SWISS-2DPAGE: a database of two-dimensional gel electrophoresis images. *Electrophoresis* **14,** 1232–1238.
32. Sanchez, J. C., Appel, R. D., Golaz, O., Pasquali, C., Ravier, F., Bairoch, A., and Hochstrasser, D. F. (1995) Inside SWISS-2DPAGE database. *Electrophoresis* **16,** 1131–1151.
33. Corbett, J. M., Wheeler, C. H., Baker, C. S., Yacoub, M. H., and Dunn, M. J (1994) The human myocardial two-dimensional gel protein database: update 1994. *Electrophoresis* **15,** 1459–1465.
34. Evans, G., Wheeler, C. H., Corbett, J. M., and Dunn, M. J. (1997) Construction of HSC-2DPAGE: a two-dimensional gel electrophoresis database of heart proteins. *Electrophoresis* **18,** 471–479.
35. Wilkins, M. R., Sanchez, J. C., Gooley, A. A., Appel, R. D., Humphery-Smith, I., Hochstrasser, D. F., and Williams, K. L. (1995) Progress with proteome projects: why all proteins expressed by a genome should be identified and how to do it. *Biotechnol. Genet. Eng. Rev.* **13,** 19–50.
36. Wirth, P. J. and Romano, A. (1995) Staining methods in gel electrophoresis, including the use of multiple detection methods. *J. Chromatogr. A* **698,** 123–143.
37. Rabilloud, T. (1992) A comparison between low background silver diamine and silver nitrate protein stains. *Electrophoresis* **13,** 429–439.
38. Rabilloud, T., Vuillard, L., Gilly, C., and Lawrence, J. J. (1994) Silver-staining of proteins in polyacrylamide gels: a general overview. *Cell Mol. Biol.* **40,** 57–75.
39. Shevchenko, A., Wilm, M., Vorm, O., and Mann, M. (1996) Mass spectrometric sequencing of proteins from silver-stained polyacrylamide gels. *Anal. Chem.* **68,** 850–858.
40. Johnston, R. F., Pickett, S. C., and Barker, D. L. (1990) Autoradiography using storage phosphor technology. *Electrophoresis* **11,** 355–360.
41. Patterson, S. D. and Latter, G. I. (1993) Evaluation of storage phosphor imaging for quantitative analysis of 2-D gels using the Quest II system. *Biotechniques* **15,** 1076–1083.

42. Appel, R. D., Palagi, P. M., Walther, D., Vargas, J. R., Sanchez, J. C., Ravier, F., Pasquali, C., Hochstrasser, D. F. (1997) Melanie II- a third-generation software package for analysis of two-dimensional electrophoresis images: I. Features and user interface. *Electrophoresis* **18,** 2724–2734.
43. Wilm, M., Shevchenko, A., Houthaeve, T., Breit, S., Schweigerer, L., Fotsis, T., and Mann, M. (1996) Femtomole sequencing of proteins from polyacrylamide gels by nanoelectrospray mass spectrometry. *Nature* **379,** 466–469.
44. Henzel, W. J., Billeci, T. M., Stults, J. T., and Wong, S. C. (1993) Identifying proteins from two-dimensional gels by molecular mass searching of peptide fragments in protein sequence databases. *Proc. Natl. Acad. Sci. USA* **90,** 5011–5015.
45. James, P., Quadroni, M., Carafoli, E., and Gonnet, G. (1993) Protein identification by mass profile fingerprinting. *Biochem. Biophys. Res. Commun.* **195,** 58–64.
46. Mann, M., Hojrup, P., and Roepstorff, P. (1993) Use of mass spectrometric molecular weight information to identify proteins in sequence databases. *Biol. Mass Spectrom.* **22,** 338–345.
47. Pappin, D., Hojrup, P., and Bleasby, A. J. (1993) Rapid identification of proteins by peptide-mass fingerprinting. *Curr. Biol.* **3,** 327–332.
48. Yates, J. R. III, Speicher, S., Griffin, P. R., and Hunkapiller, T. (1993) Peptide mass maps: a highly informative approach to protein identification. *Anal. Biochem.* **214,** 397–408.
49. Shevchenko, A., Jensen, O. N., Podtelejnikov, A. V., Sagliocco, F., Wilm, M., Vorm, O., Mortensen, P., Shevchenko, A., Boucherie, H., and Mann, M. (1996) Linking genome and proteome by mass spectrometry: large-scale identification of yeast proteins from two-dimensional gels. *Proc. Natl. Acad. Sci. USA* **93,** 14,440–14,445.
50. Mann, M. and Wilm, M. (1996) Analytical properties of the nanoelectrospray ion source. *Anal. Chem.* **68,** 1–8.
51. Eng, J. K., McCormack, A. L., and Yates, J. R., III (1994) An approach to correlate tandem mass spectral data of peptides with amino acid sequences in a protein database. *J. Am. Soc. Mass Spectrom.* **5,** 976–989.
52. Yates, J. R., III (1998) Database searching using mass spectrometry data. *Electrophoresis* **19,** 893–900.
53. Mann, M. and Wilm, M. (1994) Error-tolerant identification of peptides in sequence databases by peptide sequence tags. *Anal. Chem.* **64,** 4390–4399.
54. Annan, R. S. and Carr, S. A. (1997) The essential role of mass spectrometry in characterising protein structure: mapping posttranslational modifications. *J. Prot. Chem.* **16,** 391–402.
55. Neubauer, G. and Mann, M. (1998) Mapping of phopshorylation sites of gel-isolated proteins by nanoelectrospray tandem mass spectrometry: Potentials and limitations. *Anal. Chem.* **71,** 235–242.
56. Berkelman, T. and Stenstedt, T., eds. (1998) *2-D Electrophoresis Using Immobilised pH Gradients. Principles and Methods.* Amersham Pharmacia Biotech.
57. Link, A. J., ed. (1999) *Methods in Molecular Biology*, vol. 112: *2-D Proteome Analysis Protocols.* Humana, Totowa, NJ.

58. Marshall, T. and Williams, K. M. (1984) Artefacts associated with 2-mercaptoethanol upon high-resolution two-dimensional electrophoresis. *Anal. Biochem.* **139,** 502–505.
59. Pasquali, C., Fialka, I., and Huber, L. A. (1997) Preparative two-dimensional gel electrophoresis of membrane proteins. *Electrophoresis* **18,** 2573–2581.
60. Rabilloud, T., Adessi, C., Giraudel, A., and Lunardi, J. (1997) Improvement of the solubilization of proteins in two-dimensional electrophoresis with immobilized pH gradients. *Electrophoresis* **18,** 307–316.
61. Molloy, M. P., Herbert, B. R., Walsh, B. J., Tyler, M. I., Traini, M., Sanchez, J. C., Hochstrasser, D. F., Williams, K. L., and Gooley, A. A. (1998) Extraction of membrane proteins by differential solubilization for separation using two-dimensional gel electrophoresis. *Electrophoresis* **19,** 837–844.
62. Rabilloud, T. (1998) Use of thiourea to increase the solubility of membrane proteins in two-dimensional electrophoresis. *Electrophoresis* **19,** 758–760.
63. Hochstrasser, D. F. and Merril, C. R. (1988) "Catalysts" for polyacrylamide gel polymerization and detection of proteins by silver staining. *Appl. Theor. Electrophoresis* **1,** 35–40.
64. Hochstrasser, D. F., Patchornik, A., and Merril, C. R. (1988) Development of polyacrylamide gels that improve the separation of proteins and their detection by silver staining. *Anal. Biochem.* **173,** 412–423.
65. Herbert, B. R., Molloy, M. P., Gooley, A. A., Walsh, B. J., Bryson, W. G., and Williams, K. L. (1998) Improved protein solubility in two-dimensional electrophoresis using tributyl phosphine as reducing agent. *Electrophoresis* **19,** 845–851.
66. Jensen, O. N., Podtelejnikov, A., and Mann, M. (1996) Delayed extraction improves sensitivity in database searches by matrix-assisted laser desorption/ionization peptide maps. *Rapid Commun. Mass Spectrom.* **10,** 1371–1378.
67. Vorm, O., Roepstorff, P., and Mann, M. (1994) Matrix surfaces made by fast evaporation yield improved resolution and very high sensitivity in MALDI-TOF. *Anal. Chem.* **66,** 3281–3287.
68. Vorm, O. and Mann, M. (1994) Improved mass accuracy in matrix assisted laser desorption/ionization time-of-flight mass spectrometry of peptides. *J. Am. Soc. Mass Spectrom.* **10,** 1371–1378.
69. Sanchez, J.-C., Rouge, V., Pisteur, M., Ravier, F., Tonella, L., Moosmayer, M., Wilkins, M. R., and Hochstrasser, D. F. (1997) Improved and simplified in-gel sample application using reswelling of dry immobilized pH gradients. *Electrophoresis* **18,** 324–327.

22

Functional Genomics of *Mycobacterium tuberculosis* Using DNA Microarrays

Michael Wilson, Martin Voskuil, Dirk Schnappinger, and Gary K. Schoolnik

1. Introduction

1.1. The Postgenomic Era of M. tuberculosis *Research*

Completion of the sequence of the entire genome of strain H37Rv was a benchmark for *Mycobacterium tuberculosis* research *(1)*. This achievement ushers in the era of genome-wide functional and comparative genomics for this organism. At present, the most powerful enabling technology of the postgenomic era is microarray-based hybridization. Microarrays, by whatever means they are fabricated, contain surface-bound representations of each open reading frame (ORF) of a sequenced genome. Thus, they provide a method for parallel sampling of thousands of different genes within a complex pool of nucleic acids. Microarray gene capacity readily accommodates the number of ORFs in the relatively small genomes of bacteria and yeast and, in principle, can accommodate the entire genetic repertoire of complex multicellular animals. Below, we discuss our fabrication and use of an *M. tuberculosis* microarray, containing representations of each of the identified 3924 ORFs of this organism. We will describe two applications of this method. In the first— microarray-based gene response, i.e., transcript profiling — we ask the question: which genes are selectively expressed under a particular condition of growth, in a particular host compartment or as a result of inhibition of a metabolic or biosynthetic pathway? In the second, comparative genomics, we use a microarray containing the ORFs of one strain or species to identify ORFs deleted or absent from a second strain or species whose genome sequence may not have been determined. In this manner, microarray-based comparative genomics seeks to learn the ORF-by-ORF relatedness of two similar, but non-

From: *Methods in Molecular Medicine*, vol. 54: *Mycobacterium Tuberculosis Protocols*
Edited by: T. Parish and N. G. Stoker © Humana Press Inc., Totowa, NJ

identical organisms whose biological differences are under investigation. Examples of each application have been applied to *M. tuberculosis* *(2,3)*.

1.2. Array-Based Technologies

Recent years have witnessed a boom in the development of a variety of different technologies for producing high-density DNA and oligonucleotide arrays. The key features that characterize the different microarray formats are the type of solid support, the linkage that attaches the nucleic acids to the array surface, and the configuration of the nucleic acid elements on the array. These features are critical factors that affect the performance of the array and the types of questions that can be addressed. For detailed information about the different types of DNA microarrays, we recommend some excellent reviews on the subject *(4,5)*.

Here we present methods of microarray fabrication and use pioneered by Pat Brown and his colleagues at Stanford University *(6,7)* (*see* **Note 1**). The format consists of specific, double-stranded DNA species, each corresponding to a particular ORF or expressed sequence tag (EST) (in the case of eukaryotes), that are attached to a glass microscope slide. Thousands of different DNA species are printed onto the slide in a high-density matrix so that the position and identity of every "spot" of printed DNA is denoted and can be tracked. The two-color hybridization method employs two populations of cDNAs that have been differentially labeled with two different fluorochromes. For transcript profiling experiments, for instance, the cDNAs are derived from RNA prepared from *M. tuberculosis* exposed to two contrasting conditions. The two differentially-labeled populations of cDNAs are combined in equal masses, applied to the array surface and allowed to hybridize to the corresponding ORF-specific targets. The array is then scanned and the intensity of each label for each ORF-specific spot is quantified. These values are compared, yielding ratios that serve as a measure of the relative degree of expression or repression of each ORF for the two tested conditions.

Microarray experimental systems are an emerging technology and optimization of nearly every step is an ongoing process. Thus, currently practiced methods are subject to change and some are still awkward and punctuated with nuances and even rituals that are based more on conjecture than experimental evidence. Thus, we encourage the microarray technologist to modify and expand on the methods presented here. Nonetheless, because of the power of this method, we feel that it is timely to describe the methods that we now use and in this way provide increased access to this technique. We anticipate that broader use of microarrays by many workers in the field will yield insights into the pathogenicity, physiology, and immunologic aspects of this bacterium. And with luck, these insights should help speed the processes of drug discovery and vaccine development.

1.3. A Methodological Approach

Three general phases of conducting DNA microarray experiments are described below: (1) microarray construction, (2) preparation and hybridization of fluorescently labeled samples, and (3) data management. Although the microarray experimental system is remarkably versatile, we have focused on methods for either monitoring changes in gene expression or detecting genotypic variation.

1.3.1. Principles of Array Preparation

The construction of microarrays can be subdivided into four separate processes: creation of the DNA targets, preparation of the glass slides, printing the microarrays, and processing the printed microarrays. Beginning in **Subheading 2.** below, we present a moderate-throughput polymerase chain reaction (PCR) approach for preparing the DNA targets in microwell-plate format.

With respect to the preparation of glass slides, one area of active investigation is focused on the attachment chemistries that link DNA to a solid surface in a configuration that facilitates hybridization *(8)*. It is projected that advances in this area will lead to improved microarray consistency and sensitivity *(9)*. The method we describe for binding DNA to glass surfaces is based on the interaction of DNA with a coating of positively charged poly-lysine. The DNA is subsequently crosslinked to the surface by exposing the slides to ultraviolet light. In order to reduce nonspecific background binding of fluorescently labeled nucleic acids to lysine residues (during the hybridization step in the assay), free amino groups are blocked by treatment with succinic anhydride. The steps taken to prepare the printed slides for hybridization are referred to as postprocessing.

The performance of the printing tips that deposit the DNA onto the glass surface profoundly influences the final quality of the array. These tips affect the delivery of liquid, the spot size and consistency, and the number of slides that can be printed in a series. The tips we use resemble quill-pins because they have a fine slot machined up through the center of the sharpened tip, and the DNA solution is wicked up into the slot. Once "loaded," the tips are tapped sequentially onto separate glass slides and each tap deposits a few nanoliters of solution, without needing to be redipped into the DNA solution after each tap. Tip design and alternative means of noncontact fluid delivery are also areas of active research.

1.3.2. Principles of Sample Preparation

Sample preparation involves isolating total RNA or genomic DNA (depending on the experiment) from *M. tuberculosis* and converting those samples into fluorescently-labeled probes that will be hybridized to the array. Several methods for isolating total RNA from *M. tuberculosis* are available, and the choice of which method to use is dictated, in part, by the experimental design ***(10)***. Whichever method is selected however, a rigorous, systematic approach to RNA isolation for microarray analysis will reduce method-induced changes in transcription due to inappropriate manipulation of the organism and will diminish RNA degradation. The former issue comes from the capacity of bacteria to change their transcriptional profile within minutes of being exposed to a new condition (e.g., cells that are allowed to settle in the flask or are centrifuged in a cold centrifuge). The latter consideration is particularly important because most microarray experiments are designed to monitor the dynamic changes in expression patterns with time. Therefore, the RNA isolation method must rapidly preserve the repertoire of transcripts that is present at the moment of harvest. In practical terms, the method should provide an efficient means of harvesting and lysing the bacteria while rapidly inactivating RNases (*see* **Note 2**).

The labeling method described in this chapter employs random priming with direct incorporation of a fluorescent nucleotide analog into the polymerized product. Secondary labeling techniques and amplification techniques have been reported and are the basis of some commercial products (***[11]*** and NEN Life Science Products). We expect significant development in these areas, and we encourage the microarray technologist to test different methods in order to improve the sensitivity or versatility of this technique. Furthermore, the choice of fluorochrome used for labeling depends on the excitation and emission wavelengths that are available on the scanner that will be used for acquiring the fluorescent signal (*see* **Note 3**).

1.3.3. Principles of Data Analysis

The large-scale datasets that are generated by microarray experiments require a data management platform that enables the fundamental processes of tracking, analyzing, and interpreting the results. An effective management strategy must allow the user to store, retrieve, and interact with the data in a manner that integrates the primary microarray data with the appropriate sequence annotations and other external sources of information. It must also provide a means of feeding the data into computational algorithms that perform essential functions such as normalization, statistical analysis, and pattern finding. Several companies that produce microarray-related products or services are currently cooperating to help define a standardized microarray data platform so that microarray results can be interpreted across different laboratories or array formats (http://www.gatconsortium.org/about.html). For a more thorough coverage of the issues related to managing microarray data we refer the reader to references *(12,13)*. In **Subheading 3.3.**, we describe some of the analytical approaches that have been developed and are accessible to the academic researcher.

2. Materials

2.1. Preparation of DNA Targets

1. Clean work environment (*see* **Note 4**).
2. Multichannel pipeters or robotic dispensers.
3. Aluminum sealing tape (Beckman Instruments, Fullerton, CA).
4. 96-well PCR plates suitable for the thermocycler used.
5. Optional: 384-well polypropylene PCR plates (Corning Costar Inc., Corning, NY).
6. *M. tuberculosis* genomic DNA.
7. 5 μ*M* stocks of primer pairs to amplify the gene fragments (*see* **Notes 5** and **6**).
8. PCR buffer (1.1X) supplemented with dNTPs and acetamide: 22 m*M* Tris-HCl, pH 8.4, 55 m*M* KCl, 1.65 m*M* $MgCl_2$, 5% (w/v) acetamide, 220 μ*M* dATP, 220 μ*M* dCTP, 220 μ*M* dGTP, 220 μ*M* dTTP. Final concentration will be 20 m*M* Tris-HCl, pH 8.4, 50 m*M* KCl, 1.5 m*M* $MgCl_2$, 4.5% acetamide and 200 μ*M* each dNTP. Store in aliquots at –20°C.
9. 3 *M* Sodium acetate, pH 5.5.
10. 95% ethanol.
11. 70% ethanol.
12. Printing buffer 6X SSC: 900 m*M* NaCl, 90 m*M* sodium citrate, pH 7.0, filter sterilized.

2.2. Slide Preparation

1. Gloves, eye-protection goggles, lab coat.
2. Glass microscope slides, 1" × 3" (Becton Dickinson Gold Seal Microscope Slides).
3. Slide racks, stainless steel rack holds 30 slides/rack (PGC Scientific, Frederick, MD).
4. Slide-staining dishes.
5. Orbital shaker.
6. 95% ethanol.
7. Phosphate buffered saline (PBS) pH 7.4:1.7 m*M* KH_2PO_4, 5 m*M* Na_2HPO_4, pH 7.4, 150 m*M* NaCl.
8. NaOH-ethanol wash solution. Completely dissolve 70 g NaOH in 280 mL of distilled water. Add 420 mL of 95% ethanol slowly until completely mixed. If the solution remains cloudy, add water until it clarifies. Prepare fresh (*see* **Notes 7** and **8**).
9. Poly-L-lysine solution, supplied as 0.1% w/v in water with preservative (Sigma, St. Louis, MO) (*see* **Note 9**).

2.3. Array Fabrication

1. Microarray printing robot (*see* **Note 1** and the review by Botwell of commercially available arrayers *[14]*).
2. Aluminum sealing tape (Beckman Instruments).
3. Microwell plates containing target fragments to be arrayed (*see* **Subheadings 3.1.1.** and **3.1.2.** on target preparation).
4. *M. tuberculosis* genomic DNA.
5. Salmon sperm DNA prelabeled with Cy3 (*see* **Subheading 3.5.2.** for labeling of genomic DNA).
6. Internal standards.
7. Printing buffer: 6X SSC (*see* **Subheading 2.1., item 12**).

2.4. Post Processing

1. Slide dishes.
2. Stainless steel slide racks.
3. Hot plate for boiling water.
4. Orbital shaker.
5. Slide staining reservoir.
6. Heating block.
7. Ultra-violet (UV) illumination chamber for crosslinking DNA (e.g., Stratalinker from Stratagene, LaJolla, CA).
8. Tabletop centrifuge fitted with swinging buckets that can accommodate 96-well plates.
9. Printing buffer (*see* **Subheading 2.1., item 12**).
10. Wash Solution A: 1X SSC, 0.05% SDS.
11. Wash Solution B: 0.06X SSC.
12. 95% ethanol.
13. 1 *M* sodium borate, pH 8, filter sterilize.
14. Succinic anhydride (Aldrich Chemical Co., Milwaukee, WI).
15. 1-methyl–2-pyrrolidinone (Aldrich).
16. Succinic anhydride solution: add 6 g of succinic anhydride to 335 mL of 1-methyl–2-pyrrolidinone with stirring. As soon as the solid has dissolved, quickly mix 15 mL of 1 *M* sodium borate, pH 8. Prepare **immediately** before use (*see* **Notes 10** and **11**).

2.5. Sample Preparation and Probe Labeling

2.5.1. Synthesis and Labeling of cDNA

1. Total *M. tuberculosis* RNA: 2–8 µg per sample to be labeled (*see* **Note 12**).
2. Random primers: 1 m*M* (*see* **Note 13**).
3. Superscript II reverse transcriptase (Life Technologies, Inc., Rockville, MD).
4. 5X First-strand reaction buffer: 250 m*M* Tris-HCl, pH 8.3, 375 m*M* KCl, 15 m*M* $MgCl_2$.

5. 100 m*M* dithiothreitol (DTT), supplied by the enzyme manufacturer.
6. dNTP mixture: 5 m*M* each of dATP, dGTP, dCTP, and 2 m*M* dTTP.
7. Cy3-dUTP (Amersham Pharmacia Biotech, Piscataway, NJ) (*see* **Note 3**).
8. Cy5-dUTP (Amersham Pharmacia Biotech).
9. Microcentrifuge concentrating filters, 30 kDa cutoff, e.g., Microcon 30 (Amicon) (Millipore, Corp., Bedford, MA).
10. TE: 10 m*M* Tris-HCl, pH 7.4, 1 m*M* EDTA.
11. Optional: In vitro transcripts for internal standards (*see* **Note 14**).

2.5.2. Labeling Genomic DNA

1. Genomic DNA, free of metal chelators, detergents and organic solvents.
2. Random primers:1 m*M* (*see* **Note 13**)**Subheading 2.5.1., step 2**).
3. DNA polymerase: 5 U/µL Klenow fragment DNA polymerase I.
4. 10 × polymerase buffer: 100 m*M* Tris-HCl, pH 7.5, 75 m*M* DTT, 50 m*M* $MgCl_2$.
5. dNTP mixture: 5 m*M* each of dATP, dGTP, and dCTP and 2 m*M* dTTP.
6. Cy5-dUTP (Amersham Pharmacia Biotech) (*see* **Subheading 2.5.1., step 7**).
7. Cy5-dUTP (*see* **Subheading 2.5.1., step 8**).
8. 3 *M* sodium acetate, pH 5.2.
9. 95% ethanol.
10. 70% ethanol.

2.6. Hybridization

1. Hybridization chamber, e.g., Corning (Corning Costar Inc.) or GeneMachines (San Carlos, CA).
2. Glass coverslips, 22 mm × 22 mm, glass #1.
3. Fine-point forceps.
4. 20X SSC: 3 *M* NaCl, 0.3 *M* sodium citrate, pH 7.0.
5. Yeast tRNA: 10 µg/µL in dH_2O.
6. 2% sodium dodecyl sulfate (SDS).
7. Wash Solution A: 1X SSC, 0.05% SDS.
8. Wash Solution B: 0.06X SSC.
9. Slide staining trays and racks.

2.7. Data Acquisition and Analysis

1. Scanner — see the review by Botwell for commercially available scanners ***(14)***.
2. ScanAlyze: (Michael Eisen, 1998, http://rana.stanford.edu).
3. ProbeBrowser: (Hugh Salamon, http://molepi.stanford.edu/hugh/pb/pbbcg.html) ***(2)***.
4. Cluster and Treeview (Michael Eisen, 1998, http://rana.stanford.edu/software) ***(15)***.
5. GENECLUSTER (Pablo Tamayo, http://waldo.wi.mit.edu/MPR/software.html) ***(16)***.

3. Methods

3.1. Preparation of DNA Targets

Production of DNA microarrays is scalable so that meaningful results can be obtained from a microarray composed of a few dozen or many thousands of target fragments. Consequently, the strategies for producing the DNA target fragments are guided by the reagents and equipment available to the researcher. Here we describe a method for PCR amplification of fragments in a 96-well plate format. This medium-throughput system is amenable to manipulations using standard 8- and 12-channel manual pipeters or more sophisticated robotic liquid dispensing systems. Details of primer design are discussed in **Note 6.**

3.1.1. PCR Amplification in 96-Well Format

1. Aliquot primers into stock plates so that each well contains a pair of primers appropriate for the amplification of a unique target fragment. Add 5 μL of each primer (25 pmol) to the wells (*see* **Note 5**).
2. Create a master mix that contains PCR buffer, enzyme, and template. Calculate the amount of *M. tuberculosis* genomic DNA template and *Taq* DNA polymerase to be added to the 1.1X PCR buffer stock solution. Add the equivalent of 10 ng *M. tuberculosis* genomic DNA and 1 U *Taq* polymerase for every 65 μL reaction.
3. Add 60 μL of the PCR master mix to each well of the PCR plate.
4. Perform the PCR; select cycle times and temperatures that are appropriate for the primers and thermocycler (*see* **Note 6**).
5. Evaluate a 5 μL sample of each reaction by 2% agarose gel electrophoresis (*see* **Note 15**).

3.1.2. Preparation of the DNA for Printing

1. Add 6 μL (0.1 vol) of 3 *M* sodium acetate pH 5.2 and 165 μL (2.5 vol) of 95% ethanol to each well of the PCR plate.
2. Incubate for a minimum of 1 h at –20°C.
3. Centrifuge in a swinging bucket rotor at 5000*g* for 30 min.
4. Remove the ethanol by gently inverting the plates and blotting the excess liquid onto a bed of paper towels. Alternatively, a 12-channel aspiration tool can be used to gently remove the ethanol supernatant.
5. Wash the precipitated DNA pellets by adding 200 μL of ice-cold 70% ethanol. Centrifuge and remove the ethanol supernatant as before.
6. Dry the plates in air or use a high-speed rotary vacuum.
7. Option 1: Dissolve the pellets in 15 μL of printing buffer. The plates are ready to print, but keep and store them sealed with an aluminum sealing tape to prevent evaporation (*see* **Note 16**).
8. Option 2: to allow printing with more printing tips, the amplicons must be transferred to 384-well format. Amplicons from four 96-well plates are compressed into one 384-well plate. Dissolve the pellets in 30 μL dH_2O and redistribute 5 μL

aliquots into 5 replicate copies of the library in 384-well plates. Store the plates at –20°C. Prior to printing, dry the remaining water and dissolve the DNA in 5 μL printing buffer (*see* **Note 16**).

9. Immediately prior to printing, briefly centrifuge each plate to force the liquid to the bottom of the wells.

3.2. Slide Preparation

Preparing the poly-lysine-coated slides is a critical component in the production of high-quality microarrays (*see* **Note 9**). It is also a key variable that may be the source of background signal to the system. The goal is to create glass surfaces that are exquisitely clean for subsequent coating by poly-lysine. The recipes here are designed for preparing two slide racks (30 slides each) in the matching staining dishes.

1. Place 30 slides into each of the metal slide racks.
2. Soak slides in the NaOH:ethanol wash solution for 2 h with gentle rotation on an orbital shaker. Make sure the slides are completely submerged in the solution. Occasionally remove any air bubbles by tapping the slide rack against the bottom of the dish.
3. Rinse slides with a flowing source of dH_2O for 5 min, ensuring that the slides are completely submerged and there is good flow across the surfaces of all slides.
4. Place dH_2O filled chamber with slides on shaker for about 105 min.
5. Repeat **steps 3** and **4** (*see* **Note 17**).
6. Prepare a fresh dilution of the poly-lysine solution. Mix 30 mL of the 0.1% poly-lysine solution with 30 mL PBS and 240 mL dH_2O.
7. Soak the tray of slides in the diluted poly-lysine solution for 20–30 min. with gentle shaking (*see* **Note 18**).
8. Rinse for at least 5 min in dH_2O.
9. Spin dry the slide racks for 1–2 min at 50*g*. Place a thin bed of paper towels below the rack to absorb liquid (*see* **Note 19**).
10. Transfer the slides to a clean slide box. Dry the slides completely under vacuum for 10 min at 45–50°C.
11. Seal the slide box and store them in the airtight box for 1–2 wk prior to use (*see* **Note 20**).

3.3. Array Fabrication

Many aspects of the array printing process are specific to the type of robotic printer and software that is used. Consequently, this section focuses on the principles of successful printing that can be generalized to most types of spotting instruments. Some aspects that specifically pertain to making microarrays of bacterial genomes are emphasized in **Notes 21** and **22**.

1. Prepare a plate of controls to be printed along with the *M. tuberculosis* DNA spots on the arrays. Suggested control spots include:

a. *M. tuberculosis* total genomic DNA (*see* **Note 21**).
b. DNA for 16S and 23S ribosomal RNA genes (*see* **Note 22**).
c. Cy3-labeled salmon sperm DNA (*see* **Notes 21**, **23**, and **24**).
d. Non-*M. tuberculosis* spots containing gene fragments from other organisms.
e. Reporter genes or resistance markers that are likely to be part of recombinant strains used in the experiments.
f. Plasmids used to clone any spots that may be printed on the array.

2. Examine the surface of a few slides from each batch of the poly-lysine-coated slides. Use only slides that are perfectly clear without partially opaque patterns, scratches or water spots. These patterns are more easily visualized if water vapor is breathed onto the slide (*see* **Note 24**).
3. Pretest each of the printing tips to be used. The test printing solution should contain DNA in printing buffer at the same volume and DNA concentration that will be used for the printing session.
4. Configure an appropriate printing pattern and spot density for the dimensions of the slides, coverslips, and printing tip head (*see* **Note 25**).
5. Print the array (*see* **Note 26**).

3.4. Post Processing

3.4.1. Preparation

1. Set an aluminum heating block to 90–98°C and invert the block so that the top surface is flat.
2. Fill a slide staining chamber with water so that the slides will be suspended just above the surface of the liquid.
3. Prepare a place in the chemical fume hood for an orbital shaker, magnetic stir plate, and a hot plate.
4. Boil water in a 4 L glass beaker. Fill it to a level that allows the slide rack to be completely submerged, but the handle can extend above the surface so it can be safely grabbed.
5. Fill a slide dish with 95% ethanol.
6. Assemble the required chemicals so that they can be handled quickly.

3.4.2. Processing

1. Hydrate the DNA spots on the slides. Using a standard slide-staining chamber, hydrate slides by inverting them (array side down toward water) over the reservoir of water. Cover the chamber to create a humidified atmosphere. Let the spots of DNA on the array become glistening and beaded with moisture (approx 2–3 min) (*see* **Note 27**).
2. Snap dry by immediately but gently flipping the slide (array-side up now!) onto a heating block which has been preheated to 90–98°C. The water will evaporate away from the array spots in a rapid wave-like pattern within about 3–5 s. Remove the slide from the heating block and place it in a dust-free box. Repeat **steps 2** and **3** for each of the slides to be processed.

3. Crosslink the DNA to the slides. Place the slides, array side up, on a flat, dust-free board that fits into the UV irradiation chamber. Irradiate with 600 millijoules UV light (*see* **Note 28**).
4. Prewash the slides. Load the slides into a staining rack and plunge them into Wash Solution A for 30 s. Rinse by gentle plunging in Wash Solution B for 30 s (*see* **Note 29**).
5. Centrifuge the slides in their racks at 50*g* for 1 min to remove the excess water. Place them inside a covered staining dish until **step 5**.7.
6. Prepare fresh succinic anhydride solution (*see* **Notes 10** and **11**).
7. Pour the succinic anhydride solution into the staining dish, and plunge the slides into the solution repeatedly and rapidly for 30–60 s, keeping the slides submerged (*see* **Note 11**). Continue the mixing on a rotating platform at 60 rpm for an additional 10–12 min.
8. Remove the slide rack from the organic reaction mixture and plunge it immediately into the boiling water bath for 1 min (*see* **Note 30**).
9. Transfer the rack of slides into the 95% ethanol tray and wash briefly.
10. Spin dry the slides by centrifugation at 50*g* for 1 min. Use a counter balance with the same number of slides in a rack.
11. Transfer the slides to a dry slide box for storage (*see* **Note 31**).

3.5. Sample Preparation and Probe Labeling

3.5.1. Synthesis and Labeling of cDNA

1. Dilute the RNA sample with dH_2O to a volume of 11.2 µL. Typical labeling reactions require 2–8 µg of total RNA (*see* **Notes 12** and **14**). Keep the RNA and other reaction components on ice until instructed otherwise.
2. Add 1.5 µL of 1 m*M* random primers (*see* **Note 13**).
3. Heat samples to 70°C for 5 min, then snap cool in an ice-water bath. Centrifuge briefly to collect the contents to the bottom of the tube (*see* **Note 32**).
4. Add the following reaction components (*see* **Note 33**): 5 µL of 5X first-strand reaction buffer, 2.5 µL of 100 m*M* DTT, 2.3 µL of dNTP mixture (5 m*M* each of dATP, dGTP, dCTP, and 2 m*M* dTTP), 0.8 µL of reverse transcriptase and 1.7 µL of either Cy3-dUTP or Cy5-dUTP (*see* **Note 3**).
5. Incubate for 10 min at 25°C and then shift the incubation to 42°C for 90 min.
6. Combine the appropriate Cy3- and Cy5-labeled samples that will be co-hybridized onto the array (*see* **Note 34**).
7. Add the combined probes to a microcentrifuge concentrating filter with 400 µL filtered TE. Centrifuge at 14,000*g* (maximum microcentrifuge speed) until nearly all of the volume is pushed through the filter. Repeat the buffer exchange once by adding fresh 400 µL filtered TE and centrifuge as before. Check the volume periodically until there is only about 8–10 µL of sample remaining in the filter unit.
8. Recover the labeled cDNA by inverting the unit and placing into a fresh collection tube. Centrifuge at 4000*g* for 20 s.
9. Adjust the sample volume to 8 µL and transfer to a 0.5 mL tube.

3.5.2. Labeling Genomic DNA

1. Prepare each reaction tube by diluting 2 μg of genomic DNA with water to a final volume of 20 μL.
2. Add the following components to each DNA sample (*see* **Note 33**): 5.0 μL of 10X polymerase reaction buffer, 1.0 μL of 1 m*M* random primers, 0.5 μL of dNTP mixture, and 21 μL of dH_2O
3. Heat the sample for 3 min at 98°C, then snap cool by plunging the tubes in ice-water. Briefly centrifuge the tubes to force the condensed water back to the bottom of tube.
4. Add 1 μL of DNA polymerase and 1.5 μL of either Cy3-dUTP or Cy5-dUTP to each tube to start the reaction
5. Incubate for 90 min at 37°C.
6. Concentrate and perform **steps 6–9** according to **Subheading 3.5.1.** above. This will exchange the buffer and concentrate the sample using a micro-concentrating filter (**Subheading 3.5.1., steps 6–9**) (*see* **Note 35**).

3.6. Hybridization

1. Mix the Cy3- and Cy5-labeled samples to be comparatively hybridized to the array. Bring the total volume to 8 μL.
2. For each 8 μL of sample add 1 μL of tRNA, 2.8 μL of 20X SSC and 2 μL of 2% SDS. Final volume 13.8 μL.
3. Heat the samples to 98°C for 2 min.
4. Centrifuge for 2–3 min at 14,000*g* to pellet any particulate debris.
5. Pipet 10 μL of H_2O onto the corners of the slide, far from the array (*see* **Note 36**).
6. Carefully pipet the hybridization solution onto the array. Lay the coverslip onto the sample to spread the liquid over the array (*see* **Notes 37** and **38**).
7. Assemble the hybridization chamber with the slide inside and submerge it into a 63–65°C constant-temperature water bath. Once the slide is inside the chamber, keep it level throughout the remaining steps to prevent contact between cover glass and the top of the chamber.
8. Hybridize for 4–12 h.
9. Remove the chamber from the water bath and blot off external water while keeping the assembly level. Disassemble the chamber, pry up the slide with forceps, and place it in a slide rack for washing (*see* **Note 39**).
10. Wash off the coverslip with gentle up-and-down plunges in Wash Solution A. Continue washing for 1–2 min after the cover glass falls off (*see* **Note 40**).
11. Transfer the slide to a clean slide rack and wash for 1–2 min in Wash Solution B.
12. Remove the water droplets from the slide by centrifugation at 50*g* for 1 min. For counter-balance use a slide rack with an equivalent number of slides.
13. Place the slide in a light-proof box. It is now ready for fluorescence scanning.

3.7. Data Acquisition and Analysis

3.7.1. Data Acqusition

1. Acquire the fluorescent signals from the array. Follow the instructions provided by the manufacturer of the scanner. Store the raw data files as 16-bit TIF (tagged image format) images (*see* **Note 41**).
2. Extract the numerical data from the spot intensities. Identify and mark any spots which are flawed technically and might yield misleading data (*see* **Note 42**).
3. Store the extracted data in a database that links the spot positions (numbers) to their identification and descriptive information (*see* **Note 43**).

3.7.2. Preliminary Data Analysis

1. Subtract the local background from the intensity of each spot and both fluorescent channels. Estimate the sensitivity of the experiment (based on the internal standards and non-*M. tuberculosis* DNA spots on the array, respectively), and assign a threshold value that defines the minimal detectable signal. Depending on the subsequent calculations, spots with values that fall below the defined threshold may be omitted from further analysis (*see* **Note 44**).
2. Normalize the two channels so that the median values of both channels are equivalent. Identify the set of *M. tuberculosis* DNA spots that gave signals above background and define the median values of this gene set for each channel. Multiply the values of one channel by the factor that is requied to normalize the two channels with respect to the medians.
3. Calculate the Cy5/Cy3 ratios (channel 1/channel 2) and the $\log_2$ ratios for every spot. Assign a positive value to the $\log_2$ ratios that represent genes induced by the experimental treatment; assign a negative value to the $\log_2$ ratios that represent genes repressed by the experimental treatment (*see* **Note 45**).
4. Apply statistical tests to identify ORFs with $\log_2$ ratios that are significantly different from the population of *M. tuberculosis* genes represented on the array. Quantify the degree that each ratio is different from the population mean for all spots on the array. This is done by calculating the number of standard deviations from the mean (Z) for each spot:

$$Z = (\log_2 \text{ratio} - \text{mean})/\text{standard deviation}$$

5. Since Z values are normalized to the standard deviation of a given experiment, they can be directly compared across different experiments. Use the Z value to look up the probability (p) that a given spot is different from the population of other *M. tuberculosis* genes.

3.7.3. Advanced Options for Data Analysis

1. Analyze the values by the ORF's position on the genome to identify multigenic regions on the chromosome which have characteristic response patterns. Strand specific and location-specific expression patterns can be visualized using the *Probebrowser* software utility (*see* **Note 46**).

2. Define coregulated gene families that respond similarly across multiple experiments by clustering analysis or by self-organizing maps (*see* **Note 47**).

4. Notes

1. The microarray format that was pioneered by Pat Brown and his colleagues at Stanford University is arguably the format that is most accessible and flexible for academic exploratory research *(17)*. The high costs of commercially prepared microarrays, printing robots, scanners and full-genome primer sets, have placed significant barriers in the way of the average laboratory. In an effort to make microarray technology more affordable, members of Pat Brown's laboratory created the "MGuide" website (http://cmgm.stanford.edu/pbrown/mguide/). This project promotes a "do-it-yourself" philosophy by providing a detailed step-by-step guide for building a custom microarrayer. Included with the guide is a parts list, software for controlling the motors, and the design specifications for custom-built parts. Other excellent websites with microarray-related protocols are: http://www.nhgri.nih.gov/DIR/LCG/15K/HTML/ (National Human Genome Research Institute) and http://sequence.aecom.yu.edu/bioinf/funcgenomic.html (Albert Einstein College of Medicine).
2. The most reliable results are achieved when the experiments are carefully controlled so that RNA from the experimental condition is comparable in every way to the reference RNA sample, except for variable under investigation. Although this sounds obvious, it can sometimes be difficult to achieve for some experimental designs. The researcher must consider the dynamic nature of the RNA pool and how subtle differences in experimental handling may bias the results. Thus, an important criterion for interpreting the validity of results is the reproducibility of data from independently isolated RNA samples.
3. The choice of fluorescent nucleotide analog depends on the instrument that will be used to acquire the image. Laser-activated scanners have fixed excitation wavelengths that limit the available choices. Scanners that use xenon lamps provide a broad range of excitation wavelengths, available to excite the fluorophore. Most commercial scanners are equipped with lasers and barrier filters compatible with the Cy3- and Cy5- dyes since these have good spectral separation, high quantum efficiencies, minimal photobleaching and they fluoresce when dry. Cy3 (excitation_{max} = 550 nm; emission_{max} = 570 nm) and Cy5 (excitation_{max} = 649 nm; emission_{max} = 670 nm) are available as dCTP- or dUTP-analogs (Amersham Pharmacia Biotech).
4. Appropriate clean technique must be exercised throughout the phases of target production. This is important to reduce the introduction of dust that can interfere with subsequent steps of microarray fabrication and to eliminate cross contamination of PCR reactions that can lead to amplification of nontarget fragments. Precautions should be taken to physically segregate the preamplification materials and processes (reagent preparation and dilution of primers) from any of the materials used during or after the PCR phase. As a further precaution, we recommend using filter-plugged, disposable pipet tips for all manipulations of the primers and stock reagents.

5. For making the 5 µ*M* stock plate of primer pairs, we recommend creating two separate plates containing the individual primers (e.g., 25 µ*M* each well). The system works best if one plate contains all the 5'-primers and its partner plate contains the corresponding 3'-primers in the matching well positions. Once this is accomplished, equivalent volumes from the corresponding wells can be mixed and diluted in a third stock plate. For example, 10 µL of 5'-primers (25 µ*M*) mixed with 10 µL of 3'-primers (25 µ*M*) and 30 µL of dH_2O to yield 50 µL of solution per well with each primer at 5 µ*M*.
6. The inherent secondary structure of the G-C rich (65%) *M. tuberculosis* DNA can make for challenging PCR, especially with larger amplicons. We achieve best results if amplicons sizes are less than 1 kb and a standard PCR buffer system is supplemented with acetamide to help melt secondary structures. We prefer primers that are 20–21 nucleotides with predicted melting temperatures of 65–66°C. The primer design program "Primer 3" allows one to sequentially process batches of multiple sequence inputs according to a user-defined set of criteria. A browser-based interface is available at http://www.genome.wi.mit.edu/cgi-http://www.genome.wi.mit.edu/cgi-bin/primer/primer3_www.cgi, or the code can be downloaded and run on a UNIX platform (http://www-genome.wi.mit.edu/genome_software/other/primer3.html) [17].***(18)***. We used the following cycle profile with using a Perkin Elmer 9700 themocycler.

cycle 1:	94°C for 1 min	1 repetition
cycle 2:	94°C for 40 s	30 repetitions
	52°C for 40 s	
	72°C for 75 s	

7. Sodium hydroxide is caustic and should be handled with caution. Use gloves, safety goggles and the appropriate protective wear while handling this solution. While cleaning the slides, prevent spills by gradually adjusting orbital shaker speed until an appropriate mixing speed is reached. Use a secondary plastic basin to confine any accidental spills.
8. Prepare a dust-free workspace before starting. Use powder-free gloves for handling the slides. Throughout the procedure, avoid exposing the wet surfaces to air by keeping the slides submerged in liquid to prevent the accumulation of dust.
9. Commercial preparations of poly-lysine coated or amino-silane coated slides are available. To date, we have had inconsistent results with the commercially supplied slides we tested, so we continue to prepare our own slides as described here.
10. Exercise caution and use appropriate protection when handling 1-methyl 2-pyrolidinone and succinic anhydride. All chemical mixing and liquid transfer steps should be performed in an appropriate chemical fume hood. After the procedure, the spent organic solution must be properly disposed as hazardous chemical waste. The 1-methyl 2-pyrolidinone should be clear before use. It will develop a yellow shade after processing. Succinic anhydride is highly reactive and should be stored as directed on the reagent bottle. Maintain reagent freshness, by mixing the chemicals immediately prior to postprocessing.
11. The timing and efficiency of the chemical blocking step is critical for maintaining low background since any unblocked, positively charged amino groups will

form ionic interactions with the negatively charged DNA fragments. High background will result if either the excess spotted DNA fragments or the labeled hybridization probe bind nonspecifically to the array at unblocked sites. It is, therefore, important to have all stir-plates, reagents, glassware, and pipets ready at hand before starting the procedure. Mixing of the three reagents should be done expediently, and the slides should be plunged into the liquid as soon as mixing is complete. Once the dried spots of DNA on the microarray contact the liquid, unbound DNA fragments will diffuse away from the spot and may bind locally to other regions of the array unless the fragments are quickly dispersed and diluted by vigorous initial mixing. Therefore, the slides should initially be plunged up and down in the liquid blocking reagent as quickly and vigorously as possible without causing excessive splashing. Always plunge the slides into the prepared liquid reagents rather than pouring the reagents over the slides. Although inefficient blocking can result in a scanned image with diffuse cloudy background, a characteriztic artifact known as "pluming" often results from incomplete or slow blocking. Pluming looks much like smoke carried by prevailing winds from a smokestack as if viewed from above.

12. We have had good results labeling as little as 1 μg total RNA. Sensitivity should improve, in theory, when more labeled cDNA is hybridized to the array if the background levels can be held constant. However, we sometimes observe a trend of increased background with increasing amounts of RNA in the labeling reaction. When this happens, the sensitivity and dynamic range of the experiment suffers because the signal-to-noise ratio decreases disproportionately. In most cases, 5 μg total RNA is considered optimal for each labeling reaction.
13. In an effort to match the G+C bias of the *M. tuberculosis* genome, we use decamers which are randomized to contain a 66% G+C-content at every base position. We have had good results using a priming stock that is an equal molar mixture of the decamers and commercially prepared random hexamers (0.5 m*M* each). We have yet to optimize primer design and concentration for this labeling system.
14. If internal standards have been synthesized, they should be added to the labeling mixture along with the total RNA. Internal standards are in vitro-derived RNA transcripts of nonmycobacterial origin that do not cross-hybridize with *M. tuberculosis* DNA. They should be purified, quantified and then spiked into the labeling reaction over a range of concentrations. (Of course, the corresponding PCR products need to be printed onto the array as targets.) This allows one to obtain an estimate of the assay sensitivity and it gives a general idea of the dose-response relationship for each pool. However, internal standards are not yet reliable predictors of the concentrations of unrelated transcripts because the complexity of sequence- and length-specific hybridization dynamics produces variable signals for each transcript. In our experience, internal standards are usually unreliable sources and references for normalizing the two fluorescent channels to one another (discussed in the data analysis section). The reason is that the system is exquisitely sensitive to errors that arise from RNA quantification, pipeting inaccuracy or variations in the specific activity of the labeling reaction.

15. Gel combs are commercially available with 4.5 mm spacing that matches the distance between the wells in a 384-well plate (and half the distance between wells of a 96-well plate). Thus, rows of a 96-well plate can be loaded directly from the plate to the gel using a 12-channel pipeter. Evaluate the size and pattern of the bands on the gel and log the results into the database. This allows one to track the quality of each PCR product with the results of its amplicon on all subsequent hybridization experiments.
16. The DNA concentration should be 100–200 ng/μL in the final printing solution. For consistent printing results, it is important for the solutions in every well to have equivalent volumes and salt concentrations. If the plates are to be used for multiple printing sessions, then the accumulative effect of evaporation and changes in salt concentration need to be considered. Attempts to supplement the plates with water to account for evaporation seldom achieves satisfactory results. To avoid this problem, we redistribute the amplicon library into 384-well format (four 96-well plates per 384-well plate). We make several copies of each set by distributing the PCR products in separate sets of 384-well plates (option 2). Since evaporation from 384-well plates is relatively slow, one can print 3–4 series of arrays from each set of 384-well plates, and the extra sets are stored sealed in the freezer for future printing sessions. This also significantly reduces the printing time because a higher density printing tip configuration is used (i.e., 16 tips instead of 4).
17. It is critical to remove all traces of the NaOH/ethanol wash solution. Rinse exhaustively and keep the slides submerged in water throughout; avoid letting any part of the glass surface dry before they are rinsed completely. We typically prepare two racks of slides simultaneously, so one slide rack is kept in water on a rotating shaker while the other is flushed with fresh dH_2O.
18. Depending on the dimensions of the soaking dish being used, the mixture volumes may need to be scaled up proportionately to ensure that the slides can be completely submerged in the poly-lysine solution. We recommend using plastic trays, beakers, and measuring flasks because all glass surfaces will also be coated with the poly-lysine. To conserve solution, the racks of slides can be treated consecutively using one tray while the other rack is kept in dH_2O.
19. Centrifugation is intended to force the water droplets off the glass surfaces for rapid drying. Centrifugal forces greater than 100*g* can cause the slides to chip at the point they contact the holding rack.
20. Lysine-coated slides are thought to achieve best performance if they are stored in a dust-free environment for several days prior to using them in an experiment. Conversely, our experience suggests that slide performance decays and background increases as coated-slides age over an extended period (>3 mo). Storing unused microarrays in an inert environment may help preserve their longevity.
21. Spots containing genomic DNA are useful as reference standards for normalizing the scans of two fluorescent channels. Serial dilutions of genomic DNA should be made and printed to achieve a range of signal intensities. Salmon sperm DNA makes excellent carrier DNA for making dilutions of either genomic DNA or

ribosomal DNA since it has minimal cross-hybridization to *M. tuberculosis* DNA. The salmon sperm DNA should be sheared to the same average size as the fragments on the array and it should be at the same concentration in 3X SSC as the *M. tuberculosis* DNA being diluted.

22. Printing excess DNA corresponding to the ribosomal RNA genes can be detrimental when total RNA is the template for labeled probe. Since 95%–98% of the labeled sample corresponds to ribosomal cDNA the background levels will be exquisitely sensitive to any fragments of target ribosomal DNA which bleed onto nontarget sites of the array. For this reason, we dilute the DNA of the target fragments that contain ribosomal genes to < 10 ng/µL and limit the number of spots on the array that contain rRNA genes.
23. Prelabeled controls are used to detect carry-over contamination that may have been introduced during the printing process. They are useful to evaluate the degree of "pluming" that results during postprocessing (*see* **Note 25**). We recommend salmon sperm DNA for making Cy3-labeled control spots. The same procedure for making labeled genomic DNA can be used to prepare these as well (*see* **Subheading 3.5.2.**). Prepare a 1:100 dilution (Cy3-labeled:unlabeled) to reduce the specific activity of labeled sample since this reagent has the potential to contribute to background if minor pluming does occur. When setting up the control plate the prelabeled spots should be followed immediately in the printing order by wells containing only printing buffer. This allows one to assess the level of possible carry-over contamination that results if DNA is transferred to neighboring wells by quill-type printing tips that are improperly rinsed or dried between cycles. This is normally fixed by adjusting the drying station so that sufficient suction is applied to all printing tips.
24. Test printing is important for three reasons. First, the user can select a set of printing tips that delivers consistent spot sizes. Second, the fluid delivery characteristics of the quill-type printing tips can be evaluated to help the user decide how many slides can be reliably printed during that day's setup. Third, by using fluorescently prelabeled DNA controls, one can test the washing and drying system for possible carry-over contamination (*see* **Note 15**).
25. The printing configuration is determined by the dimensions of the slide, coverslip, and printing tip holder that are part of the system. For example, a 20 mm × 20 mm array can be printed onto a standard microscope slide with either a 4-tip (when printing from 96-well plates) or a 16-tip print head (used for 384-well plates). With this configuration an array of 5000 spots should be printed with a spot density of 225 µ*M* (center-to-center spacing).
26. It is helpful to keep a checklist to ensure that the correct order and orientation of the plates is maintained throughout the printing session. If the plates have been stored in the refrigerator or freezer, allow them to warm to room temperature, and, before removing the sealing tape, centrifuge them to push the condensed liquid down to the bottom of the wells. Do not allow plates to stay open to the air for any longer than is essential for printing.

27. The slides are suspended above the surface of the aqueous reservoir with the array side facing downward. Avoid moving the slide chamber, creating waves that slosh up onto the surface of the array. The time it takes to rehydrate the slides can be accelerated if the 2X SSC is heated slightly (35–40°C). However, it is important not to let the slides become overly beaded with water since this can cause the spots to form water channels between each other, effectively mixing the contents of merged spots.
28. Maintain a dust-free environment during the steps when the slides are open to the air. The UV crosslinking increases the amount of DNA that remains attached to the slide. It also reduces the lateral spread of target DNA that might merge with adjacent spots when excess DNA is printed onto a spot.
29. Prewashing the slides in a SDS-containing buffer before postprocessing reduces the amount of DNA that bleeds onto nontarget sites on the array. This reduces background and improves the overall signal-to-noise ratio.
30. Submerging the slides in boiling water serves to melt and release DNA fragments that are not covalently crosslinked to the slide or the matrix of DNA within the spot. We imagine that the boiling step generates an open single-stranded conformation that facilitates hybridization to the target DNA.
31. It is not clear whether postprocessing alters the shelf-life of the array. Our current assumption is that arrays are more stable as dried salt deposits on the surface of the glass, and that the performance is best if slides are recently postprocessed. Therefore, we customarily process slides in batches that will be used for hybridization within 1–2 wk.
32. Good quality RNA tolerates heating to 95°C for 5–10 min prior to snap cooling on ice. This results in moderate RNA degradation, but the sample still labels and hybridizes nicely to the array. This treatment has the advantage of thoroughly melting secondary structure before labeling and it completely inactivates any DNAse activity that may have been introduced as part of the RNA isolation procedure. Additionally, we suspect that the smaller fragments generated by this procedure may improve hybridization to the array, but more testing is needed to determine the extent of this potential benefit *(4)*.
33. To obtain better consistency when more than two samples are prepared, make a master mix of the reagents, without the Cy3 or Cy5 dyes. Then split the master mix into two equal batches, add the appropriate fluorescent dye and dispense 12.3 µL of the master mix into the RNA samples to begin the reaction.
34. It is sometimes advantageous to concentrate the Cy3- and Cy5-labeled samples separately before combining the correct proportions of each for the hybridization. Adjust the volumes accordingly so that the combined probe mixture is 8 µL.
35. An alternative to concentrating the sample over a filter is to precipitate in ethanol as follows: add 5.5 µL of 3 *M* sodium acetate pH 5.5 and 140 µL of 100% ethanol, chill on ice and centrifuge for 30 min at > 12,000*g*. Remove the ethanol, and rinse the labeled DNA pellets in 70% ethanol. Centrifuge again for 7–10 min, remove the ethanol and dry the pellets. Dissolve the pellets in 8 µL of water or TE in preparation for the hybridization described in **Subheading 3.6.** If the Cy3- and

Cy5-labeled samples were precipitated separately then dissolve each in 4 μL and combine as appropriate.

36. Water is added to the slide to supply a source of humidity and prevent evaporation of the sample during hybridization. Most commercial hybridization chambers are designed with wells in the bottom plate for the addition of water. Avoid placing more than 30 μL of water in the chamber because excess water can form condensation droplets within the chamber that drop onto the coverslip and wick into the sample.
37. Samples should not be applied to the array while still hot. When this happens a characteriztic circular pattern of high background forms where the droplet first touched the array. Conversely the samples should not be snap cooled on ice after heating because the SDS will precipitate out of solution.
38. It is important to practice the technique of laying the coverslip down onto the array. Significant damage can be done to the array if this step is done in a clumsy manner. Take care to avoid forming bubbles or touching the surface of the array with the pipet tip or the cover glass. Avoid trapping bubbles under the cover glass by gently laying it down at an angle so that all the liquid is pushed in one direction as the cover glass descends. Some find it helpful to position the slide on the edge of a bench top so that the knuckles of the hand holding the forceps can drop below the plane of the slide. Never tap down on the cover glass once it is laid down onto the array.
39. Work quickly through **steps 9** and **10** to prevent significant cooling of the slide before it is plunged into the wash solutions.
40. Sometimes the cover glass sticks to the slide as it is being washed. Once the cover glass starts to move off the slide, keep it from touching the bottom of the tray because this will scratch the array.
41. Maximize the sensitivity by boosting the laser intensity (or signal acquisition time if a CCD device is used) to the point at which some spots on the array are saturated. Then adjust the photomultiplier gain settings to help normalize the two channels while maintaining a low overall background. Spots containing genomic DNA can be used to help normalize the two fluorescent channels at the time of scanning. (The photomultiplier gain is an electronic amplification that scales the signal and does not participate in the amount of fluorescent light that is emitted or acquired by the instrument.) Decide on scan settings quickly and avoid rescanning the slide multiple times since photobleaching will reduce the signal with each subsequent scan. The Cy5 dye is more vulnerable to bleaching and fading than the Cy3-labeled sample.
42. Extracting numerical data from the spot intensities can be done using a number of different programs. We recommend Scanalyze 2.1 (free for nonprofit and academic use) which was written by Mike Eisen and can be downloaded at http://rana.Stanford.EDU/software/. Manufacturers of scanners are now offering software that extracts the data from the images as well. We expect improvements in this area in the near future, which should improve the speed and accuracy of this process.

43. The database for managing gene expression data can be a simple set of tables containing the array results (spot position, fluorescence data) that are linked to the descriptive information about the amplicons. Most applications, however, require more elaborate strategies to accommodate multiple users, complex queries, web-based servers, and links to external and complex queries.databases. The microarray project sponsored by the National Human Genome Research Institute, offers the software modules and schematic layout for the database that they use (http://genome.nhgri.nih.gov/arraydb/). A centralized data repository and retrieval network, patterned after the Genebank model for DNA sequence data, has also been proposed for array-based expression data ***(12)***.
44. The minimum specifically detectable signal is arbitrarily defined. For example it could be the level that is two standard deviations above the background values for all spots on the array ***(7)***. Another choice is one standard deviation above the average signal of all spots containing non-*M. tuberculosis* DNA ***(3)***. Finally, if there is adequate coverage of the low concentration range by internal standards, one can calculate a dose-response curve for the experiment and use it to guide selection of the sensitivity threshold.
45. Calculations using log-transformed values are suitable for comparing ratios because the distance on the positive scale is equivalent to the distance of the inverse ratio on the negative scale. Log_2 ratios are chosen for intuitive convenience since each integer represents a twofold increase in the ratio value. For example, a fourfold induction is +2 ($\log_2$ ratio) and a fourfold repression is –2 ($\log_2$ ratio). Using simple ratios, a fourfold repression is 0.25 because ratio values that represent repression are compressed on the scale between 0 and 1.
46. Written originally for viewing data generated by the *M. tuberculosis* microarray project at Stanford, Probebrowser presents the results in the context of the ORFs and their positions on the chromosome. Probebrowser was created by Hugh Salamon, and it can be downloaded from http://molepi.stanford.edu/hugh/pb/pbbcg.html. The user supplies the results file for each experiment. Then the experimental ratio data is plotted on the *y*-axis and the corresponding ORF positions presented on the *x*-axis. Probebrowser enables the user to scroll along the genome and zoom into specific regions of interest. Each ORF is linked to a descriptive database that includes the gene name, putative functional assignment, and position on the genome. Although a default database of *M. tuberculosis* ORFs and annotations is provided, the user can supply a custom database of annotations, thereby making Probebrowser a versatile tool for analyzing microarray data for any microorganism.
47. The "Cluster" program described by Eisen, et. al., uses a hierarchical clustering method to organize a matrix of correlation coefficients that measure the pairwise similarity of expression patterns between genes ***(15)***. Other clustering methods are available (e.g., K-means) that may be equally useful for this approach. Clustering can be done on two dimensions (based on similarity between genes and similarity between experimental treatments) so that one gets an impression of the relationship between experimental treatments in the context of the cell's overall

response profiles. The program "Treeview" presents the results as a dendogram and a graphical table. It uses a coloring scheme that is calibrated for $\log_2$ ratio values. Self-organizing maps is an alternative method for finding related genes according to their expression patterns over multiple experiments ***(16,19)***. This method has the advantage over hierarchical clustering method in that it allows the user to impose partial structure on the clusters. Furthermore, the computational properties of self-organizing maps more easily scale to accommodate large data sets. Undoubtedly, both these methods will be useful for discovering biologically relevant patterns in the data.

References

1. Cole, S. T., Brosch, R., Parkhill, J., Garnier, T., Churcher, C., Harris, D., Gordon, S. V., Figimejer, K., Gas, S., Barry, C. E., 3rd, Tekaia, F., Badeock, K., Basham, D., Brown, D., Chillingworth, T., Connor, R., Davies, R., Devlin, K., Feitwell, T., Gentles., S., Hamlin, N., Hoiroyd, S., Hornsby, T., Jagels, K., Barrell, B. G., et al (1998) Deciphering the biology *of Mycobacterium tuberculosis* from the complete genome sequence. *Nature* **393,** 537–544.
2. Behr, M. A., Wilson, M. A., Gill, W. P., Salamon, H., Schoolnik, G. K., Rane, S., and Small, P. M. (1999) Comparative genomics of BCG vaccines by whole genome DNA microarray. *Science* **284,** 1520–1523.
3. Wilson, M., DeRisi, J., Kristensen, H. H., Imboden, P., Rane, S., Brown, P. O., and Schoolnik, G. K. (1999) Exploring drug-induced alterations in gene expression in *Mycobacterium tuberculosis* by microarray hybridization. *Proc. Natl. Acad. Sci. USA* **96,** 12,833–12,838.
4. Southern, E., Mir, K., and Shchepinov, M. (1999) Molecular interactions on microarrays. *Nat. Genet.* **21,** 5–9.
5. Lipshutz, R. J., Fodor, S. P., Gingeras, T. R., and Lockhart, D. J. (1999) High density synthetic oligonucleotide arrays. *Nat. Genet.* **21,** 20–24.
6. Schena, M., Shalon, D., Davis, R. W., and Brown, P. O. (1995) Quantitative monitoring of gene expression patterns with a complementary DNA microarray. *Science* **270,** 467–470.
7. DeRisi, J. L., Iyer, V. R., and Brown, P. O. (1997) Exploring the metabolic and genetic control of gene expression on a genomic scale. *Science* **278,** 680–686.
8. Beier, M. and Hoheisel, J. D. (1999) Versatile derivatisation of solid support media for covalent bonding on DNA-microchips. *Nucleic Acids Res.* **27,** 1970–1977.
9. Duggan, D. J., Bittner, M., Chen, Y., Meltzer, P., and Trent, J. M. (1999) Expression profiling using DNA microarrays. *Nat. Genet.* **21,** 10–14.
10. Mangan, J. A., Sole, K. M., Mitchison, D. A., and Butcher, P. D (1997) An effective method of RNA extraction from bacteria refractory to disruption, including mycobacteria. *Nucleic Acids Res.* **25,** 675–676.
11. Lockhart, D. J., Dong, H., Byrne, M. C., Follettie, M. T., Gallo, M. V., Chee, M. S., Mittmann, M., Wang, C., Kobayashi, M., Horton, H., and Brown, E. L. (1996) Expression monitoring by hybridization to high-density oligonucleotide arrays. *Nat. Biotechnol.* **14,** 1675–1680.

12. Ermolaeva, O., Rastogi, M., Pruitt, K. D., Schuler, G. D., Bittner, M. L., Chen, Y., Simon, R., Meltzcr, P., Trent, J. M., and Boguski, M. S. (1998) Data management and analysis for gene expression arrays. *Nat. Genet.* **20,** 19–23.
13. Bassett, D. B., Jr., Eisen, M. B., and Boguski, M. S. (1999) Gene expression informatics — it's all in your mine. *Nat. Genet.* **21,** 51–55.
14. Bowtell, D. D. (1999) Options available—from start to finish—for obtaining expression data by microarray. *Nat. Genet.* **21,** 25–32.
15. Eisen, M. B., Speliman, P. T., Brown, P. O., and Botstein, D. (1998) Cluster analysis and display of genome-wide expression patterns. *Proc. Natl. Acad. Sci. USA* **95,** 14,863–14,868.
16. Tamayo, P., Slonim, D., Mesirov, J., Zhu, Q., Kitareewan, S., Dmitrovsky, E., Lander, E. S., and Golub, T. R. (1999) Interpreting patterns of gene expression with self-organizing maps: methods and application to hematopoietic differentiation. *Proc. Natl. Acad. Sci. USA* **96,** 2907–2912.
17. Brown, P. O. and Botstein, D. (1999) Exploring the new world of the genome with DNA microarrays. *Nat Genet.* **21,** 33-7.
18. Steve Rozen, H. J. S. (1996, 1997) Primer3. Whitehead Institute for Biomedical Research http://www-genome.wi.mit.edulgenome_software/other/primer3.html.
19. Toronen, P., Kolehmainen, M., Wong, G., and Castren, E., (1999) Analysis of gene expression data using self-organizing maps. *FEBS Lett.* **451,** 142–146.

23

Storage of Mycobacterial Strains

Kristin Kremer, Tridia van der Laan, and Dick van Soolingen

1. Introduction

The storage and maintenance of mycobacterial reference strains and clinical isolates are important parts of good laboratory practice in a mycobacterial laboratory. The storage of reference and control strains facilitates a reliable control on intra- and inter-test reproducibility *(1,2)*. Furthermore, to study various aspects of the epidemiology of tuberculosis it is important to be able to study serial isolates of individual patients *(3)* or of patients associated with particular place or time factors *(4)*.

It is possible to maintain mycobacterial cultures by reculturing on solid medium, like Löwenstein–Jensen medium. There are, however, many examples of significant genetic rearrangements in mycobacterial strains during in vitro culturing *(5,6)*. It is therefore of the utmost importance to preserve reference strains and clinical isolates under circumstances with the lowest metabolic activity.

In the past, lyophilization has been the most frequently used approach to preserve cultures. However, because the viability of the lyophilized bacteria drops dramatically within a few years, storage of cultures in –70°C freezers is increasingly applied. In the Netherlands 15 years of experience with the latter method for storage has shown that this method is highly efficient for maintaining the viability of mycobacterial cultures.

This chapter describes how to establish and maintain a mycobacterial strain collection and how strains can be stored at –70°C in glycerol.

2. Materials

2.1. Establishing a Mycobacterial Strain Collection

1. Sticker machine (e.g., the Brady LS2000, WH Brady N.V., Zele, Belgium) (*see* **Note 1**).

From: *Methods in Molecular Medicine*, vol. 54: *Mycobacterium Tuberculosis Protocols*
Edited by: T. Parish and N. G. Stoker © Humana Press Inc., Totowa, NJ

2. Culture media tubes containing either solid or liquid medium (*see* **Note 2**).
3. Solid medium: Löwenstein–Jensen medium or Löwenstein-Jensen medium supplemented with pyruvate *(7)* (*see* **Note 2**).
4. Liquid medium: 5 mL Middlebrook 7H9 medium *(7)* (*see* **Note 2**).
5. Inoculating loops.
6. Plugged pipets (2 mL).
7. Incubator 30°C, 35.5°C, and 42°C (*see* **Note 3** and **Table 1**).
8. Freezer, –70°C (*see* **Note 4**).

2.2. Storing Mycobacterial Cultures in the –70°C Freezer

2.2.1. For Cultures from Solid Media

1. Sticker machine (*see* **Note 1**).
2. Cryovial tubes, with screw thread on the outside and a content of about 2 mL, e.g., cryovials, (Simport Plastic, Quebec, Canada).
3. Dry-ice-mixture; prepare the following mixture (*see* **Note 5**): mix 100 mL of crushed dry-ice, 100 mL of 80% ethanol and 50 mL of tap water. Mix well and store in a polystyrene box.
4. Storage medium; mix 3 g Tryptone Soya Broth (Oxoid, Basingstoke, UK), 20 mL of glycerol and 80 mL of distilled water. Autoclave and store at 4°C for up to 6 mo.
5. Inoculating loops.
6. Freezer, –70°C (*see* **Note 4**).

2.2.2. For Liquid Cultures

1. 2X storage medium; add 6 g of Tryptone Soya Broth (Oxoid) and 40 mL of glycerol to 80 mL of distilled water. Autoclave and store at 4°C for up to 6 mo.
2. Plugged pipets (2 mL).
3. Freezer, –70°C (*see* **Note 4**).

2.2.3. Storing a Large Batch of a Strain

See **Subheadings 2.1.**, **2.2.1.**, and **2.2.2.**

2.3. Reculturing Strains from the –70°C Freezer

1. Sticker machine (e.g., the Brady LS2000, WH Brady N.V., Zele, Belgium) (*see* **Note 1**).
2. Culture media tubes containing either solid or liquid medium (*see* **Note 2**).
3. Solid medium: Löwenstein–Jensen medium or Löwenstein-Jensen medium supplemented with pyruvate *(7)* (*see* **Note 2**).
4. Liquid medium: 5 mL Middlebrook 7H9 medium *(7)* (*see* **Note 2**).
5. Inoculating loops.
6. Incubator 30°C, 35.5°C, and 42°C (*see* **Note 3** and **Table 1**).
7. Dry-ice-mixture (*see* **Subheading 2.2.1., step 3**).

Table 1
Optimum Temperatures to Grow Mycobacteria

Species	Temperature (°C)
M. tuberculosis complex	35.5
M. avium complex	30
M. malmoense	30
M. xenopi	45
other mycobacterial species	35.5

3. Methods

Caution: All strain of *M. tuberculosis* may be pathogenic to humans and should always be handled in the appropriate containment facilities.

3.1. Establishing a Mycobacterial Strain Collection

1. Label each mycobacterial isolate that arrives at the laboratory with a unique strain number (*see* **Notes 1** and **6**).
2. Label the patient data or other information belonging to that isolate with the same strain number and enter it in a strain collection database (*see* **Note 7**).
3. Label at least two fresh culture media tubes for each isolate and set up (*see* **Notes 1**, **2**, and **8**).
4. Incubate the cultures at the appropriate temperature (*see* **Note 3** and **Table 1**).
5. Store each strain in the –70°C freezer as described below.

3.2. Storing Mycobacterial Cultures in the –70°C Freezer

Three methods to store mycobacterial strains in the –70°C freezer are described, one for mycobacteria grown on solid media, one for liquid mycobacterial cultures, and one for storing a large batch of a certain strain (*see* **Notes 2**, **4**, and **9**).

3.2.1. Storing from Solid Cultures

1. Select a well-grown (noncontaminated) culture of each of the mycobacterial strains that should be stored (*see* **Note 2**).
2. Label two cryovial tubes, both on the top and the side, for each strain (*see* **Note 10**).
3. Prepare a fresh dry-ice-mixture.
4. Add 2 mL storage-medium to the slope with a pipet.
5. Resuspend the mycobacteria with a loop (*see* **Note 11**).
6. Pipet the bacterial suspension from the slope and divide it between the two labeled cryovial tubes.
7. Put the cryovial tubes containing the suspension as quickly as possible on the dry-ice-mixture (*see* **Note 12**).

8. Allow the suspensions to freeze completely and store at –70°C(*see* **Note 4**).
9. Register the storage of the cultures on an appropriate form or in the strain collection database.

3.2.2. Storage from Liquid Cultures

1. Select a well-grown (noncontaminated) culture of each of the mycobacterial strains that should be stored (*see* **Note 2**).
2. Label two cryovial tubes, both on the top and the side, for each strain (*see* **Note 10**).
3. Prepare a fresh dry-ice-mixture.
4. Add 1 mL of 2X storage medium to a cryovial tube labeled with the strain number.
5. Add 1 mL of the mycobacterial culture to be frozen.
6. Homogenize the bacterial suspension by carefully pipetting up and down a few times (*see* **Note 11**).
7. Transfer 1 mL of this suspension to the other labeled cryovial tube.
8. Put the cryovial tubes containing the suspension as quickly as possible on the dry-ice-mixture (*see* **Note 12**).
9. Allow the suspensions to freeze completely and store at –70°C (*see* **Note 4**).
10. Register the storage of the cultures on an appropriate form or in the strain collection database.

3.2.3. Storage of a Large Batch of a Strain (see **Notes 13** and **14**)

1. Inoculate twelve culture medium tubes with the appropriate strain and incubate them at the appropriate temperature until they are well-grown (*see* **Notes 2** and **3**, and **Table 1**).
2. Label 24 cryovial tubes with the strain number, both on the side and the top (*see* **Note 10**).
3. Transfer as many bacteria as possible to 24 mL storage medium (*see* **Note 15**).
4. Homogenize the suspension by swirling.
5. Distribute 1 mL volumes of the suspension to the labeled cryovial tubes.
6. Prepare a fresh dry-ice-mixture.
7. Put the cryovial tubes containing the suspension as quickly as possible on the dry-ice-mixture (*see* **Note 12**).
8. Allow the suspensions to freeze completely and store at –70°C (*see* **Note 4**).
9. Perform a quality control on the batch by checking the growth and the biochemical and/or molecular characteriztics of the respective strain.

3.3. Reculturing Strains from the –70°C Freezer (see Note 16)

1. Label two culture media tubes with the strain name (*see* **Note 2**).
2. Prepare a fresh dry-ice mixture.
3. Remove the cryovial tube from the freezer and place it on the dry-ice-mixture.
4. Scrape some of the frozen suspension from the tube with a loop, while keeping the suspension frozen. Place the cryovial tube back into the freezer as soon as possible.

5. Inoculate two culture media tubes (*see* **Notes 2** and **17**).
6. Incubate the cultured tubes at the appropriate temperature (*see* **Note 3** and **Table 1**).

4. Notes

1. To label the tubes it is convenient to use a sophisticated sticker machine. Such a machine can prepare several stickers with the same number at once, and in addition prepare series of stickers with incremental numbers or date. Alternatively, a more basic sticker machine can be used, such as a supermarket sticker machine (e.g., Meto 826, Esselte Meto bv, Nieuwegein, The Netherlands).
2. For various (mainly practical) reasons it may be more convenient to use either a solid or a liquid culture. Generally, you can choose the culture medium you are accustomed to. The procedure to store liquid media can be executed faster and is therefore recommended if many strains are to be stored. Solid media have the advantage that it is more easy to see whether the culture is contaminated or not, whereas this is difficult to see when liquid media are used.
3. Different mycobacterial species require different optimal growth conditions. *See* **Table 1** for the optimal incubation temperatures for the various mycobacterial species.
4. It is recommended to prepare the culture collection in duplicate. Therefore, use two –70°C freezers, and store the two cryovial tubes of each strain in different freezers. Preferably the two freezers should be in different locations, and depending on different power supplies. In this way, in case of an accident (e.g., fire in the laboratory, or long periods of time without electricity) the culture collection is still maintained. For practical reasons, one freezer should be kept in the working laboratory. When frozen mycobacteria have to be transported out of the laboratory to another location use a biohazard-safety-carrier. Both freezers should be maintained under the appropriate containment conditions.
5. The dry-ice-mixture is well-prepared when it looks mushy. In this case the cryovial tube has immediate contact with the ice everywhere, and therefore freezes most efficiently.
6. Each strain should have a unique strain number. The patient data and the patient's isolate should be linked to this number. Preferably this strain number should be used for all the procedures in the laboratory in which the culture is handled. The advantage of a numbering code consisting of a year and a serial number is that one more or less knows when the sample was received, but the disadvantage is that writing errors may occur more easily.
7. We recommend using a strain collection database (e.g., Microsoft Access) or a dedicated laboratory information management system to store all the patient- and experimental data of the patient's isolate in, simultaneously linking the patient data to a unique strain number.
8. We recommend subculturing each new isolate in at least two culture media tubes. One tube can then be used for storing the isolate in the –70°C freezer, the other tube (or tubes) for laboratory procedures. In addition, the tube(s) used for labora-

tory procedures can be kept at room temperature for about 3 to 6 mo. In case additional tests are required using this tube may be quicker than reculturing the strain from the –70°C freezer.

9. It is useful to prepare a large batch of reference or other strains that are taken from the freezer more frequently. A less time consuming protocol to store many vials of such strains is described here.
10. Use stickers that do not come off after thawing, or cover the sticker with tape. If a culture collection is maintained in duplicate it may be convenient to label the two cryovial tubes with different colors. For this purpose plastic labels that fit into the top of the lid of the cryovial tubes are commercially available.
11. Resuspend the mycobacteria carefully, avoid the forming of aerosols.
12. The suspensions should be frozen as quickly as possible in order to keep the storage medium homogeneous and to damage the bacteria as little as possible.
13. When a large batch of a strain is to be stored, it is recommended to grow the strain on solid medium because now it is especially important to know that the culture is pure (not contaminated). This protocol describes the use of 12 grown cultures. Of course, if desired, this number can either be increased or decreased. If so, then the number of cryovial tubes and the volume to suspend the bacteria in should be adjusted accordingly.
14. It is also possible to use a liquid culture, but besides the disadvantage of the worse recognition of contaminations, it is also difficult to estimate the volume of storage medium that is to be used to dissolve the bacteria in. If a liquid culture is preferred, then use the following protocol: (a) grow the strain on, e.g., 50 or 100 mL liquid medium; (b) When the culture is well-grown, centrifuge at 1200*g* for 15 min, and discard the supernatant; (c) dissolve the pellet in 5 to 10 mL storage medium, depending on the size of the pellet; (d) continue with **Subheading 3.2.4., step 4**.
15. The volume of storage medium and the number of cryovial tubes to distribute the homogenized suspension in can be increased if the growth on the culture tubes was abundant.
16. It may be useful to reculture certain reference strains regularly (e.g., each month) from the –70°C freezer, so that there is always a fresh culture of that strain available.
17. If a cryovial tube from the collection is almost empty or defrosted, then subculture a new culture medium tube and repeat the procedure described in **Subheading 3.2.**, to store the strain again. Register the replacement on an appropriate form or in the strain collection database.

References

1. Van Embden, J. D. A., Crawford, J. T., Dale, J. W., Gicquel, B., Hermans, P., McAdam, R., Shinnick, T., and Small, P. M. (1993) Strain identification of *Mycobacterium tuberculosis* by DNA fingerprinting: recommendations for a standardized methodology. *J. Clin. Microbiol.* **31,** 406–409.

2. Kremer, K., van Soolingen, D., Frothingham, R., Haas, W. H., Hermans, P. W. M., Martin, C., Palittapongarnpim, P., Plikaytis, B. B., Riley, L. W., Yakrus, M. A., Musser, J. M., and van Embden, J. D. A. (1999) Comparison of methods based on different molecular epidemiological markers for typing of *Mycobacterium tuberculosis* complex strains: Interlaboratory study of discriminatory power and reproducibility. *J. Clin. Microbiol.* **37,** 2607–2618.
3. Van Rie, A., Warren, R., Richardson, M., Victor, T. C., Gie, R. P., Enarson, D. A., Beyers, N., and Van Helden, P. D. (1999) Exogeneous reinfection as a cause of recurrent tuberculosis after curative treatment. *N. Engl. J. Med.* **341,** 1174–1179.
4. Doveren, R. F. C., Keizer, S. T., Kremer, K., and van Soolingen, D. (1998) A tuberculous micro-epidemic caused by endogenous reactivation eight years after infection demonstrated by DNA fingerprinting (in Dutch). *Ned. Tijdschr. Geneesk.* **142,** 189–192.
5. Steenken, Jr., W. and Gardner, L. U. (1946) History of H37 strain of tubercle bacillus. *Am. Rev. Tuberc.* **54,** 62–66.
6. Behr, M. A. and Small, P. M. (1999) A historical and molecular phylogeny of BCG strains. *Vaccine* **17,** 915–922.
7. Allen, B. W. (1998) Mycobacteria: general culture methodology and safety precautions, in *Methods in Molecular Biology*, vol. 101: *Mycobacteria Protocols* (Parish, T. and Stoker, N. G., eds.) Humana, Totowa, NJ, pp. 15–30.

24

Safety in the Laboratory

Heidi Alderton and Debbie Smith

1. Introduction

The worldwide resurgence of tuberculosis (TB) has resulted in a rapid expansion in research efforts directed at a deeper understanding of the disease, the efficacy of vaccines, and improved drug targets. This has required the establishment of multiple new facilities to contain the pathogen and to protect staff from accidental infection. In addition, much of the research effort has been due to the emergence of multidrug resistant (MDR) strains which offer increased levels of hazard in the event of laboratory infection and focus the need for stringent working practices. This chapter presents an overview of the recommendations and regulations for working with *Mycobacterium tuberculosis*, and suggests some ideas based on our experience in setting up and using Category 3 facilities.

2. Classification of Biological Hazards

It became clear in the 1960s and early 1970s that a system of classification was needed to separate harmless organisms from those that needed containment or special handling procedures. This idea was pioneered in the United States in 1969 and evolved through the 1970s and early 1980s *(1,2)* and was developed by the Godber working party in the UK *(3)*. In addition, the WHO has developed a similar system of classification. Nowadays there is a reasonable agreement about grouping of organisms and risk assessment, though wording of the different documents differs. Those who need further information are directed toward the relevant texts for their own country and in the absence of specific guidelines the WHO publication is available *(4)*.

The categorization is based on the following criteria:

1. Is the organism pathogenic to man?
2. Is it a hazard in the laboratory?

From: *Methods in Molecular Medicine*, vol. 54: *Mycobacterium Tuberculosis Protocols*
Edited by: T. Parish and N. G. Stoker © Humana Press Inc., Totowa, NJ

3. Is it transmissible in the community?
4. Is effective prophylaxis or treatment available?

People involved in research on mycobacteria need to understand the criteria for Hazard Group 2 categorization also known as Category 2. These are defined as biological agents that can cause human disease and may be a hazard to laboratory workers, but are unlikely to spread to the community. Laboratory exposure rarely produces infection and effective prophylaxis or treatment is usually available. Of greater importance to this review and *Mycobacterium tuberculosis* is Hazard Group 3 (Category 3) which includes infectious agents that can cause severe human disease and present a serious risk to employees. Category 3 organisms present a risk of spreading to the community, but there is usually effective prophylaxis or treatment available. This may be complicated by the emergence of increasing multidrug resistance.

Mycobacteria retained at Category 2 level in the UK 1990 definition *(5)* are those that cause localized nonpulmonary infections, and include the BCG strains of *M. bovis* which have been used in vaccines (**Table 1**). Since the vaccine strains of *M. microti* can, if mishandled, give rise to abscess formation, these are placed in Hazard Group 3 with allowances for the type of work to be undertaken. Other important mycobacterial species include those that are generally not pathogenic to humans but can cause infection in immunocompromised hosts either due to illness or medication with steroids or immunosuppressants. These in fact include a number of commonly used laboratory strains and opportunistic bacteria, such as *M. avium* which was upgraded to a Category 3 pathogen in the UK in 1990. The mycobacterial species listed in Hazard Group 3, those capable of causing serious disease which requires a prolonged course of treatment, include *M. tuberculosis* and *M. leprae*, which are both pathogenic to humans and have been used in containment level 3 facilities for some time.

In this chapter we will address some of the issues related to safe working with *M. tuberculosis* in particular, discuss methods of containment and procedures for training staff, the instigation of universal procedures, the understanding of the risks, and risk assessment for procedures. In addition we have included protocols which have allowed us to develop safe working practices such as for the transfer of uninfected material out of or between Category 3 facilities on and off site. We will also address the safe collection of samples, their transportation and examples of protocols for tested techniques for containment, storage, and disposal, since all materials and samples leaving the laboratory need to be adequately contained, disinfected, or autoclaved. We will comment on practices to ensure that viable tubercle bacilli cannot leave the laboratory through clothes, personal items or stationery, i.e., "what goes in cannot come out" unless disinfected, autoclaved, or contained.

Table 1
Hazard Grouping of Mycobacteria

Hazard Group 2 (Category 2)	Hazard Group 3 (Category 3)	
M. bovis BCG	*M. tuberculosis*	*M. africanum*
M. paratuberculosis	*M. leprae*	*M. malmoense*
M. fortuitum	*M. avium/intracellulare*	*M. xenopi*
M. marinum	*M. bovis*	*M. kansasii*
M. chelonae	*M. simiae*	*M. scrofulaceum*
	M. ulcerans[a]	*M. szulgai*
	M. microti[a]	

[a]Hazard Group 3 with facility for derogation.

3. Risk of Infection

Approximately one-third of the world's population is infected with tuberculosis. The 1997 WHO bulletin reported 3.3 million new cases worldwide *(6)*. However, 90% of infected individuals control the infection with little clinical consequence. The remaining 10% proceed to various stages of clinical disease with a significant annual mortality of three million. Progression to clinical disease and mortality rates are much higher in HIV infected populations.

Typically, *M. tuberculosis* is spread/contracted by the respiratory route, and people are usually infected with *M. tuberculosis* by inhaling a particle of sputum-containing bacteria. This is called the droplet nucleus and contains between 1–10 bacteria. It can land anywhere in the lung, and if it gets past the cilia and mucus in the trachea and bronchi may be engulfed by alveolar macrophages. The number of tubercle bacilli reported to be infective is very low, less than 10 *(7a)*. Rarely, infection is by injection or ingestion of infected food or drink. The creation of aerosols is therefore the major risk to laboratory workers. As such all procedures which may create aerosols should be carried out with care and in containment such as in Class I/III or Class II cabinets, which will be described.

4. Risks in the Laboratory

In the early 1960s, it was reported that laboratory workers handling material infected with *M. tuberculosis* were at a threefold increased risk of acquiring infection relative to the general population. Since then there has been an increase in the stringency of legislation and improvement of working practices designed to protect the worker, and the development and use of appropriate safety cabinets. Because workers, particularly in diagnostic laboratories, are increasingly handling MDR strains for follow-up culture and drug sensitivity testing, this increases the risk assessment of accidental infection. Thus important considerations include the availability of effective pre- and postgap-exposure vaccination, and of antibiotic and chemotherapeutic agents. However, particularly in countries where tuberculosis is endemic, there is the view that there is little point in placing an organism in a high risk category requiring special precautions in the laboratory, if the workers are extensively exposed during the 16 or so hours that they are out of the laboratory. Apart from the risk of aerosol infection there are a number of necessary experimental procedures, for example, intravenous inoculation of mice, where *M. tuberculosis* is transmissible directly as the result of needlestick, and therefore requires stringent safety precautions.

5. Containment

There are basically two levels of containment; primary containment is designed to protect the laboratory staff and the immediate environment, whereas secondary containment aims to provide protection to those outside the laboratory. Protection of staff is achieved by the use of dedicated cabinets and contained laboratory procedures, and secondary containment is provided by an independent facility working at best at negative pressure to the surrounding environment. The levels of containment specify the kind of environment, i.e., architectural, equipment and technical requirements for working with microorganisms within each of the hazard groups.

6. Microbiological Safety Cabinets

There are three types or levels of safety cabinet used for work with *M. tuberculosis*. Class II cabinets were designed for tissue culture and operate basically to protect cell cultures from infection. They also afford a degree of protection to the worker and may be used with low doses of bacteria and for procedures that involve little risk of aerosol generation. Although they are designed to protect both the work and the operator they are more prone to the disruptive effects of air movements across the front of the cabinet and require careful control and testing.

All operations which involve infectious or potentially infectious material are best carried out in a Class I safety cabinet. This cabinet is designed to pull air across the face of the cabinet at a minimum face velocity of 0.7 m/s. This air is exhausted through a high efficiency particulate air (HEPA) filter. The design affords a high degree of protection to the worker, but may lead to contamination of opened containers and thus bacteriological cultures or sterile tissue cultures inside the cabinet. Our experience is that with good culture techniques and a clean external environment this is a small level of risk. Thus the cabinet is often used for work including the sterile culture of cells in the presence of mycobacteria.

If a face plate is fitted to the front the cabinet can be turned into Class III mode, operating entirely under negative pressure with the air supply being filtered. The exhaust air is usually filtered through two HEPA filters in series. This type of cabinet is completely self contained and offers maximum protection to staff.

There are guidelines as to placement of these cabinets and recommended distances between other cabinets and walls and between opposite cabinets in the British Standard *(8)*. They need routine operator protection testing in accordance with BS-5726 at 6-mo intervals (the UK requirement is every 14 mo) for which commercial apparatus is available (Ki-Discus, Watson and Watkins Medical Air Technology, Manchester, UK). There has been much discussion over the last decade about which tests best measure cabinet performance and safety and which cabinets provide best protection. However, it is likely that with proper testing, maintenance, location, and staff understanding of how they function and how to work properly within them that both Class I and Class II are suitable *(9)*.

Class I or III cabinets should be used for all procedures where there is a risk of creating infectious aerosols or splashes where possible. For this reason personnel need to be aware of the process of droplet formation and the risk associated with procedures including vortexing, centrifugation, sonication, homogenization, electroporation, pipeting, opening containers such as centrifuge tubes and plating.

7. Category 3 Specifications and Operational Measures

Some of these have already been mentioned and others will be covered in the course of this article. Generally Category 3 laboratories should be separated from other sites in the building, with sealed or lockable external windows, and it is recommended that internal viewing windows are included to allow observation of laboratory staff. Intercom systems are useful for communication. These laboratories are maintained at negative pressure to the atmosphere with HEPA filtration of extract air. Airlock access to the laboratory is recommended, or at least a foyer independent from neighboring corridors or laboratories. Since regular fumigation is necessary, rooms need to be sealable for decontamination. All surfaces, benching and floors thus need to be impermeable to water and resistant to cleaning agents, acids, bases, solvents and disinfectants. Handbasins are needed in each room and showers are recommended where practical, but the problem with this is that any such facility requires separate effluent treatment. This is because any waste or products leaving the room must be filtered, decontaminated or securely contained.

Before starting work the room needs to be tested for containment capability and the cabinets need to pass the relevant operator protection tests. Ideally these procedures will need to be repeated at least annually. The entrance doors need to be labeled with biohazard signs and a list for access to authorized users. Protective clothing and gloves need to be provided, and emergency plans need to be drawn up, especially in the event of a spillage of infectious material both internal and external to the cabinets. The appropriate equipment needs to be provided for the safe storage and containment of infectious material.

8. Equipment

This should be dedicated for use in the containment facilities, and includes the microbiological safety cabinets described, centrifuges (with sealable buckets) and appropriate equipment such as fridges, freezers, and microbiological and/or tissue culture incubators. It is a good idea to situate the gas cylinders for incubators external to the suite so that no decontamination is required prior to changing cylinders. In an ideal world there would be autoclaves that could be loaded in the room and unloaded externally, but at the very least these should be nearby, for which procedures need to be instigated for the safe transport of autoclave boxes in sealed secondary containment. No effluent from the runs should be released in the drain until the whole cycle is completed and has been sterilized.

9. Clothing

The use of dedicated and differently colored gowns or coats is required. These should be stored separately from general laboratory coats, preferably in a foyer or anteroom where they should remain after work and prior to disinfection. General laboratory coats should not enter the Category 3 area. Dedicated gowns should be autoclaved and laundered after any procedure that involves high levels of risk, or routinely at least once a week. Gloves must be worn and additional protection may be afforded by the use of disposable protective sleeves (which we use routinely to cover the lower arm exposed in the cabinet), and in some situations a head cover. In the UK, personnel protection through the usage of face mask or HEPA-filtered face masks is not generally applied, as the UK Health and Safety Executive (HSE) prefer that all bacteria should be contained, i.e., in a Class I or III cabinet. It is worth mentioning here that latex gloves present in the room when it is being fumigated can become weakened by the effect of formaldehyde and may have undetectable holes develop. In addition, these gloves are prone to aging and it helps to have a regular turnover. It has been noticed that plasticware may become brittle with repeated formaldehyde fumigation and thus it is preferable not to keep large stocks of gloves or other consumables in the laboratory.

10. Access and Procedures

Access is the responsibility of the supervisor in charge, and requires successful completion of training to ensure that individuals work to high and equal standards and have confidence that the rooms and cabinets have been left safe. Access should be restricted by locking the door. The legal requirement for biohazard notices is one stating that the laboratory is a Category 3 laboratory, and a list of authorized users, but it is helpful to list personnel, pathogen, person in charge, and emergency contacts. Biosafety information in the form of a manual and methodological details need to be available both in the laboratory and outside for reference. One of the most important parts of training ensures that all personnel are aware of emergency procedures. It is important to remember that material such as paper and pens may not leave the laboratory and therefore a computer or fax line may be installed within the Category 3 area. Like plasticware, equipment with digital rather than mechanical function is prone to the effects of fumigation, and in our experience we have had difficulties with computer function as a result of this.

11. Health Screening of Laboratory Workers

This differs from institute to institute but there is general agreement that a system of screening new workers should take place before commencement of work with Category 3 pathogens. Often most of the information on individual health status is obtained once employment has commenced. In countries where BCG vaccination is administered throughout the population at school age, screening may include checking for a BCG scar, chest X-ray and Heaf testing for response to tuberculin. In other countries such as the United States, the Heaf test is used to monitor exposure, since BCG vaccination is uncommon. Personnel should be informed of early manifestations of tuberculosis.

12. Training

Laboratory personnel need specific training not only in the general areas of handling dangerous organisms, but in addition in development of individual risk assessments for each technique used. Section 7 of the Health and Safety at Work Act (1974) ***(10)*** reads:

> It shall be the duty of every employee while at work: a) to take reasonable care for the health and safety of himself and of other persons who may be affected by his acts or omissions at work; and b) as regards any duty or requirement imposed on his employer or any other person by or under any of the relevant statutory provisions, to cooperate with him so far as is necessary to enable that duty or requirement to be performed or complied with.

Within this institute it is felt that senior laboratory staff experienced in specific techniques should be involved in hands-on training of new workers. The techniques that workers are required to become familiar with are split into areas of expertise. Therefore, one individual may be involved in training for techniques associated with molecular biology and mycobacteria, another with animal usage, and another with tissues culture techniques. There is information to indicate that protocol drift is common in laboratories where supervision is poor and Standard Operating Procedures are not under continuous review. Evans et al. ***(11)*** identified inappropriate behavior, flawed techniques, mouth pipeting, and failure to wear gloves as contributors to accident and infection. Thus, it is a good idea to have a local policy on refresher training and to reassess all risk assessments on a regular basis (*see* **Appendix 2**).

13. Transport

All containers containing *M. tuberculosis* should be designed to prevent leakage during transport or storage. There are strict Post Office ***(12)*** and Airline ***(13)*** guidelines about the appropriate packaging and transport of dangerous pathogens, and other guidelines are available ***(14,15)***. Generally these samples must be sent from a qualified medical practitioner or nurse, veterinary practitioner or a recognized laboratory or institution. Packages containing infectious organisms or samples must arrive at their destination in good condition and present no hazard to people or animals during transport. The Post Office requires transport to be at ambient temperatures with no means of refrigeration used in the packing. Guidelines exist for the maximum volumes or weights that may be transported, and in the case of the Post Office this is that the primary vessel should contain no more than 50 mL, this being the total volume that may be transported in secondary packaging. A watertight primary receptacle contains the sample, which is surrounded by watertight secondary packaging. For liquid samples an absorbent material of sufficient quantity to absorb the entire contents of all primary receptacle must be placed between the primary and secondary container. If multiple primary receptacles are placed in a single secondary packaging they must be wrapped individually to ensure contact between them is prevented. An itemized list of contents needs to be placed between the secondary packaging and the outer packaging. Increasingly couriers insist on their own handlers packing pathogens and may have limitations on the amount of material that they will handle. The use of dry ice represents an additional hazard and again there are guidelines for its usage, the most accessible being the airline guidelines ***(13)***.

14. Transport In-House

The above guidelines also form the basis of transport and storage between laboratory facilities on-site, since it is not always possible to complete all aspects of a piece of work in one containment area. For example, the housing of animals may be separated from the laboratory where the processing of samples takes place. Material that needs to be transported around an institute should be contained in an unbreakable primary container, within secondary containment sufficient to contain hazardous material in the case of breakage or accident. In this institute, we also have transport containers with handles that are autoclavable and lockable. These are clearly labeled on the outside identifying the hazard and the responsible person and should never be left unattended outside a Category 3 room.

15. Decontamination

Decontamination is not only required between procedures in the disposal of waste but also to make laboratories safe for untrained staff or contractors (who have not been through health screening procedures) to enter for routine checks, cleaning, and maintenance. All individual items of equipment should be decontaminated prior to repair or maintenance. For larger items such as centrifuges, the easiest way to decontaminate them is to leave the equipment open and fumigate the room. Some problems have been found in repetitive room fumigation when equipment has digital displays, and thus the older style, more mechanically controlled equipment may be better. For surface decontamination and disinfection using hycolin, a phenolic disinfectant, at 5% and made fresh on a daily basis, is appropriate. As hycolin is corrosive, surfaces are often wiped over with 70% alcohol after use but 70% alcohol does NOT substitute for hycolin as it is not effective against mycobacteria. Discards are soaked overnight before being removed to the autoclave, and it is helpful to contain them in a container with a lid that is still accessible to steam penetration in an autoclave. Formaldehyde boxes have sometimes been used for the external disinfection of samples or slides, but all these disinfection and disposal procedures need to be validated on-site. Formaldehyde boxes are sealed boxes with tissue soaked in formaldehyde in which the specimens can be put and exposed to the vapors overnight. There is increasing demand to render material safe for work outside the Category 3 facility in those institutes where expensive shared equipment cannot be dedicated solely for Category 3 usage (*see* **Appendix 1**).

Cabinets may need to be fumigated at regular intervals, and this is done by the use of 15 mL of formaldehyde (40% w/v) solution (HCOH) per 0.86 m^3 of volume to be fumigated, mixed with an equal volume of water. Thus for a cabinet which is 1.2 m wide, dispense 22 mL of formaldehyde solution (40% w/v) together with an equal volume of water into a vaporizer. Generally, as with room fumigation, this is best performed at the end of the day to allow overnight exposure. It is also possible to buy commercially prepared formaldehyde bombs. There are no recommendations for the minimum or maximum number of room or cabinet bombings to be done each year outside of those necessary to allow the entry of engineers and maintenance people. However anecdotal evidence exists to suggest that continued bombing of rooms may lead to problems, particularly with cell function in assays involving tissue culture.

16. Safe Working Practices

The use of sharps such as syringe needles is discouraged unless there is no alternative. In as far as is practicable, laboratoryware should be disposable thus avoiding the need for disinfection and washing. Sharps disposal boxes should contain appropriate disinfectant and be autoclaved before disposal by incineration.

There is often discussion about high and low levels of risk. Although it is true to say that different procedures involve varying degrees of risk, if the infectious dose of mycobacteria is really from 1–10 bacilli, it is safe to assume that risk is inherent in working with these pathogens. However, it is obvious that there are certain techniques such as the large-scale culture of mycobacteria for research purposes that involve extremely high risk elements and thus procedures should be well designed to protect the worker. For an example of a risk assessment (*see* **Appendix 3**).

17. Animal Usage

Animal work is also done under Category 3 conditions and special consideration needs to be given to health surveillance, and immunization of animal staff. Protective clothing, for example, gloves, may need to be more robust. Facilities need to be organized for the safe housing and infection of laboratory animals. The optimal situation is for the animals to be housed in protective isolators that are reached through ports in the side of a Class I/III cabinet. This allows for all feeding and housing material to be fed into the isolators and for waste products to be formaldehyde fumigated before exiting from the cabinet. The dispersion of airborne organisms from the animals, their cages and their bedding should be minimized. Engineering features include housing cages in secondary containment or isolators and directional ventilation of caging, i.e., negative to the surrounding environment. Thus the isolator operates at negative pressure to the room, fed via HEPA-filtered air, and extracts via double HEPA filters. Working with animals is performed by bringing them from the isolator into the cabinet via a double-door port. Many procedures such as harvesting tissue, inoculation by intravenous, subcutaneous or intraperitoneal route, autopsy and disposal of mice carry increased levels of risk because of either the high pathogen doses involved or the unavoidable usage of sharps such as needles. For this reason procedures and practices need careful consideration, for example, the fact that autopsies on animals invariably generate aerosols and need Class I or III mode. Risk assessments should be written for each procedure. Thus all procedures involving laboratory animals should be performed in a Class I or III cabinet.

Appendices

These appendices include some of the protocols we have checked in-house for mycobacterial killing. In addition included here is a draft document for training of personnel and an example of a risk assessment. Finally the reference lists additional documentation which may be helpful in determining local rules outside the UK.

Appendix 1: Tested Methods for Killing Bacteria

A. Disinfection

The most commonly used and approved methods for killing bacteria include autoclaving and the use of hycolin. Fumigation with formaldehyde is also accepted as the most common method for surface disinfection, for example, within the cabinet. The use of cabinets for containment means that other areas of the laboratory should be unexposed to pathogen. There have been some instances within this institute where, to allow for work to continue external to the Category 3 facility, protocols have been developed and methods checked to ensure that all bacteria are killed prior to removal of samples from the laboratory. The most obvious is the storage of samples 200 mg in size in formol saline (40% Formaldehyde 100 mL, NaCl 9 g, water 900 mL) for processing for histology. These samples which are in bijoux containing formol saline are formaldehyde-fumigated in the cabinet, for external decontamination, before being removed to the main laboratory.

B. Filtration

For samples such as tissue culture supernatants, filtration through 0.22 μm filters is sufficient, followed by exposure of tubes to formaldehyde to render the external surfaces sterile. These have been used subsequently for ELISA in conditions where it was not possible to dedicate a plate washer to be kept in the Class I cabinet. Filtration has been used in our laboratory to sterilize supernatants from homogenized tissues for further analysis by gel electrophoresis in the normal laboratory. However extreme caution should be taken, since pressure build-up behind the filter could lead to serious aerosol formation, thus a prefilter and/or centrifugation stage is employed. Prior to removal from the laboratory a formaldehyde fumigation step is included to remove risk of bacteria on the outside of tubes.

C. Toxic Substances

Here we list a few examples of substances that have been tested in house for killing of mycobacteria:

1. Extraction of RNA — we have found that storage of tissue samples in RNAzol at –70°C and subsequent extraction as per suppliers instructions killed mycobacteria, when RNA samples were tested post extraction on plates, slopes, and in liquid media.

2. Immunohistochemistry — Staining of sections has been restricted to the use of tissues harvested into formol saline overnight before processing and embedding in paraffin wax. This involved the use of antigen-unmasking protocols.
3. In a previous book in this series, chloroform-methanol extraction was referred to as being fatal for mycobacteria ***(16)***. We have tested this and found it to be true for the conditions stated.

This brings us to the point that any of these techniques should be validated in thc places where employed, and specific guidelines for conditions, length of time, temperature, and so on, drawn up. For example, outgrowth of *M. avium*, five plaques from an initial inoculum of 1×10^6 was found even after overnight incubation in 4% paraformaldehyde prior to washing and plating on 7H11 plates.

Appendix 2: Training

This is an example of a training document to give an idea of the types of issues which need to be covered by newcomers to working with mycobacteria at Category 3 level.

Draft documentation for training procedures.

Name:
Trainer:
Starting Date:
Completion Date:
Signature of Trainer:

Copies to go to the trainer, the trainee and the safety officer.

Organisms and risk assessment:

The pathogens currently in use in the Category 3 laboratories are *Mycobacterium tuberculosis*, *Mycobacterium leprae*, *Mycobacterium avium*. For all these pathogens infection is known or believed to occur primarily by the respiratory route as well as by ingestion, contact, or inoculation. **The creation of aerosols therefore represents the major risk to laboratory workers.**

Clinical samples which are also used may contain other pathogens including HIV and/or Hepatitis B for which the major risk of infection is from inoculation via accidental injection or via cuts and abrasions.

The facilities covered by these training procedures are rooms X, Y and Z as well as the dedicated facility in the Biological Services Unit.

Training Procedures for Laboratory Personnel working in Category 3 areas

Training of staff will address the following issues:

1. Infectious hazards; routes of infection; classification of infectious agents on the basis of hazard; assessment of risks and levels of containment.

2. Aerosols and infectious airborne particles.
3. Design, testing, and proper use of microbiological safety cabinets including fumigation.
4. Transport and storage of infectious material both within and outside the Category 3 facilities.
5. Decontamination procedures; dealing with spillages; fumigation procedures.
6. Personal protection; hygiene and protective clothing; health and medical surveillance.
7. Emergency procedures in the event of an accident or breakdown of equipment; procedure to follow in the event of a fire or other evacuation alarm.

This document is to be used in conjunction with the local Category 3 Safety Code plus the specific *M. tuberculosis* Code of Practice which covers or exceeds the safety requirements needed to work with the pathogens listed above. Workers need to have a thorough understanding of all procedures that create aerosols, the correct disinfection protocols and how to dispose of waste safely.

Approval to work in Category 3 facilities:

To work alone in any of the Category 3 areas, individuals will need to be deemed competent in all aspects listed in section a) training requirements for all Category 3 laboratories by the trainer and the academic in charge of the laboratory. In addition, individuals will need to be approved for each of the techniques they wish to use in section b) selected procedures. Individuals wishing to add further techniques or organisms or to work in additional areas must discuss their requirements and obtain approval (and additional supervision or training if necessary) from the designated trainer. Anyone who does not abide by this procedure will not be permitted to use the Category 3 facilities.

A) Training Requirements for all Cat 3 Laboratories

Details of housekeeping procedures may vary between laboratories. Individuals trained in one laboratory, who wish to carry out procedures in another, should discuss these procedures with the person responsible when obtaining permission to work in the second laboratory. It is required that the following areas are covered and understood.

1. Risk assessment and the creation of aerosols: awareness of the process of droplet formation and the risk associated with procedures including vortexing, centrifugation, sonication, homogenization, electroporation, pipeting, opening containers.
2. Administrative: booking and access; alarm systems for cabinets and room pressure; closure of doors; logging of procedures; logging of fridges, freezers and incubators.
3. Laboratory practices *(7)* gowns and gloves; documentation and transfer of records out of the laboratory, responsibility for general cleaning; how the laboratory should be left. Concept of one way flow of material into Category 3 laboratories.
4. Laboratory practices *(7)*: use of the cabinets; transfer and containment of material between cabinets and incubators, fridges etc; precautions for infectious material in fridges and incubators.

5. Disinfection: preparation of disinfectant; decontamination of surfaces and equipment. Appropriate disposal of HIV/hepatitis B risk samples.
6. Storage and transport: how to prepare samples for storage; where to store; logging; transport of infectious material outside the laboratories, i.e., from an animal facility.
7. Waste: choice and preparation of disinfectants; use of disinfectants and disposal of disinfected items; autoclaving; transport of waste outside laboratories to autoclaves. Regular disinfection of gowns.
8. Use of centrifuges.
9. Accidents and emergencies: how to deal with spillages both inside and outside the safety cabinet; who to contact in the event of and emergency, procedure for reporting accidents.
10. Where to get help or advice on practical procedures.

B) Selected Procedures, for Use of Which Individuals Must be Specifically Trained

Individuals will be trained in the procedures they require for the work they propose to carry out. If they wish to undertake additional techniques they should seek the necessary additional training or approval. For new techniques, the procedure to be used should be planned in discussion with the person responsible for the laboratory to be used. Defined procedures within our institute are organized into key groups such as molecular microbiology, basic microbiology, cell and tissue culture, and divided into mouse and human studies. The development of procedures and training in these and related procedures is allocated to key individuals who are specifically responsible for the training of personnel. Such techniques and disciplines might include:

Microbiology
Bulk culture of mycobacteria
Dilution and plating for colony counts
Mycobacteriophage infections

Molecular microbiology
Mycobacterial DNA preps
Genetic manipulation of mycobacteria
Electroporation
Methods for diagnostic PCR
RT-PCR from infected material

Cell culture and Immunology
Homogenization of infected tissues
Tissue culture
ELISA from infected material
Use of microscopes/slide preparation/handling
Use of Cryostat
Cell Harvester/Use of radioactive material/cytotoxicity assays

Clinical studies
Shipping of infected material
Handling of clinical specimens
Handling and separation of human blood from infected donors
Cell separation from infectious material
Freezing and thawing of samples/cells.

Use of Biological Services Unit/Animal Facility
Infection and housing of infected animals.

Appendix 3: Summary Protocol and Risk Assessment

To be read in conjunction with the Category 3 Code of Practice.

Title:	Bulk Culture of Mycobacteria for in vivo and in vitro use
Organism:	*M. tuberculosis* H37Rv/Ra; *M. avium*
Laboratory:	X
Project Supervisor:	Dr. John Smith
Routes of Infection:	Infection occurs predominantly via the respiratory route as well as by ingestion, contact and inoculation
Disinfectants:	5% hycolin overnight/autoclave

Summary of Procedures and Precautions:

Procedure	**Precautions**
Culture of Mycobacteria	Wear two pairs of gloves and disposable sleeve protectors over gown. Sterile media inoculated in Class I cabinet. Maximum volume in one container 100 mL. Use of disposable tissue culture flasks retrained in external rack. After inoculation wipe external surfaces of flask with 5% hycolin before transfer to incubator. No shaking.
Harvesting of mycobacteria	Transfer flasks to Class I cabinet. Aliquot into 50 mL centrifuge tubes in centrifuge tube rack using 10 mL pipet maximum — work over Biohazard tray with disposable cover, on tissue soaked with 5% hycolin inside cabinet. Seal culture flasks, swab with hycolin and transfer to autoclave box for disposal.
Centrifugation	Tubes transferred to centrifuge buckets in cabinet, buckets fitted with lids, transfer to centrifuge after surface decontamination with 5% hycolin. Spin, check centrifuge for breakages. Remove buckets, open in cabinet. Remove supernatant to waste container containing hycolin to

	final volume or 5%. Resuspend bacteria using pastette. Add media — aliquot
Storage	Samples aliquoted in 1 mL volume in cryovials, held in polypropylene autoclavable boxes. Individual vials swabbed with hycolin. Lids put on boxes put inside ziplock bag. Label with biohazard tape and details of organism, concentration and user. Transfer to racks in dedicated Category 3 lockable –70°C freezer.

References

1. CDC (1976c) *Classification of Etiological Agents on the Basis of Hazard.* 4th ed. Washington: Government Printing Office.
2. CDC (1981) Classification of Etiological Agents on the Basis of Hazard. *Federal Register* **46,** 59,379–59,380.
3. DH (1975) *Report of the Working Party on the Laboratory Use of Dangerous Pathogens.* Cdmnd. 6054. London, The Stationary Office.
4. WHO (1993) Laboratory Biosafety Manual, 2 nd edn, Geneva: World Health Organisation.
5. ADCP, (1990) Categorization of Pathogens According to hazard and categories of Containment. Advisory Committee on Dangerous Pathogens, London: The Stationary Office.
6. WHO, 1997 bulletin.
7. Lurie, M. B. (1964) *Resistance to Tuberculosis: Experimental Studies in Native and Acquired Defense Mechanisms.* Harvard University Press, Cambridge, MA.
8. BS, 5726 (1992) *Microbiological safety Cabinets.* Part 1. Specification for design, Construction and performance prior to installation. Part 2. Recommendations for information to be exchanged between purchaser, vendor and installer and recommendations for installation. Part 3 Specifications for performance after installation. Part 4. Recommendations for selection, use and maintenance. London: British Standards Institution.
9. Osbourne R., Durkin, T., Shannon, H., Dornan, E., and Hughes, C. (1999) Performance of open-fronted microbiology safety cabinets: the value of operator protection tests during routine servicing. *J. Appl. Micro.* **86,** 962–970.
10. Health and Safety at Work Act (1974) London: The Stationery Office.
11. Evans, M. R., Henderson, D. K., and Bennett, J. E. (1990) Potential for laboratory exposure to biohazardous agents found in blood. *Am. J. Public Health* **80,** 423–427.
12. Royal Mail. *The Post Office Packaging and Labeling Specification for the Safe Transport of Diagnostic Samples, including Infectious Substances.*
13. IATA (1994). *Dangerous goods regulations.* Montreal: International Air Transport Association.
14. United Nations (1996) *Committee of experts on transport of Dangerous Goods, Division 2 Infectious substances* 10th ed. revised New York: UN
15. WHO guidelines for the safe transport of infectious substances and dangerous goods 1997.

16. Belisle, J. T. and Sonnenberg, M. G. (1998) Isolation of genomic DNA from mycobacteria, in *Mycobacterial Protocols, Methods in Molecular Biology*, vol. 101, Parish, T. and Stoker, N. G., eds., ISBN 0-89603-471-2.

In addition to published documents, there are many sources of Health and Safety information available on the internet. Four starting points for information are:

1. Health and Safety Information Service
   http://www.open.gov.uk/hse.hsehome.htm
2. Institute of Occupational Health and Safety and Health — Global OSH links
   http://www.iosh.co.uk/links. htm
3. Index of Occupational Safety and Health Resources
   http://turva.me.tut.fi/~oshweb/
4. Silver Platter and Safety World
   http://www.silverplatter.com/oshinfo. htm

Other Reading

1. Collins, C. H. and Kennedy, D. A. (1999) *Laboratory-Acquired Infections: History, Incidence, Causes and Preventions*. 4th ed. Butterworth and Heinemann ISBN 0 7506 4023 5.

Index

D

N

O

P